Sustainable Development Goals Series

The **Sustainable Development Goals Series** is Springer Nature's inaugural cross-imprint book series that addresses and supports the United Nations' seventeen Sustainable Development Goals. The series fosters comprehensive research focused on these global targets and endeavours to address some of society's greatest grand challenges. The SDGs are inherently multidisciplinary, and they bring people working across different fields together and working towards a common goal. In this spirit, the Sustainable Development Goals series is the first at Springer Nature to publish books under both the Springer and Palgrave Macmillan imprints, bringing the strengths of our imprints together.

The Sustainable Development Goals Series is organized into eighteen subseries: one subseries based around each of the seventeen respective Sustainable Development Goals, and an eighteenth subseries, "Connecting the Goals," which serves as a home for volumes addressing multiple goals or studying the SDGs as a whole. Each subseries is guided by an expert Subseries Advisor with years or decades of experience studying and addressing core components of their respective Goal.

The SDG Series has a remit as broad as the SDGs themselves, and contributions are welcome from scientists, academics, policymakers, and researchers working in fields related to any of the seventeen goals. If you are interested in contributing a monograph or curated volume to the series, please contact the Publishers: Zachary Romano [Springer; zachary.romano@springer.com] and Rachael Ballard [Palgrave Macmillan; rachael.ballard@palgrave.com].

John Paul Sánchez • Donald Rodriguez
Editors

Latino, Hispanic, or of Spanish Origin+ Identified Student Leaders in Medicine

Recognizing More Than 50 years of Presence, Activism, and Leadership

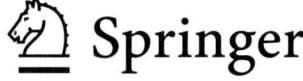 Springer

Editors
John Paul Sánchez
Diversity, Equity, and Inclusion
University of New Mexico Health
Sciences
Albuquerque, NM, USA

Donald Rodriguez
Pritzker School of Medicine
University of Chicago
Chicago, IL, USA

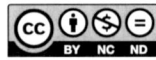

ISSN 2523-3084   ISSN 2523-3092   (electronic)
ISBN 978-3-031-35019-1   ISBN 978-3-031-35020-7   (eBook)
https://doi.org/10.1007/978-3-031-35020-7

Color wheel and icons: From https://www.un.org/sustainabledevelopment/
Copyright © 2020 United Nations. Used with the permission of the United Nations.
The content of this publication has not been approved by the United Nations and does not reflect the views of the United Nations or its officials or Member States.
The Latino Medical Student Association

This Springer imprint is published by the registered company Springer Nature Switzerland AG
The registered company address is: Gewerbestrasse 11, 6330 Cham, Switzerland

Foreword

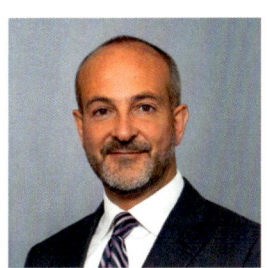

Joseph Betancourt, MD, MPH, President, Commonwealth Fund, Associate Professor of Medicine at Harvard Medical School

It was a new world. I had achieved my lifelong dream of beginning the path to becoming a doctor. So much sacrifice from my family, support from friends, and advice from the rare mentor led to this moment, one equally intimidating and inspiring. As a Latino medical student, I quickly noticed three things. First, given my lived experience, it was clear our community had difficulty accessing the health care system, and suffered from it, with higher rates of chronic conditions as one of many prices they paid. This was confirmed not only by the research I reviewed early in my medical education, but also by what I saw firsthand with the Latino patients I began to see in the clinical setting. Second, I realized that by the simple fact that I was bilingual and understood our culture, I had an advantage over my peers. Even without advanced clinical knowledge, my simple and natural ability to communicate with patients of different backgrounds—and especially Spanish-speaking Latino patients—made me an asset on the care teams I was assigned to. Third, and finally, we as a community of Latinos were drastically underrepresented in medical education, and medicine in general. This was clear as day as I looked around at my medical school peers and saw few who liked like me and came from where I came from.

These experiences weren't unique to me; more importantly, many Latino medical students before me felt of all these things much more acutely, particularly being underrepresented in medicine. There were many trailblazers whose shoulders I stood on, who were the many "firsts" not only in their family like many of us were, but literally were the "first" Latinos in their medical school classes. These courageous students made many sacrifices, often at great personal costs, so that my experience years later would be better as a Latino medical student, and doctor. They worked hard to change medical education so that all students knew how to better care for our community, while also rooting out much of the inherent racism, bias, and stereotypes that were taught about and against our community. In addition, they were tireless in their efforts to assure our communities lived in a social context in which they could thrive and be healthy; that they had equal access to care; and that they received, high-quality, culturally and linguistically competent care in any and all clinical settings.

The Boricua Health Organization (BHO) was one such pioneering effort that I benefitted from greatly. As a medical student BHO made me feel part of a community. BHO gave me the reassurance I needed that the issues I faced I wouldn't face alone, and the issues I saw and was committed to addressing—including Latino health disparities—would be tackled with the help of others. BHO was inspiring, simply by its existence, and the knowledge that those that came before me thought of creating such an important, meaningful, and worthwhile effort. With this appreciation also came a great sense of responsibility. The responsibility to add my part to the movement and move forward in addressing the challenges that our communities and our patients faced. BHO and similar sister organizations across the country that represented the diversity of Latino medical students did this for all of us, and the evolution and consolidation of these organizations in the Latino Medical Student Association (LMSA) was also a crowning moment for all of us who had been part of the struggle. LMSA was a sign of success, strength, and unity.

This book aims to capture all this and more. It looks at 50 years of Latino presence, activism, and leadership by providing the history, stories, and data that come together to make this compelling movement come alive. Not only do we review the past, and learn about the heroes of those moment, but we review the data, and reflect on the future and where we need to go. It is a major addition to our history, our journey, and our story. Long overdue.

I'll end by dedicating this foreword to one such pioneer and hero—one of the co-founders of BHO and my close friend and mentor—Dr. Emilio Carrillo. It is through benefitting from his wisdom and mentorship that I am where I am today, and so many are where they are. He, BHO, and all of LMSA have done so much good, and touched so many lives, and we need to learn that history and build on it with dedication and commitment. This book will serve as the foundation for that in a time when our communities need us most and we should all be grateful for those who put this together and did the work and sacrificed so much to make us better, and our communities healthier.

UMDNJ-New Jersey Medical   Joseph R. Betancourt, MD, MPH
School (Alumnus)
Newark, NJ, USA

Massachusetts General Hospital
Boston, MA, USA

Sustainable Development Goals Series

The **Sustainable Development Goals Series** is Springer Nature's inaugural cross-imprint book series that addresses and supports the United Nations' seventeen Sustainable Development Goals. The series fosters comprehensive research focused on these global targets and endeavors to address some of society's greatest grand challenges. The SDGs are inherently multidisciplinary, and they bring people working across different fields together and working towards a common goal. In this spirit, the Sustainable Development Goals series is the first at Springer Nature to publish books under both the Springer and Palgrave Macmillan imprints, bringing the strengths of our imprints together.

The Sustainable Development Goals Series is organized into eighteen subseries: one subseries based around each of the seventeen respective Sustainable Development Goals, and an eighteenth subseries, "Connecting the Goals," which serves as a home for volumes addressing multiple goals or studying the SDGs as a whole. Each subseries is guided by an expert Subseries Advisor with years or decades of experience studying and addressing core components of their respective Goal.

The SDG Series has a remit as broad as the SDGs themselves, and contributions are welcome from scientists, academics, policymakers, and researchers working in fields related to any of the seventeen goals. If you are interested in contributing a monograph or curated volume to the series, please contact the Publishers: Zachary Romano [Springer; zachary.romano@springer.com] and Rachael Ballard [Palgrave Macmillan; rachael.ballard@palgrave.com].

Goal 4: Quality Education

Latina/o/x/e, Hispanic, or of Spanish Origin+ (LHS+) Identified Student Leaders in Medicine: More Than 50 Years of Presence, Activism, and Leadership contributes to several SDGs, with the most pertinent being Goal 4: Quality Education. The mission of this goal is to ensure inclusive and equitable quality education and promote lifelong learning opportunities for all.

The chapters included in this book contribute to SDG4—specifically, Target 4.7—by discussing opportunities for enhancing U.S. medical education and including detailed accounts of the efforts by the stakeholders of the Latino Medical Student Association (LMSA) and antecedent organizations. This national non-profit organization exists to unite and empower current and future physicians through service, mentorship, and education, to advocate for the improved health of LHS+ communities in the U.S. While this work most directly addresses Target 4.7, we hope that, as the SDGs continue to expand, our book will also contribute to new and/or revised indicators under Targets 4.3 and 4.5. Contributions to the specific targets and indicators of SDG4, previously mentioned, are described in Tables 1 and 2.

Table 1 SDG4 Main Target and Indicator Contributed to by the Book

Target	Indicator
4.7: By 2030, ensure that all learners acquire the knowledge and skills needed to promote sustainable development, including, among others, through education for sustainable development and sustainable lifestyles, human rights, gender equality, promotion of a culture of peace and non-violence, global citizenship and appreciation of cultural diversity and of culture's contribution to sustainable development	4.7.1: Extent to which (1) global citizenship education and (2) education for sustainable development are mainstreamed in (a) national education policies; (b) curricula; (c) teacher education, and (d) student assessment

Table 2 SDG4 Additional Targets and Indicators This Book May Contribute to in the Future

Target	Indicator
4.3: By 2030, ensure equal access for all women and men to affordable and quality technical, vocational, and tertiary education, including university	4.3.1: Participation rate of youth and adults in formal and non-formal education and training in the previous 12 months, by sex
4.5: By 2030, eliminate gender disparities in education and ensure equal access to all levels of education and vocational training for the vulnerable, including persons with disabilities, indigenous peoples, and children in vulnerable situations	4.5.1: Parity indices (female/male, rural/urban, bottom/top wealth quintile and others such as disability status, indigenous peoples and conflict-affected, as data become available) for all education indicators on this list that can be disaggregated

Open Access Acknowledgment

Open Access of this book was made possible by the generous donations of individual co-authors and the organizations listed below. Our sincerest gratitude for allowing this book to be available to every learner around the globe.

Institutions/Organizations:
Association of American Medical Colleges (AAMC)
Individuals:
David Acosta, MD
Emilio Carrillo, MD, MPH
Edgar Figueroa, MD, MPH
Alvaro Galvis, MD, PhD
Francisco Lucio, JD
Aneeta Mehta, DO
Sunny Nakae, PhD, MSW
Pilar Ortega, MD
Norma Poll-Hunter, PhD
Hector Rasgado-Flores, PhD
Elena Rios, MD, MSPH
Franklyn Rocha-Cabrero, MD
Valerie Romero-Leggott, MD
John Paul Sánchez, MD, MPH
Debora Silva, MD, MEd
Orlando Sola, MD, MPH
Jeff Uribe, MD
Larissa Velez, MD

Contents

List of Contributors

David Acosta

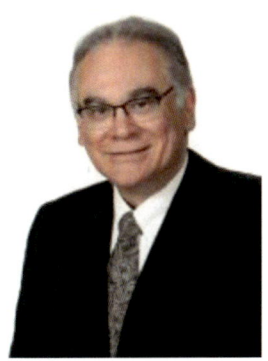

Association of American Medical Colleges, Washington, DC, USA

Emilio Carrillo

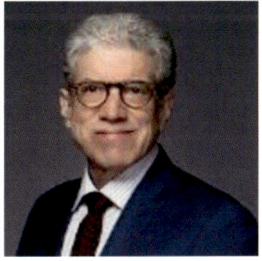

Weill Cornell Medical College, New York, NY, USA

Victor Cueto

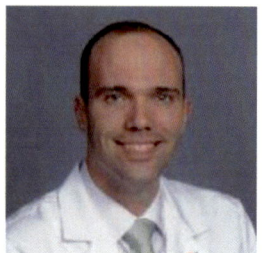

Department of Pediatrics and Internal Medicine, University of Miami, Miller School of Medicine, Miami, FL, USA

Karina Diaz-Davis

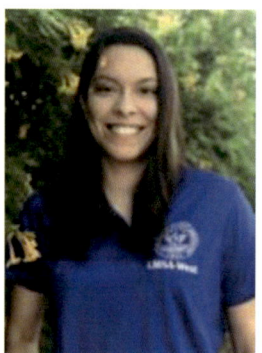

University of Colorado Pediatrics Residency, Aurora, CO, USA

Deion Ellis

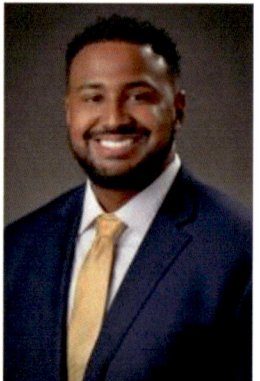

Diversity, Equity, and Inclusion, University of New Mexico Health Sciences, Albuquerque, NM, USA

Edgar Figueroa

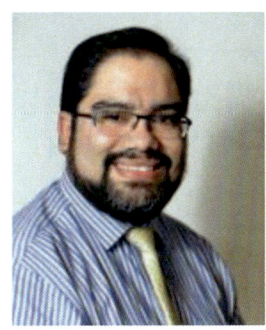

Weill Cornell Medical College, New York, NY, USA

Alvaro Galvis

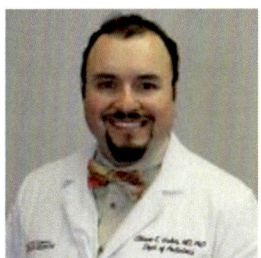

Department of Pediatrics, Division of Pediatric Infectious Diseases, Loma Linda University Children's Health, Loma Linda, CA, USA

Glenn E. García Jr.

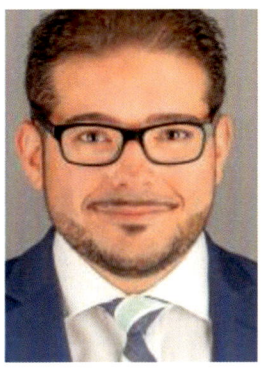

HCA Healthcare/USF Morsani College of Medicine GME: Bayonet Point Hospital, Hudson, FL, USA

Jorge Girotti

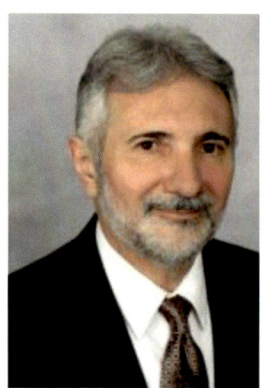

Hispanic Center of Excellence, University of Illinois College of Medicine, Chicago, IL, USA

Amanda Lynn Hernandez

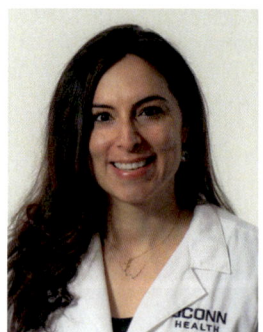

Department of Neurology, University of Connecticut School of Medicine, Farmington, CT, USA

Elizabeth Homan Sandoval

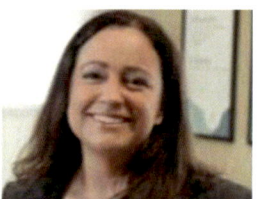

Ashland Memorial Medical Center, University of Iowa Hospitals and Clinics, Iowa City, IA, USA

Francisco Lucio

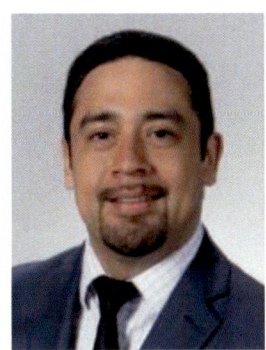

Obstetrics and Gynecology, University of Arizona College of Medicine-Phoenix, Phoenix, AZ, USA

Pedro Mancias

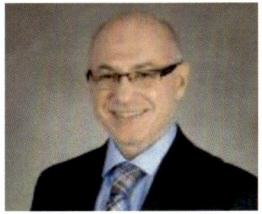

McGovern Medical School, Houston, TX, USA

Denise Martinez

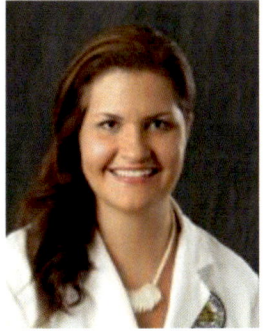

University of Iowa Carver College of Medicine, Iowa City, IA, USA

Nicole McManus

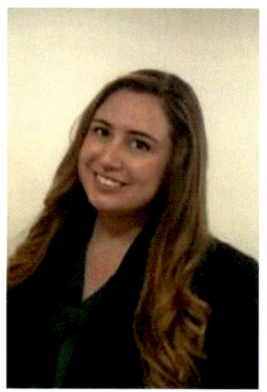

Philadelphia College of Osteopathic Medicine, Philadelphia, PA, USA

Ankeeta Mehta

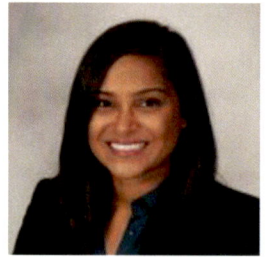

UT Southwestern Medical Center in Dallas, Dallas, TX, USA

Eric Molina

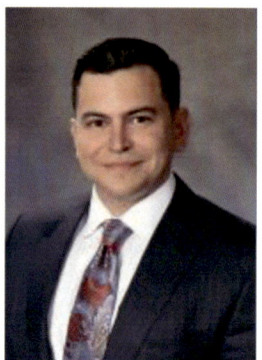

Massachusetts General Hospital – Mass General Brigham, Boston, MA, USA

Francisco Moreno

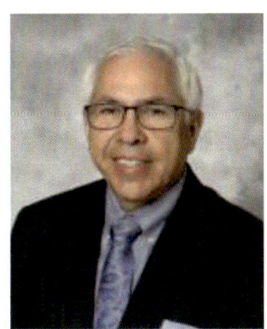

The University of Arizona College of Medicine Tucson, University of Arizona Health Sciences, Tucson, AZ, USA

Sunny Nakae

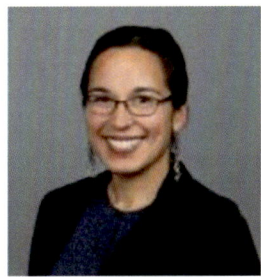

California University of Science and Medicine School of Medicine, Colton, CA, USA

Emma B. Olivera

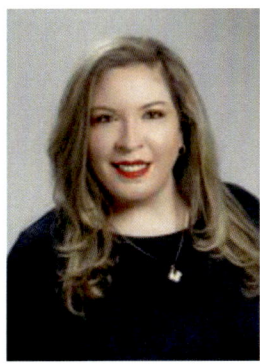

College of Medicine - Rockford General Pediatrics, Advocate Children's Hospital, Advocate-Aurora Health, University of Illinois, Rockford, IL, USA

Pilar Ortega

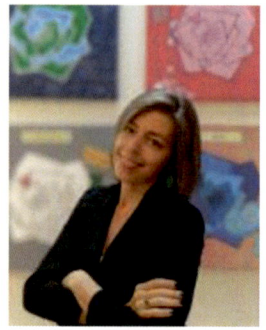

Department of Medical Education, Department of Emergency Medicine, University of Illinois College of Medicine at Chicago, Chicago, IL, USA

Norma Poll-Hunter

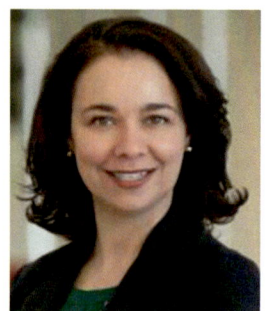

Association of American Medical Colleges (AAMC), Washington, DC, USA

Hector Rasgado-Flores

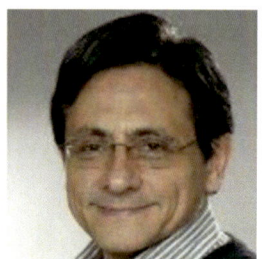

Outreach and Success Chicago Medical School, School of Graduate and Postdoctoral Studies, College of Health Professions, Chicago, IL, USA

Franklyn Rocha-Cabrero

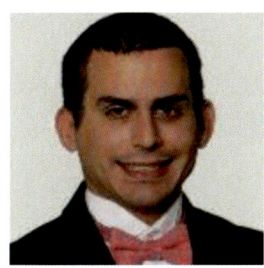

Adult General Neurologist & Clinical Neurophysiologist (Epilepsy/NIOM), Diplomate of the American Board of Psychiatry and Neurology, Long Beach, CA, USA

Donald Rodriguez

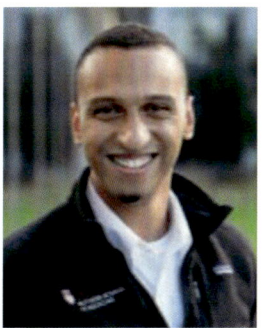

The University of Chicago Pritzker School of Medicine, Chicago, IL, USA

José E. Rodríguez

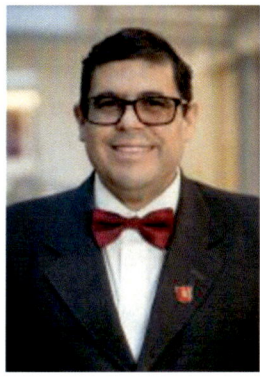

University of Utah Health, Salt Lake City, UT, USA

Victor H. Rodríguez

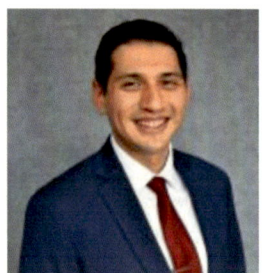

Tulane University School of Medicine, New Orleans, LA, USA

Minerva A. Romero Arenas

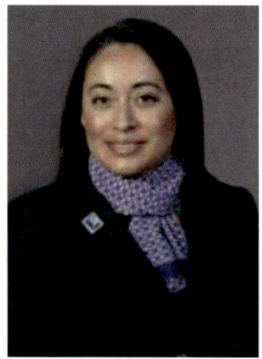

New York Presbyterian Brooklyn Methodist Hospital, Weill Cornell Medicine, New York City, NY, USA

Valerie Romero-Leggott

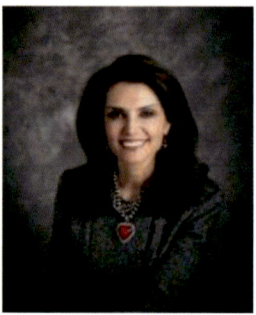

UNM SOM Combined BA/MD Program, Albuquerque, NM, USA

Fidencio Saldana

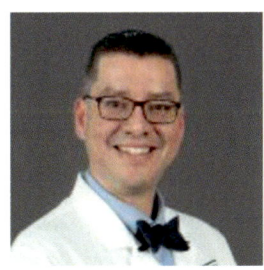

Harvard Medical School, Boston, MA, USA

John Paul Sánchez

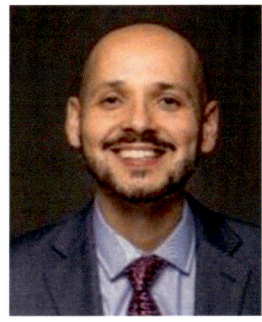

Diversity, Equity, and Inclusion, University of New Mexico Health Sciences, Albuquerque, NM, USA

Maria Santos

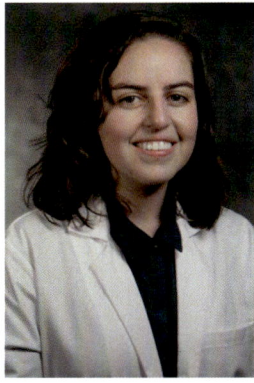

Family Medicine, Duke Family Medicine and Community Health, Durham, NC, USA

Debora Silva

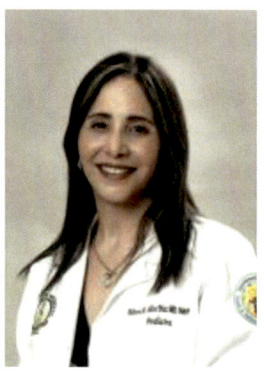

Department of Pediatrics, School of Medicine, University of Puerto Rico, San Juan, PR, USA

Orlando Sola

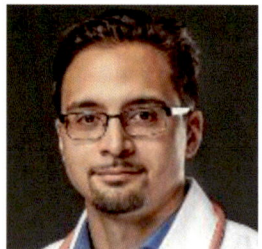

Department of Family Medicine, Chase Brexton Health Services, Baltimore, MD, USA

Sylk Sotto-Santiago

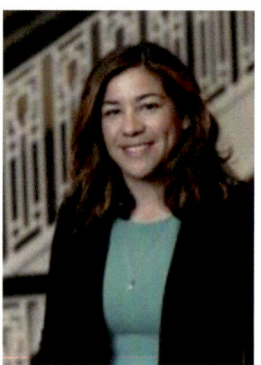

Department of Medicine, Indiana University School of Medicine, Indiana CTSI, Indianapolis, IN, USA

Julia Su

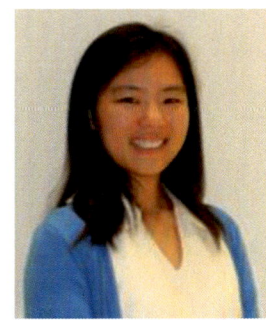

Donald and Barbara Zucker School of Medicine at Hofstra/Northwell, Long Island, NY, USA

Jeffrey Uribe

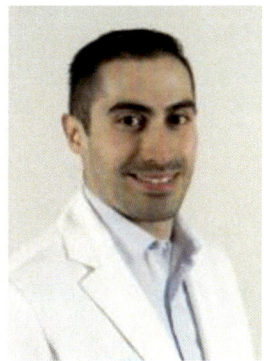

Georgetown University School of Medicine (GUSOM), Washington, DC, USA

Monica Vela

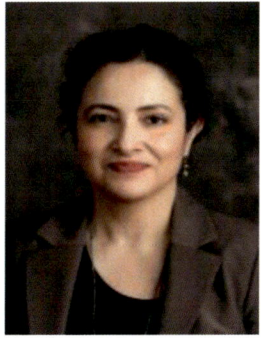

Center of Excellence at the University of Illinois College of Medicine, Chicago, IL, USA

Larissa Velez

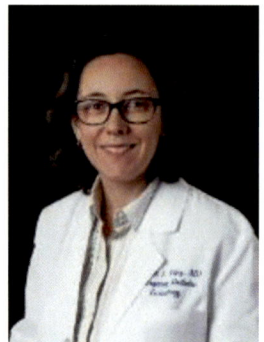

UT Southwestern Medical Center, Dallas, TX, USA

John Paul Sánchez, Donald Rodriguez, Deion Ellis, and Monica Vela

Latina/o/x/e, Hispanic or of Spanish Origin + (LHS+) Identified Student Leaders in Medicine: More Than 50 Years of Presence, Activism, and Leadership was written by stakeholders of the Latino Medical Student Association (LMSA), a national non-profit organization that exists to unite and empower current and future physicians through service, mentorship, and education to advocate for the improved health of Latina, Latino, Latinx, Latine, Hispanic, or of Spanish Origin+ (LHS+) communities in the United States (U.S.). Throughout this book we use the umbrella term LHS+ to be reflective of communities with our common geographic (e.g. Caribbean; North, Central, and South America; and Spain) and Spanish language ancestry; to recognize historical terms Latino, Latina, Hispanic, or of Spanish Origin (e.g. used on standardized surveys such as the AAMC Matriculating Student Questionnaire, AAMC Graduation Questionnaire, U.S. Census, etc.), emerging generational/non-binary terms (e.g. Latine, Latinx), with the plus '+' acknowledging other terms linked to national or social identity (e.g. Mexican, Afro-Latin, Nuyorican, etc.). Throughout the book a variety of terms are used to recognize, respect, and honor historical and current individual and communal identities. Timewise, the book primarily focuses on activism since the 1960s, a time of empowerment to battle social injustices, till the present, with mention of some seminal events affecting LHS+ diversity, inclusion, and equity in medicine as early as the 1900s.

For over 50 years, LMSA and its antecedent organizations have worked on behalf of thousands of learners and alumni across 180+ allopathic and osteopathic medical schools, providing the resources needed to promote the recruitment, retention, and promotion of diverse physicians. Notably, today's LMSA grew out of the efforts of medical students in distinct pockets across the U.S., who recognized a need to make such resources available to historically underrepresented groups in medicine. This book chronicles the successes and struggles of students, faculty, and staff, and organizational leaders in supporting LHS+ advancement within medicine over the last half-century, along with the ways in which this success can be built upon over the next 50 years.

J. P. Sánchez (✉)
Diversity, Equity, and Inclusion, University of New Mexico Health Sciences, Albuquerque, NM, USA
e-mail: exec.director@lmsa.net

D. Rodriguez
The University of Chicago Pritzker School of Medicine, Chicago, IL, USA

D. Ellis
National Center for LMSA Leadership and Advancement, Office for Diversity, Equity, and Inclusion, University of New Mexico Health Sciences Center (UNM HSC), Albuquerque, NM, USA

M. Vela
University of Illinois College of Medicine, Chicago, IL, USA

© The Author(s) 2024
J. P. Sánchez, D. Rodriguez (eds.), *Latino, Hispanic, or of Spanish Origin+ Identified Student Leaders in Medicine*, Sustainable Development Goals Series, https://doi.org/10.1007/978-3-031-35020-7_1

The 1960s and 1970s, served as a period for LHS+ learners to critically evaluate the ill-equipped landscape of medical education to address the unique challenges facing diverse medical trainees, as well as the critical health issues disproportionately affecting communities of color in the U.S. In mirroring the principles and tactics of ongoing labor movements throughout the U.S, LHS+ medical students in different regions of the country began to create chapters with formalized infrastructure. Akin to unions, these chapters supported their members, made their grievances known to medical school administrators, and advocated for basic rights for themselves, their patients, and their communities. As time passed, student organizers increasingly recognized the importance of developing a single unified national voice to call for change for the benefit of diverse trainees, faculty, staff, patients, and their communities. In chapters two through seven, we review the history of student organizing across five U.S. regions; the transition from smaller groups to a larger national entity; and the sociopolitical, cultural, and educational factors that influenced the development of LMSA and its members.

Importantly, many of the factors that affected medical trainees in the 1960s persist to the modern day. Among these factors is the continued underrepresentation of LHS+ individuals among the physician workforce. LHS+ individuals represented less than 6% of the U.S. physician workforce in 2021 [1], with lower proportions characterizing the presence of LHS+ individuals in positions of leadership within U.S. academic medical centers [2]. In contrast, based on the 2022 U.S. Census, those identifying as Hispanic or Latino comprised 18.9% of the overall population, underscoring this group's status as underrepresented in medicine (UIM) [1–3]. As patient care improves when the lived experiences of healthcare providers match those of their patients, diversity-related workforce inequities compromise the U.S. healthcare system's ability to mitigate health disparities [2, 3]. To address this, LMSA has steadily developed infrastructure to support those already in medicine, to bolster the pipeline to medical education, and to leverage partners in the quest to increase diversity, equity, and inclusion within osteopathic and allopathic medicine. Chapters eight through fifteen synthesize these efforts and provide opportunities for medical schools, national organizations, and LMSA to work together to meet their shared mission of improving health and well-being for all.

While this book highlights challenges that continue to affect LHS+ learners in medicine, this book is intended to serve as a celebration of the accomplishments realized in the face of adversities. As noted throughout, student, faculty, staff, and organizational leaders—alongside dozens of alumni—came together to recount their stories firsthand. Names of hundreds of students, advisors, and alumni and their distinct contributions, service, and sacrifices are listed throughout the book. The chapters of this book were comprised by 39 authors, spanning from medical students to full professors with tenure and chancellors/presidents, whose presence has spanned over 50 years (since 1972). All of the chapters' co-authors identify with nationalities of the LHS+ diaspora and other groups underrepresented in the health professions—sexual and gender minorities, ethnic and racial minorities, women, first-generation, etc. Their diverse voices and eloquent descriptions of the history of LHS+ presence, activism, and leadership in medicine and LMSA is conveyed through personal narratives and may resonate with your own lived experiences. We encourage readers to not only bear witness to the lived experiences of co-authors but also to continue championing progress for LHS+ and other underrepresented in medicine (UIM) groups for the betterment of our patients and communities. The book is filled with lessons learned and promising and best practices to support LHS+ and other minoritized communities' inclusion in medicine.

Personal Perspective: Donald M. Rodriguez, PhD (MD Candidate)

As I reflect on the creation and content of this book, I find it incredibly heartening to see these stories being told. Relatively few narratives or scholarly works have emphasized the journey and experiences of LHS+ individuals in medicine. However, our voices are critically needed to ensure that no one is left behind by the U.S. healthcare system, especially as the LHS+ population in the U.S. continues to grow.

In particular, it excites me to see this book come to fruition, as I firmly believe its unique composition—consisting of historical overviews, personal accounts, and actionable guidance—can provide meaningful insights to a wide range of readers. For administrators and senior leaders at academic medical centers, this book sheds light on the issues with which many of your learners grapple. Addressing these issues and learning from the experiences of your trainees and their predecessors are key steps to building inclusive learning environments and positioning UIM individuals for *success*. For faculty members and other professionals, this book highlights the importance of consistent engagement with colleagues and trainees. LMSA arose from the desire to build a community "by us, for us." Herein, we state how leveraging this community not only increases the number of visible role models for the next generation of diverse clinicians, but also leads to your advancement and fulfillment throughout your professional career. For LMSA alumni, this book showcases your legacy in building an organization that has helped countless individuals pursue their dreams of a more equitable society. Moreover, this book highlights both the progress that has been achieved and the work that remains to be accomplished in furthering the development of LMSA, its student members, and the LHS+ pipeline in medicine. Lastly, for current and future LHS+ physicians-in-training, this book hopefully shows you that *you are not alone*, that the challenges you may face are surmountable, and that there is a community in LMSA that exists to support you as you work to become the physician the world needs you to be.

In my own journey, I decided to pursue medicine following family health emergencies, through which I was thrust into the world of hospitals and clinics. In helping my grandmother overcome language barriers to care, or supporting my sister as she advocated for her needs during her appointments, I recognized the need for caring physicians exhibiting shared backgrounds and lived experiences to those of my family. While a desire to address this need drove me towards a career in medicine, I have kept along this path by the desire to make academic medicine more accessible to diverse learners whose stories, like mine, are not told enough in medicine. Sharing our stories is a critical first step to understanding how—together—learners, physicians, administrators, and partners can enhance the presence of LHS+ individuals in medicine and remind them that they belong.

Personal Perspective: Monica Vela, MD

This book is for all those students who do not have a parent able to guide them through the complex higher educational system in the United States and/or could not afford the very basic necessities to forward their education. It is for any learner who enters classrooms or other learning experiences hoping to see someone who looks or speaks like them and does not. The authors of this book want you to know that we see you, we acknowledge you and we hope to support you. We hope that our experiences will not only inform you but uplift and inspire you to believe that you belong, that you can accomplish your dreams, and that you can flourish. We also hope that you will, in turn, share your experiences, insights, and wisdom to uplift others.

Personal Perspective: Deion L. Ellis, MD, MMS

The importance of diversity, equity and inclusion in medicine is well known. For minorities in medicine, the lack of proper representation is a constant reminder to continue the work to support our students and make the healthcare provider population more reflective of the patient population. What can be lost in the progression towards this goal, is the celebration of the individuals who help pave the way up to this point. Although the LHS+ community comprises 18.9% of the U.S population, only a small subset of that percentage is reflected in the healthcare community. An even smaller subset of those individuals is celebrated and broadcasted to all for their accomplishments and contributions to increasing and supporting diversity in medicine.

To witness individuals, from similar cultural backgrounds, achieving at the highest levels in their respective positions, while also giving back to the advancement of our communities is nothing short of inspiring. Having these role models makes any notion of self-doubt decrease because a member of *la familia* has made it to their position, laying the foundation for future generations. That is why this book is so meaningful and important. The book is another opportunity to celebrate leaders of our LHS+ community who contributed to the formation of the Latino Medical Student Association (LMSA) through their activism and leadership.

Celebrating our rich heritage and LHS+ communities in medicine helps us embed the lessons of the past, so we don't repeat any pitfalls. It helps us understand the evolution of our communities and the journey we are on so we are more prepared for what may come. But most importantly it brings us joy and pride in who we are. I take pride in being able to learn about the outstanding role models that we have in our communities for our communities.

The following is a summary of the book chapters:

Chapter 2: LHS+ Medical Student History and Heritage of the U.S. Northeast Region

The Northeast region has the third-largest LHS+ population in the country. Harvard Medical School, with its formation of the Boricua Health Organization (BHO), in 1972, stakes claim to the oldest LHS+ regional medical student organization of the Latino Medical Student Association. The foundation and evolution of BHO to the Boricua Latino Health Organization (BLHO) and

then National BLHO in the 1990s, was a reflection of LHS+ youth, gathering into a critical mass to succeed in their dream of becoming health professionals and addressing health inequities in their underserved communities. As they entered an unfamiliar homogenous, hierarchical culture, often with limited resources for academic success and defying stereotypes to maintain a positive LHS+ identity, the constant inner whisper of 'Pa'lante, Siempre Pa'lante'[1] has led to generations of LHS+ Northeast physician leaders.

Chapter 3: LHS+ Medical Student History and Heritage of the U.S. Southeast Region

The purpose of this chapter is to highlight the history and rapid growth of LHS+ communities in the southeast region. The vast immigration to this region from outside the U.S. and the surrounding events are the context in which the students of the LMSA were raised and planted the seeds for LHS+-identified individuals in medicine. As the region continues to grow, there is hope and evidence that the tide of progress will continue to rise in the Southeast region.

Chapter 4: LHS+ Medical Student History and Heritage of the U.S. Midwest Region

The focus of this chapter is to highlight the path towards the empowerment of Latinos in the U.S. Midwest — both in general and in medicine — through reviews of published literature, statistics, and oral history. Through migration, education, and self-determination, Latinos grew from being an impermanent fixture of the Midwestern labor force in the mid-1800s to a driver of diversity, equity, and inclusion efforts within medicine regionally and nationally in the late 1900s and early 2000s. This chapter recounts the key sociopolitical and cultural factors that brought Latinos to the Midwest, shaped this community's presence within the region, and catalyzed activism within this community for increased representation in the physician workforce and improved health outcomes. Lastly, this chapter chronicles the trainee-driven grassroots efforts that culminated in the formation of official medical student organizations. The Latino Medical Student Association (LMSA) that exists as of this chapter's writing reflects the hard work of Midwest students and physicians and will rely on continuation of these efforts in order to promote a healthier Latino community and a stronger healthcare system for all.

Chapter 5: LHS+ Medical Student History and Heritage of the U.S. Southwest Region

This chapter highlights the unique experiences with access to health care and medical education by LHS+ identified individuals in the U.S. Southwest Region. Since the annexation of the southwest regions' constitutive states, LHS+ individuals, primarily of Mexican heritage, have endured unique forms of marginalization and discrimination that led to disparities in illness, injuries and deaths in comparison to White individuals. As LHS+ individuals entered the physician workforce, despite academic success, they often faced unique roadblocks in seeking employment. The Chicano movements in the 1960s, in particular students' demands for educational equity in high schools and colleges in Texas, served as inspiration for medical students to seek similar equity within Southwest medical schools. Over several decades, LHS+ medical students and physicians were able to grow local medical student groups and organize on the regional and national level to ensure LHS+ student specific issues were met.

Chapter 6: LHS+ Medical Student History and Heritage of the U.S. West Region

The history of LMSA West begins in the 1960s with a small group of first-generation premedical Chicano students with a vision of serving those in need and dedicating their lives and careers to ensure everyone has access to basic human necessities including healthcare. When those same students started to enter medical school, they found few students like themselves and no role models. They had to pull themselves up by their bootstraps. They were the change they wanted to see. They created a new organization to provide a safe space for mentorship, support, and professional development for future generations of medical students like themselves. The organization evolved from a strong presence in California and other Western states to a unified network that could support students across the region. Influenced by their Latino heritage, generations of LMSA members have shared the values of comunidad, valor, liderazgo, conocimiento and compromiso. This is the story of the LMSA familia in the West region.

Chapter 7: A Unified National Organization: The Budding of LMSA

Decades before the creation of a national organization, medical students across the country formed Latino medical student groups at their respective medical schools, and started to collaborate with other similar groups at the local, state, and regional levels. Eventually, a loose network of engagement began between these regional Latino medical student organizations that evolved into a thriving national 501(c)(3) non-profit organization called the Latino Medical Student Association (LMSA). This chapter tells the story of some of the medical students who stepped up as leaders to unify and advocate towards a shared dream of supporting a national community and identity. The existence and growth of the organization has been consistently borne out of student-led grassroots efforts, characterized by incremental successes despite the impermanence of leadership tied to the short time period leaders spend in medical school. The organization has also existed as a dynamic amalgamation of personal, professional, regional and Latin American ethnonational and social identities. The organization known today as LMSA is in so many ways the realization of past dreams and the fruit of seeds planted decades ago. In 2022, the organization recognized its oldest originating chapter (Boricua Health Organization Chapter, Harvard Medical School, 1972) while celebrating its 17th annual national conference, 19 years of 501(c)(3) non-profit status, and its 24th national coordinator/president and board of directors.

Chapter 8: Tu Lucha es Mi Lucha: The Evolution of a Student-Driven LHS+ Health Policy Initiative

The rich Latino history in different American continents, including the United States, has been a constant fight for resources to meet the community's basic needs while preserving our ethnic background, culture, traditions, and values. Through the centuries of colonialism, forced assimilation and imperialism, multiple prominent Latino leaders and organizations have dedicated their lives to health equity and social justice. Advocacy and grassroot organizational skills are essential to instill transformative changes in healthcare, however these are rarely taught in traditional academic medical curriculum. In this chapter, we explore the complex process of creating a Latino health-driven organizational structure that teaches students how to effectively advocate for their patients, community and profession. In response to those needs, student leaders created the Latino Medical Student Association Policy Summit (LMSA-PS). Using the Kern model and the CDC Policy Development Framework, LMSA students created an annual policy conference composed of student-led rallies, legislative visits, policy-related lectures and a legislative session called the Congress of Delegates. In describing the LMSA-PS we contextualize LMSA student advocacy through historical perspectives of Latino community advocacy, healthcare advocacy, and medical student mobilization. These best practices can be used to help students from marginalized and underrepresented minority populations develop effective health policy training and advocacy programming.

Chapter 9: LMSA Faculty/Physician Advisors: A Critical Partner in Supporting LHS+ Medical Students

LHS+ physicians and faculty have had the dual role of advising LHS+ medical students and assisting in the initiation, maintenance, and growth of medical student groups at medical school campuses and leadership on the regional and national levels. This chapter describes the historical and emerging role and challenges, faced by Latino/Hispanic physicians and faculty, in supporting a primarily student-led medical association while ensuring their own promotion to senior academic health center positions.

Chapter 10: Student Affairs Offices and the LHS+ Medical Student

This chapter seeks to review activities, innovations, and research of the Offices of Student Affairs (OSA) in supporting medical students of LHS+ identities. For this chapter, we are using LHS+ as an umbrella term to include Latina, Latino, Latinx, and other words associated with ancestry from a Spanish-speaking country. In 2016, the AAMC Group on Student Affairs (GSA) developed a GSA Performance Framework to describe the eight areas of expertise that student affairs professionals should develop for the successful performance of specific roles, functions, and services within student affairs [4]. In this chapter, we use this framework to describe current and potential future efforts to support LHS+ students. We will focus on the three areas most relevant to the OSA role - student wellness and mental health, academic progression, and professional and career development. Also, we will address areas that the OSA collaborate closely with such as Student Diversity and Inclusion, Medical School Recruitment & Admission, Student Records Management, Financial Assistance, and Unit Operations Management.

Chapter 11: The Role of Medical Education Offices in Preparing the Physician Workforce to Care for LHS+ Individuals

This chapter discusses the role of medical education offices in the advancement of health equity for LHS+ communities. Medical education must evolve to reflect the needs of the patient population to ensure that physicians are prepared to equitably care for their communities. LHS+ medical students and faculty at U.S. medical schools have made significant contributions to the development of educational strategies for medical students and physician preparedness to care for the growing LHS+ population. In this chapter, we discuss the gradual integration of LHS+ health and health disparities into medical education, including the curriculum content standards of accrediting institutions. We present examples of Latino/Hispanic-focused cultural competency education in the context of medical education. We also discuss the development of medical Spanish educational programs to build a language-concordant physician workforce with the skills to address the communication needs of Spanish-speaking Hispanics with non-English language preference. Finally, we propose the next steps needed in medical education systems that prioritize health equity, cultural competency, and language access for the LHS+ population.

Chapter 12: LHS+ Individuals in Graduate Medical Education

According to the Accreditation Council on Graduate Medical Education (ACGME), in the 2018–2019 year, Hispanics consisted 5.3% of residents and fellows [5]. More concerning are specialty areas where the percentage of Hispanics is critically low, such as radiology, orthopedic surgery, and otolaryngology. Some tout Latin American graduates as a potential solution, but the data is scarce. The Educational Commission for Foreign Medical Graduates does not release regular reporting on the racial and ethnic compo-

sition of internationally trained physicians aspiring to enter residencies and fellowships. Beyond recognizing USMLE and clerkship grades as biased, institutional leaders should consider the question "How ought GME Program Directors best assess the LHS+ medical student?" The answer is to do so the same way we should evaluate all candidates—holistically.

Chapter 13: LHS+ Faculty Development and Advancement

Current and future faculty member development is an essential catalyst to expand impactful LHS+ scholarship of discovery, education, and service in pursuit of health equity for the 63 million (18.9%) Americans identified as Hispanic or Latino by the U.S. Census Bureau [6]. This chapter seeks to address two relevant aspects of faculty development: (1) developing skills and values in faculty from all backgrounds to best equip LHS+ trainees; and (2) optimize success of current and future LHS+ faculty.

Chapter 14: The Role of Offices of Diversity, Equity & Inclusion to the LHS+ Community

Academic health science centers (AHSCs) in the United States (U.S.) are positioned as leaders in health professions education, clinical care and biomedical health science research. AHSCs often comprise a medical school, other health professions programs (e.g. pharmacy, nursing, physician assistant, etc.), teaching hospital(s), and faculty heavily involved in biomedical, clinical, and medical education research [7]. Whether private or public, these institutions represent societal hubs that provide enormous benefits for the health and well-being of the communities that they serve. As LHS+ communities in the U.S. continue to expand in size and geographical distribution, so too does the social obligation to provide meaningful, culturally responsive, and equitable care for and engagement with this population. At many AHSCs, this engagement is often facilitated and led by offices of diversity, equity and inclusion (ODEIs). This chapter highlights several strategies and opportunities for ODEIs to enact positive change for LHS+ communities within and around AHSCs.

Chapter 15: Looking Forward

In this book, we bring together the work completed through LMSA as a community, and an organization over the past 50+ years. We highlight the changes that have occurred in medicine because we are here to advocate for the LHS+ community. With every year, we become more robust, and with every year we continue to see the ways in which the medical community still needs to change to provide better care and support for the LHS+ students, trainees, and patients. Although the future of LMSA is bright and built on a strong foundation of the past 50 years, there remain legal and political threats that could stymie progress. The authors in this book have covered in depth the underrepresentation amongst LHS+ physicians and trainees in the U.S. Ongoing developments in the legal and political landscape threaten to exacerbate an already dire situation.

References

1. Diversity among Hispanic/Latinx US Physicians - AAMC. https://www.aamc.org/media/56736/download.
2. Jones N. "2020 Census Illuminates Racial and Ethnic Composition of the Country." Census.gov, 10 June 2022, https://www.census.gov/library/stories/2021/08/improved-race-ethnicity-measures-reveal-united-states-population-much-more-multiracial.html.
3. Table 3: U.S. Medical School Faculty by Rank and Race/Ethnicity ... - AAMC. https://www.aamc.org/media/9681/download?attachment.
4. GSA Performance Framework. AAMC 2016. https://www.aamc.org/system/files/2019-08/gsaframework-overview.pdf. Accessed 5 Jan 2023.
5. Data Resource Book Academic Year 2018-2019. PDF. Accreditation Council for Graduate Medical Education; 2018. https://www.acgme.org/Portals/0/PFAssets/PublicationsBooks/2018-2019_ACGME_DATABOOK_DOCUMENT.pdf
6. U.S. Census Bureau QuickFacts United States. https://www.census.gov/quickfacts/fact/table/US/PST045221. Accessed 10 Jan 2023.
7. Anderson G, Steinberg E, Heyssel R. The pivotal role of the academic health center. Health Affairs. 1994;13(3):146–58. https://doi.org/10.1377/hlthaff.13.3.146.

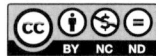

LHS+ Medical Student History and Heritage of the U.S. Northeast Region

John Paul Sánchez, Amanda Lynn Hernandez, Edgar Figueroa, Jeffrey Uribe, and Emilio Carrillo

1960s to 2020s: LHS+ Migration, Identity, and Socioeconomic Trends

Migration

The Northeast (NE) currently represents the third largest regional population of Hispanics in the U.S., with 7.7 of 56.6 million U.S. Hispanics in 2015 [1]. Between 1970 and 2015 the populace of Hispanics in the Northeast increased from 1.9 million to 7.7 million, with 71% of the region's Hispanics living in two Northeastern states—New York and New Jersey. Initially, NE Hispanics resided in metropolitan cities, however after 2000, there has been greater parity with Hispanics residing in suburbs and cities [1].

The national origin of Hispanics in the Northeast is quite distinct from other regions of the United States. The Northeast houses a significant portion of Hispanics from the Caribbean, from islands such as Puerto Rico, the Dominican Republic, and Cuba. In the 1970s, Puerto Ricans represented 2/3 of all Hispanics in the NE, followed by Cubans (roughly 11% of the population), and all other Hispanic groups individually represented single digits in proportion [1]. The large Puerto Rican influx to the mainland was attributed to seeking economic opportunities among a cohort that uniquely held citizenship status. By 2015, Puerto Ricans became 1/3 of the Hispanic NE population, and other groups represented double-digit proportions (Mexicans—12.1% and Dominicans—17.4%) [1].

Identity

Hispanic identity is often influenced and rooted in Spanish, Indigenous, and/or African cultures. Northeast Hispanics, because of the large proportion from Spanish-speaking countries in the Caribbean, have a greater influence of African culture. This contribution is largely due to Caribbean countries importing slave labor from Africa to support the large plantation economy in the Caribbean. Massey and colleagues, point out that race among Caribbean Hispanics "is not perceived as a black-white dichotomy, but more of a continuum." [1]

J. P. Sánchez (✉)
Diversity, Equity, and Inclusion, University of New Mexico Health Sciences, Albuquerque, NM, USA
e-mail: exec.director@lmsa.net

A. L. Hernandez
Department of Neurology, University of Connecticut School of Medicine, Farmington, CT, USA

E. Figueroa · E. Carrillo
Weill Cornell Medical College, New York, NY, USA

J. Uribe
Georgetown University School of Medicine (GUSOM), Washington, DC, USA

© The Author(s) 2024
J. P. Sánchez, D. Rodriguez (eds.), *Latino, Hispanic, or of Spanish Origin+ Identified Student Leaders in Medicine*, Sustainable Development Goals Series, https://doi.org/10.1007/978-3-031-35020-7_2

For NE Caribbean Hispanics, indication of racial categorization on surveys is more likely as "mixed origin" rather than a fixed category of White, Black, Asian, or American Indian.

Socioeconomic Trends

Numerous socioeconomic factors have influenced Hispanic attainment of medical degrees—including completion of high school and college degrees, resources to serve as competitive applicants and a network of role models, mentors and champions. First and foremost, graduation from college is a pre-requisite to attending medical school. In the 1970s, nearly 70% of NE Hispanics had less than a H.S. diploma; in 2015, that proportion dropped to roughly 30% [1]. Over the same time period, the proportion of individuals having some college education rose from 6% to 23% and college graduation rates increased from 6% to 19% [1]. In terms of college graduates, there was also variability within Hispanic country of origin, with Cubans and South Americans achieving college graduation at a higher proportion (respectively 37% and 27%) than Mexicans, Dominicans, Puerto Ricans, and Central Americans (ranging from 15% to 17%) [1].

In terms of financial resources, in 2015, Dominicans, Mexicans, and Puerto Ricans displayed the highest rates of poverty (approximately 25%), whereas Central Americans were approximately 18% and South Americans and Cubans were approximately 12% [1]. Lack of financial resources makes it difficult for pre-medical applicants to access test preparation materials to have an equitable chance of scoring competitively on standardized exams and the opportunity to apply to multiple medical schools.

Beyond high levels of poverty and low rates of college graduation, isolation and segregation placed Hispanics in the NE "at a distinct disadvantage in American society" in achieving graduate education, in particular medical education [1].

In reflecting on her own journey to medical school Sylvia M. Ramos, M.D., M.S., F.A.C.S., Clinical Professor of Surgery, University of New Mexico School of Medicine (Albert Einstein College of Medicine (AECOM), 1969–1974) shares:

> I was born in Puerto Rico and arrived in the South Bronx at age 12 in 1959. I lived there during the decades beginning with the great white flight and ending with the burning of the Bronx. An aptitude test in high school, where I did well in Math and Science, led me to the library to explore careers in those fields. I was drawn to Medicine though I didn't know any doctors or what such a career entailed. Nor did anyone at school suggest that path for me. At Hunter College in the Bronx, where I was a Thomas Hunter Honors Scholar, I remember being told by my pre-med advisor that he didn't think I could become a physician. I took my own road and sought support from a professor who knew my abilities and believed in me. While a student at the Albert Einstein College of Medicine (AECOM), I adopted my niece when my sister died and took a year-long leave of absence to care for her. I graduated in 1974 and undertook a surgery residency in AECOM and affiliated NYC hospitals program. My struggles and triumphs guided me as I became the inaugural Educational Programs Coordinator of the Office for Under-Represented Students at Einstein from 1978–1982. We served as a primary location for students to express concerns about academic challenges, minority student retention, and family related issues. The office provided academic enrichment programs to enrolled students and successfully engaged in recruitment activities to increase the number of non-traditional students at Einstein. I retired from a fulfilling career in general and breast surgery in 2015.

Norma Villanueva MD, Associate Professor and the Regional Director of Medical Education A.T. Still University's School of Osteopathic Medicine (Albert Einstein College of Medicine, 1981–1986) shares:

> Growing up in the South Bronx in the 70s was tough. We were on welfare and like many youth in the neighborhood we suffered from malnourishment. We never had a primary care physician and would go to the emergency department for care. I would see white teachers and principals and ask myself why weren't we running institutions. I would see doctors on TV and would think about being that doctor who made house calls…that's what I wanted to be for families in the South Bronx.

Sociopolitical Activism

The increased migration by Hispanics to the NE occurred during a time of increased sociopolitical consciousness and growing unrest by youth and young adults over unemployment, lack of housing and lack of access to policy-making structure. Numerous groups emerged during the 60s and 70s to support Hispanic youth during these counterculture times. Since 1961, ASPIRA has been a well-known organization "dedicated to serving NYC youth and their families, providing opportunities that would otherwise not be available to them, serving as an effective advocate, and fighting to improve education in the Puerto Rican and Latino communities." [2] The Young Lords Party, was another group that emerged to address social and health inequities in the late 60 s. The Young Lords gained recognition for organizing sectors of the community around health care issues, with demands that included access to quality health care and education and subsequent recruitment of Latinos into health care fields [3].

Elizabeth Lee-Rey MD, MPH, private practice physician (University of Pittsburgh School of Medicine, 1984–1990) notes,

> My political activism and my love for my Latina Puerto Rican heritage was rooted by involvement with ASPIRA of New York back during the 1970–1980s. True to the vision of Dr. Antonia Pantoja at that time there existed the early Pre Health program that involved leadership development, activities for building self esteem and confidence, medical school tours led by medical students of color, writing workshops for our personal statements, MCAT prep and most importantly, not knowing at that time that I would have lifelong friendships and colleagues in medicine. This early exposure to the opportunities, resources and witnessing those like me who succeeded and were making a difference—kept my aspirations alive.

Health Issues and Disparities

For Hispanics in the Northeast, reproductive health and family planning, access to culturally competent health care and environmental health were dominant topics [3, 4]. In the 1950s–1970s, salient to the large proportion of Puerto Ricans in the Northeast, was reproductive health and family planning. During that time the U.S. strategized to achieve population control on the island, through encouraging migration off the island and promoting sterilization services among Puerto Rican women residing on the island; this period is well narrated in the documentary "La Operación" [5]. Additionally, U.S. companies and governmental officials, in their efforts to develop and test birth control pills, had implemented numerous early clinical trials among Puerto Rican women, without proper informed consent. Nearly one-fifth of these women eventually reported regretting their decision [5–7].

The passage of the 1964 Civil Rights Act and the 1965 Social Security Act opened access to hospital employment and medical care for everyone [8]. Health care systems were now confronted with the responsibility of providing quality, comprehensive care for a Hispanic community, diverse by Spanish and English language preference, degree of acculturation, and social determinants of health. Unfortunately, the medical workforce at the time lacked a critical mass of Hispanic physicians and there was little if any medical education content or instruction dedicated to caring for Hispanic patients.

Concurrently, Hispanic leaders like Dr. Helen Rodríguez-Trías and community groups like the Young Lords Party were calling for greater attention to environmental and institutional factors contributing to the poorer health of Hispanic, especially in urban areas [9]. The Young Lords Party launched various programs to combat public health and medical inequalities including—street clean-ups, food kitchens, and health screenings. One of their most notable efforts was the 'Lincoln Offensive' of 1970, where members took over Lincoln Hospital in the South Bronx and demanded infrastructural upkeep (e.g. to manage the high levels of lead content in the walls), preventive health services, drug addiction care, and maternal and child care services [9].

Medical Student Activism Emerges and Coalesces

The emergence of social activism in the throes of the 1969 demonstrations and calls for national reform of civil rights and inequities served as the backdrop for Latino/Hispanic medical students to stand, speak, and assume a new role in medical education and the health care systems. LMSA-Northeast arose from the Boricua Health Organization (BHO), which was founded in 1972 by Harvard medical students Jaime Rivera and Emilio Carrillo [10, 11]. At the time, the medical students were motivated to mobilize in response to the rampant discrimination both inside and outside educational institutions. Moreover, they had been deeply involved in social activism and were experienced and skilled in organizing and communication. These pioneers understood first-hand that the health status of the Latino/Hispanic communities was poor and that it suffered from substandard health care. The quest for health equity inspired the resolve of these student organizers, who at times imperiled their studies, to serve a higher purpose.

Emilio Carrillo, Clinical Associate Professor of Medicine, Weill Cornell Medical College, (Harvard Medical School, 1972–1976) shares,

> Doing tenant organizing and participating in student government during college prepared me for the big job ahead. One of the first things I did, even before buying my medical books, was to start organizing and talking to people about a student organization. Our class was the first to have even a handful of Latinos. Jaime Rivera and I were the only two Latinos from the East Coast. There were a few Latinos from the West Coast. This small number was in fact huge. Earlier classes had at most one and rarely two Latinos who were mostly children of Latin American families that could pay tuition and other expenses in full.

The name Boricua Health Organization was reflective of the mission of the organization to improve the health status of 'Boricuas' or Puerto Ricans. Prior to Spanish colonization, the native Taíno Indians referred to the island of Puerto Rico as Boriken and the inhabitants were named Boricua. The term Boricua in the name Boricua Health Organization recognized the predominant make-up of Hispanics in the Northeast, at the time, to be of Puerto Rican ancestry, and the great sense of pride Puerto Ricans had of their identity. The three areas BHO focused on were: (1) to recruit more Hispanics into medical school, (2) to retain Hispanics in medical school by understanding their cultural issues and their academic foundation, and (3) to maintain Hispanic students' focus on the health needs of their community—"recruitment, retention, and education".

The initial mission of the Harvard group stated:

> Every person has certain inalienable rights. Foremost among these is the right of every person to live as free from illness and harm as the current status of knowledge and technology will permit. But health statistics show a strong association between the highest morbidity and mortality rates with the poorest members of our society.
> We are students, providers and consumers of healthcare services, who direct our attention to the inadequacies engendered with our community in combating the ills of today's society, we have come together as an organization in search of knowledge and common strength. We seek progressive and equitable institutionalized changes, and advocate for human rights as they apply to health care for our community [11, 12].

Early on, the Harvard students turned to several strong supporters and mentors, Dr. Alvin Poussaint, Dr. Leon Einsenberg, Dr. Furshpan, and Dr. Kravitz, as they shaped their argument that minority students had a place in medicine and a place at Harvard. The medical students shared their own experiences with the administration and highlighted examples of when the school had failed Latino/Hispanic students. One notable example was the loss of a peer and friend Luis Garden Acosta [13]. Emilio Carrillo recounts:

> A joint MIT-Harvard accelerated B.A.-M.D. 6-year program had been started to recruit promising minority students—African American, Native American, immigrant, Latinos, Puerto Ricans, and Chicanos. They recruited one Latino student, Luís Garden Acosta who was an activist in New York, and he had done a lot of work with the Young Lords (former Minister of Health, New York Chapter, Young Lord's Party). He did very poorly in this program. The program was very well-intentioned, but in taking students who may not have all the required background, the necessary foundation in the medical sciences and

biochemistry, and putting them through a 6-year accelerated program, that's a lot for a student. Luis, because of his poor academic performance, was about to be removed from the program. I remember organizing the students to protest and call for him to be given another chance. The protest was on the local news channels and a group of community activists ended up protesting at the admissions committee. Eventually a decision was made to allow Luís to be re-accepted into the class, but he would basically have to perform at the same level as any other student. Unfortunately, despite a lot of support he got from the students, and tutoring, and the school, he fell off after the first semester.

During the 1970s, BHO built a significant infrastructure. In 1972, Jaime and Emilio reached out to Latino/Hispanic leaders in New York City, including Dr. Helen Rodríguez-Trías, to form a steering committee composed of representatives from several medical schools, as well as, practicing physicians and allied health care professionals. This led to the 1st Boricua Health Organization Conference, in 1973, at Lincoln Hospital, in New York City. Between 1973 and 1980, an active chapter continued at Harvard Medical School (led by Juan Albino, Mike Muñoz, Robert Taylor) and new chapters emerged in Boston (led by Sandra Palleja and Concha Mendoza at Boston University School of Medicine), New York City (led by Mariano Rey and Ernie Ferran at the New York University College of Medicine and led by George Friedman Jiménez and Luis Estevez at the Albert Einstein College of Medicine), Newark (led by Ambrosio Romero and Tom Ortiz at University of Medicine and Dentistry of New Jersey (UMDNJ)), and others in New Haven and Philadelphia. The organization was not just a Boston phenomenon, but an East Coast phenomenon. The member chapters became a way to sustain and grow their base of Latino/Hispanic trainees. Carrillo states "It wasn't just being altruistic, but basically, by working with others and helping others, we were helping ourselves. It was a very lonely time. I mean, very few of us had role models in our own family." In 1978, BHO drafted and adopted its first constitution. In the Fall of 1982, BHO with partners, launched a new journal entitled Journal of Latin Community Health. The journal was an innova-tive scholarly format but due to limited financial means lasted for only two issues.

Many Latino/Hispanic medical students didn't have a BHO chapter at their school, but were fortunate to tap other networks. Others had to weather the storm and survive on their own till a critical mass arose.

Susana Morales MD, Associate Professor, Clinical Medicine, Vice Chair, Diversity, Department of Medicine, Director, Diversity Center of Excellence of the Cornell Center for Health Equity, Weill Cornell Medicine (Columbia College of Physicians and Surgeons, 1982–1986) shared that her career was directly impacted by her community experiences:

During my undergraduate years at Harvard, I worked at Brookside, a community health center in Jamaica Plain MA, as a family health worker, which strengthened my commitment to medicine. My mentors at Brookside included a Puerto Rican primary care physician, Dr. Juan Albino, a Harvard Medical School graduate and an early member of the Boricua Health Organization. I also encountered BHO at Harvard Medical School at that time, and got to know minority medical students who mentored me, including Lydia Rios, who was incredibly supportive.

My medical school experience at Columbia was complex. We had a very strong student organization named BALSO (the Black and Latin Student Organization) and tremendous support from Dr. Margaret Haynes, our Dean for Minority Affairs, and other faculty like Dr. Jean Smith, Dr. John Lindenbaum and Dr. Gerald Thomson. The fact that our school was in Washington Heights and that one of our teaching hospitals was Harlem Hospital led to our involvement in community activities. We also advocated for linguistically and culturally competent care. Unbelievably at that time, there was no interpreter service in our hospital though it served a huge Latino community. I was frequently the only Spanish speaking provider available, and patients would sigh with relief at being able to communicate, given the absence for many years of any interpreter system. The inequities and system related structural discrimination were so stark.

Another significant urban challenge during medical school and residency years was the confluence of HIV, crack, tuberculosis, gun violence and homelessness epidemics in New York City. All of these problems disproportionately impacted communities of color. AIDS was first described to us in our first years of medical school, and we cared for HIV patients at a time when there was initially no HIV test, no treatment, and intense fear. We saw many people, including many young people, die of HIV in tragic ways. The federal government's early inaction in the face of the AIDS crisis is legendary and the entire catastrophe is in part an example of a failure of the public health system which had been systematically starved of resources and leadership for years, a punitive criminal justice system, and a drug treatment apparatus that was woefully inadequate for the needs of the community. My experiences during this tumultuous time influenced my decision to enter primary care and work on issues of health equity, access to care, advocacy around HIV, and diversity in medicine.

For Kenneth Domínguez MD, MPH, Captain U.S. Public Health Service, (Columbia College of Physicians and Surgeons and Columbia Mailman School of Public Health, 1983–1988), an awareness of Latino/Hispanic Health in the classroom and through family, pipeline programs, and mentors:

I first learned about the detailed educational pathway towards becoming a physician during a 7th grade class assignment where I interviewed my pediatrician about his career choice. I admired his vast knowledge base and ability to reassure my mom about ailments I experienced as a child. I gained a greater appreciation of Hispanic social determinants of health through stories shared by my dad at the dinner table about equity issues facing Hispanic federal workers and the importance of having union representation to address those issues particularly as they related to equal opportunity for jobs and promotions. I also learned about health issues facing migrant farm workers and the need for occupational health protections by reading leaflets on César Chávez and the grape boycotts during college at Harvard. During winter college breaks, I attended Health Careers Opportunities Program (HCOP) seminars focused on career development and health equity sponsored by the State of California and met several Hispanic physicians with joint MD/MPH degrees. This helped lay the groundwork for my goal of obtaining a joint MD/MPH... During my undergraduate years, I eagerly sought out Hispanic physician role models and enrolled in a special elective with Dr. Emilio Carrillo, an internist at Cambridge City Hospital and associate professor of medicine, who has always been passionate about serving the health needs of the local Hispanic community with a focus on culture and public health. Among the assignments was going to the community and writing down what we saw and thought was putting the health of Hispanic communities at risk; it included mapping out burned-out abandoned buildings and other potential health hazards. This work helped to

support a tool to study social and cultural determinants of health which was called the Social and Environmental Relations Profile (SERP) [which eventually led to Health Care Access Barriers Model (HCAB) [14].

As a medical student at Columbia College of Physicians and Surgeons, I found myself in a greater role as a cultural informant/teacher for peers and faculty about Hispanic health. Despite being in Washington Heights, part of Manhattan's 'little D.R.', there were no Spanish interpreters at the hospital. It gave me the impression that the health of Latinos and their special needs weren't being properly addressed. Two weeks after I co-organized an educational workshop about the value of medical interpreters for students, hospital staff, and senior administrators, with the help of Dagmaris Cabezas, the Director of Community Affairs at P&S, the hospital administration hired 5 new interpreters.

Elizabeth Lee-Rey MD, MPH describes,

I grew up in a multilingual, multiracial family on the Lower East Side of NYC—known then as Alphabet City—now as Loisada. My father was born in Shanghai, China and my mother was from Arecibo, Puerto Rico. I chose the University of Pittsburgh School of Medicine because of the frequent calls from African-American and Chinese faculty who sought out my attendance at the school. However throughout my years at Pittsburgh I did not have any Latina/o medical student peers, no Hispanic advisors, and there was no Hispanic medical organization; but there was the Student National Medical Association. I knew I was different and others viewed me differently because of the way I looked and spoke; more so, others knew each other and I didn't know anyone. The experience of being the only one and being told I only got in because of affirmative action drove me to prove myself and take action. I worked in the admissions office for four years and served as a medical student peer interviewer, casting votes like the other committee members.

Despite the physical distance I didn't feel alone because I spoke often to 'sisters' from ASPIRA and other pipeline programs who did have BHO, like Daisy Otero—Harvard Medical School, Bianca Gamboa—Boston Medical College, Alina Valdez—New York Medical College and Susana Morales—Cornell Medical College.

Norma Villanueva recounts,

After starting a family and taking pre-med night classes at Hostos Community College I entered medical school (Einstein) in 1981. In the summer biochemistry review class, I met Nellie Correa,

Diana Burgos, Diana Torres, Marcus Maldonado, and Jerry Maldonado. Seeing other Hispanic medical students gave me a sense of belonging. The black students were well organized through SNMA but when I started there was no BHO. Hispanics were struggling as a group to ensure that we ALL succeeded academically and worked to prevent any of us from being dismissed. Beyond Dr. Sylvia Ramos, who was extremely busy, we didn't have mentors. The administrators in the diversity office were not able to help us with academic or personal challenges, they simply weren't trained or prepared. There were a few Hispanic faculty, but they had completed their training in Spain or Colombia and didn't seem to appreciate the Hispanic American experience. SNMA had great black role models and leaders. I didn't feel like we had that and it was tough for me as a Latina coming from the community.

Ana E. Núñez, MD, Ana Núñez, MD, FACP is a Professor of General Internal Medicine and Vice Dean for Diversity, Equity and Inclusion at the University of Minnesota (Hahnemann Medical College, 1982–1986) explains,

> I grew up in Altoona, a small city in central Pennsylvania. We were the only Latino family in Altoona and the way to survive was acculturation. In one medical school interview—I was told I was "Hispanic enough" because my fluency was subpar. Walking in the streets of Philly for medical school was quite different than growing up in Altoona. Actually, for me, entering into medical school was entering into three worlds—what it meant to be Latina in Philly, a Latina in medical school, and also as part of the LGBT community. As a medical student, in 1982–1986, it was weird being inaccurately stereotyped as 'a Latina from the Philly barrios' or as an oppressed minority.
>
> In medical school, the expectation that came with scholarship support was engagement in support sessions. In our class, there were far more black students than Latino students. The 'default' approach for advising minority students was harsh tough love. "They don't want you here" "They want to get you to fail out". For me as a Puerto Rican from Altoona this approach was foreign, made me paranoid, and was oppressive at times. Attending those mandatory meetings, viewing myself from a deficit approach, reinforced an imposter syndrome. It was a very 'fifty shades of gray'-like culture, tough, and perpetuated a sense of isolation. That being said, being able to speak Spanish to patients, and having others ask me for help in caring for Spanish speaking patients, did grant me a counter-balance of self-worth. I had a unique skill that helped me connect, decode and understand and then broker

issues to the medical team in ways they could understand.

> I didn't have a Hispanic medical student organization at Hahnemann Medical College. When I was chief resident and as an attending, our students, who consisted largely of West Coast Chicano students and East Coast Puerto Rican students started to galvanize to develop a medical student group. BHO or BLHO didn't work for us at the time, because of the diversity of our students so our first group named themselves the Latino Medical Student Association (circa 1990–1991). Jessy Sandaval Barrett, MD, now a child psychiatrist in Philadelphia was the founding president and I had the privilege of serving as faculty advisor. This group grew, held events and talking circles, engaged community and became an integral group within the medical school.

As more Latinos/Hispanics from different states and backgrounds joined and strengthened the organization, BHO evolved into the Boricua Latino Health Organization (BLHO); the board and membership voted in this name change in 1992. In 1993, BLHO changed its name to the National Boricua Latino Health Organization (NBLHO). "National" in the name was adopted in reference to the founders' idea of eventually forming a national student organization.

Arturo P. Saavedra, MD/PhD, MBA, Dean and VP for Medical Affairs, Virginia Commonwealth University (University of Pennsylvania School of Medicine, 1993–2000) shared what he gained from being involved with NBLHO:

> I was part of BLHO, first as a chapter member, then as a member of the executive team, becoming treasurer in 1994, at the University of Pennsylvania School of Medicine. The strong sense of community and support allowed me to confidently run for, and become, National Parliamentarian in 1998. Throughout my time with BLHO/NBLHO, I had the opportunity to learn more about my interest in medicine by serving in volunteer activities in various settings including Migrant Health work. This continues today as I participate in many events for the LHS+ community and served as the LMSA advisor for UVA School of Medicine.
>
> I have benefited greatly from the wisdom and talent of my mentors and hope to do the same for others. Formal mentorship programs and national conferences expanded my network and allowed me to learn about future opportunities. This organization, along with other faculty members such as Dr. Ernesto Gonzalez at Massachusetts General

Hospital, increased visibility around other success-ful Latino/a leaders that inspired me to get to the position I have today at VCU.

Luz M. Ortiz PhD, MA (Former Assistant Dean, Office of Diversity and Minority Affairs at Jefferson Medical College; Formerly Program Administrator; Minority Recruiter Counselor for Minority Disadvantaged Students at UMDNJ-Robert Wood Johnson Medical School) recounts her initial encounter with NBLHO Board members:

In April 1991, I joined the UMDNJ—RWJMS family as Recruiter Counselor for Minority and Educationally/Economically Disadvantaged Students. On my second week at the medical school, I was asked by Maxine Lisboa, MS from (UMDNJ—NJMS) to get involved with NBLHO and attend a Board meeting at Temple School of Medicine. Maxine was Director, Recruiter Counselor at UMDNJ-NJMS. I knew Maxine for well over 15 years prior to coming to UMDNJ-RWJMS. She was a champion for Latino students, faculty and administrators. She was instrumental in identifying Latinos for administrative positions at the medical schools in the Northeast. At the time, Maxine was in the process of leaving NJMS to continue her doctoral studies and asked me to attend the meeting so that I could meet the Board members and get involved with the organization. Little did Hilda Luiggi and I know when we attended that meeting that her plan from the incep-tion was to leave National BLHO in our hands.

At the meeting, I met Hilda Luiggi, MS from Temple School of Medicine. Both of us were Faculty Advisors of our local BLHO chapters at our respective medical schools. At that Board meeting, the outgoing President and Vice President of NBLHO, asked us to serve as their official Faculty Advisors. Both Hilda and I agreed to do so. We were handed a box with information on BLHO. To our surprise, some chapters had dis-banded, others were basically hanging on with lit-tle membership and, yet others, were not participating fully. At that meeting, elections were held and Bobby Ortiz from Temple School of Medicine became President; Belkis Pimentel of UMDNJ-RWJMS became Vice President.

As for the infamous box that Hilda and I were handed at the Board meeting, after the meeting ended, Hilda and I went through the contents of the box. We sat in disbelief that this was the only infor-mation available on the organization and that these students carried this box yearly, from one school to another, as the presidency changed. We laughed at the idea of the contents of this box being the only records that represented an entire organization.

Que Bochorno!!!! We were in disbelief and total shock!

A few weeks later, due to personal reasons, Bobby resigned from his position as NBLHO President and Belkis ascended to the Presidency. Since we now had the presidency held by Belkis, one of my medical students from UMDNJ-RWJMS, I decided to request office space and funding for the organi-zation. The thought of NBLHO not having a physi-cal office in any medical school was quite alarming. At the time, our Dean was Norman Edelman, MD and the Associate Dean for the Office of Special Academic Programs was Florence Kimball, PhD. They were both in agreement that NBLHO should be headquartered at our respective medical school and provided NBLHO with a fully fur-nished office, computers, phone and financial sup-port. To my knowledge, it was the first and only physical office that existed for NBLHO. When I left UMDNJ-RWJMS to join Jefferson Medical College to become the Assistant Dean for the Office of Diversity and Minority Affairs, Jefferson agreed to provide office space for the NBLHO Board.

Once Maxine left UMDNJ-NJMS to pursue her doctorate, Nancy Vega, MS was hired to fill that position. Nancy worked for many years at ASPIRA in Newark. After her first year at UMDNJ-NJMS, Nancy joined us in advising NBLHO as did Nilda Soto, MSEd, AECOM. While Hilda and I remained the official Faculty Advisors to NBLHO on paper, Nancy and Nilda helped us immensely throughout the years.

The journey for establishing NBLHO at a medi-cal school was not a given and at times precari-ous. Beyond the administrative work associated with establishing a chapter, sometimes existing minority diversity leaders were uncertain of the value of having a new Hispanic student group at the medical school or the need to separate them from the Student National Medical Association, which was primarily for African-American/Black students. As Hispanic students increased in num-bers, so did the resolve and confidence of a criti-cal mass to be heard.

Luz Ortiz remembers,

It was difficult for some to understand the unique experience and needs of Hispanic students. Most Minority/Diversity Affairs Offices were pushing to grow SNMA and there wasn't often an interest to emphasize or open NBLHO chapters on their respective campuses. Often students were told, 'What are you complaining about? We have an SNMA chapter here to represent you'. Many times, the students requesting to open a chapter on their campus were given an emphatic "No" and told that there was no funding available for another student organization. However, as the number of Hispanic students grew, their unified voices called for fairness in allowing them to have an organization that could address their unique needs; an organization that could represent them as students who come from diverse Hispanic backgrounds and subgroups. They also pressured the administration further by telling them what other medical schools had done for their Hispanic students. Some students went directly to the Dean of Student Affairs or found themselves going to the Dean of the Medical School, circumventing the Minority/Diversity Affairs Office, in an effort to request permission to open a chapter of NBLHO at their respective medical school. Most were asked to explain the need for an NBLHO chapter in their request. The students persisted until they were allowed to open a chapter at their respective medical school.

With the evolution of the chapters there was constant networking to champion the recruitment, retention, and education of LHS+ students. A major remaining challenge was developing student leaders and transitioning leadership.

Growth of Latino/Hispanic Identified Minority/Diversity Affairs Administrators

Along with the growth of Latino/Hispanic medical students was a concurrent growth of Latino/Hispanic identified—Minority /Diversity Affairs Administrators. Latino/Hispanic administrators were slowly emerging at medical schools and coalescing in a similar way as the medical students to support themselves and build "una familia" for their students. Not uncommonly these staff were strong Latina/Hispanic women and over time several became advisors to and fixtures at NBLHO events, so much so they were dubbed by some NBLHO members and other Minority/Diversity Affairs Administrators as "Las Comadres".

Luz Ortiz, one of Las Comadres, states.

> Hilda Luiggi, MS (Temple School of Medicine; UPenn School of Medicine), Maxine Lisboa, MS, Doctoral Candidate (UMDNJ-NJMS), Nancy Vega, MS (UMDNJ-NJMS hired after Maxine left NJMS), Nilda Soto, MSed (AECOM) and I were

some of the very few Hispanics in these Minority/Diversity Affairs Offices at medical schools across the nation at that time. We realized early on that we needed to form a "united front" and find a way to work together in a concerted effort to create a pipeline of qualified Hispanic students for our respective medical schools. Our decision to work closely together to advise, nurture and educate students on demystifying the admissions process and preparing them adequately for entrance into medical school became our mission. We became known by students and colleagues as, "The Comadres (The Godmothers)." From 1990–2000, we were the only four Hispanics involved in medical school recruitment. It was a priority for us to show our strength and union in recruiting Hispanics to our respective medical schools. It was not a competition for us, rather it was about guiding and getting students into the system. Students followed suit and applied to all four of our schools. Our colleagues knew that nothing was going to come between our relationship and people marveled at our strength. We were in four different schools but we planned our recruitment trips together, presented workshops for underrepresented students nationally, recruited together, and shared our resources. We would sometimes interact with 250–500 students at an event. Eventually students were being advised by their pre-health advisors or faculty from their respective colleges/universities to seek our help and advice. Looking back, we can all safely say that we needed each other because we rarely had anyone else to turn to. The lack of Hispanic representation at our level, within the administration at medical schools nationally and within our own administration, clearly helped us to see that it was imperative for us to formulate this cohesive group of like-minded Hispanic women. It empowered us in meeting the many obstacles and challenges we dealt with on a professional level and in carrying out the mission and goals for our respective medical schools. To this day, Hilda, Nilda, Maxine, Nancy and I remain best friends.

Nilda Soto shared,

> Las Comadres shared the same mission which was to assist Latino premedical students to become competitive applicants to medical school. Even though we may have wanted a particular premedical student to attend our individual institution, we shared with them the contact information of the other Comadres so the student would know who they could reach out to at that medical school.

The impact of Las Comadres was felt by hundreds of students. Romeo Morales MD (Clinical Educator Associate Professor, Department of Dermatology, School of Medicine, University of

New Mexico, Boston University School of Medicine, 1992–1996) noted,

> In 1991, I met Ms. Hilda Luiggi while interviewing at Temple University School of Medicine for a spot in that school. My first impression of Ms. Luiggi was offering nothing less than frank, supportive, calm, and unyielding commitment to advance the agenda of not only Latino/Hispanic groups, but underrepresented minority individuals.
>
> In 1992, I entered Boston University School of Medicine, where there was no representation of medical students of Hispanic/Latino origins. By 1994, the Association of Latin Medical Students at Boston University was a chapter of the National Boricua/Latino Health Organization, which I presided following the capable leadership of Belkis Pimentel.
>
> At the time, one of the accomplishments derived from the National Boricua/Latino Health Organization was the 1994 Annual Convention, "Preparing for the 21st Century" which brought over 150 participants from the Northeast to Boston University. One of the main goals was simply to highlight the contributions and impact Hispanic/Latinos had in medicine. At the time the guest speakers were, Drs. Ernesto Gonzalez-Martinez and Miguel Ondetti.
>
> The common denominator in the success and advancement of the Hispanic/Latino agenda in the Northeast were the four pistons—Hilda, Luz, Nancy, and Nilda. To those 4 pistons, I will always humbly tip my hat—por esa convicción y mentalidad siempre vanguardista!

Forming a National Identity Beyond the Northeast

In the 1990s, amidst rumors that the nascent National Hispanic Medical Association was contemplating starting its own parallel student organization and with increasing recognition among leaders of Latino/Hispanic medical student organizations throughout the U.S. of a need to collaborate more regularly, in 1999, NBLHO agreed in principle to join the National Network of Latin American Medical Students (NNLAMS). NNLAMS would have a two-tiered board, with one tier made up of the leaders of the regional organizations and a second tier of selected (as opposed to elected) officers—specifically not a president. In March 2000, NNLAMS drafted a constitution and in April 2000, NBLHO updated

their constitution to indicate membership in NNLAMS. As Edgar Figueroa, M.D., M.P.H., FAAFP, Director of Student Health, Associate Professor of Family Medicine in Clinical Medicine, Weill Cornell Medicine.

Student Health Services and NBLHO President in 1999–2000 wrote in a manual to incoming officers in May 2000:

> NNLAMS is a consortium formed by five regional Latino student groups throughout the United States. It was founded as an organization to represent Latino medical students with one voice, as a national Latino organization. It was formed with the hopes that the five regions would ultimately come under one name, one logo, in essence one organization.

This decision was met with some resistance—some of the student members from the NE chapters as well as some of the advisors were concerned about what this unification would mean—there were concerns about loss of history, loss of autonomy and financial implications. These themes would recur frequently over the subsequent decade.

From NNLAMS to Union Under LMSA

The decision for NBLHO to join LMSA as LMSA Northeast was an even more contentious decision. It meant moving NBLHO members and alumni from participation in a network based in the Northeast to become a part of a national organization, with governance by a national board and responsibility to four other regions. For many prior generations of NBLHO leaders and members, there was a concern of a loss of history of Puerto Rican activism, a reduction of focus on Northeast health, and a diffusion of investment in on-going Hispanic student recruitment, retention and promotion challenges in the Northeast.

Gezzer Ortega MD, MPH, Lead Faculty for Research and Innovation for Equitable Surgical Care at the Center for Surgery and Public Health, Instructor in Surgery, Department of Surgery, Brigham and Women's Hospital, Harvard Medical School (Howard University College of

Medicine, NBLHO Co-Chair, 2008–2009) shares,

> In 2008, I remembered working with the other Co-Chair, Raj Sawh, to consider whether we would remain the National Boricua Latino Health Organization (NBLHO) or join a new national group named Latino Medical Student Association (LMSA). The Boricua Health Organization was founded at Harvard Medical School in 1972, and then became the Boricua Latino Health Organization and eventually the National BLHO. We eventually decided to move forward with LMSA. We were seeking something more. The name LMSA, with the word 'Latino' seemed more inclusive, and it was simpler; four letters like AMSA and SNMA. But for a short period, LMSA wasn't a given. The West leaders were concerned that sharing their name with other regions on a national level might negatively impact their brand and reputation. At that time, the West had the largest membership and active alumni base. After several conversations, West extended the use of their name, and NBLHO joined as LMSA-NE.

Luz Ortiz PhD, MA (co-faculty advisor NBLHO, 1994–2013) recalls,

> While we, as Chapter Advisors, understood the rationale and importance of having all regional Hispanic organizations under one name, we were not in favor of the name being changed to LMSA for several reasons.

1. Continuity in Leadership was imperative. It took us about 10 years to build our chapters back up and maintain continuity in leadership. The regional board members changed yearly. The students could only commit a small portion of their time to the activities of the organization. Experience had taught us that we could not depend on the students to keep the organization thriving. As advisors, we had to step up to the plate and invest many hours to it, to ensure that the organization would not fall apart, like in the late 1980s and early 1990s. By the late 1990s, we had over 40 chapters and needed to keep them functioning well.

2. For faculty advisors, it was difficult to maintain our chapters at a regional level, let alone a national level. Who would be responsible for each region and serve as their advisor? Would there be a National Advisor who could take on all of the regions and ensure continuity and keep chapters from disbanding?

3. Legacy of the Organization: We were worried that future students would lose the legacy of Puerto Rican leadership that built BHO/BLHO/NBLHO organization from the ground up.

4. History, Mission and Goals of the Organization: We were also worried that there would be a loss of the history, mission and goals of the organization. The change would not represent the Northeast perspective any longer.

It was not an easy decision to make. It took years to come to an agreement. However, as we began to see the climate change for our respective Minority/Diversity Affairs offices, nationally, it soon became apparent to us that all regional organizations needed to merge and unify in order to have a stronger voice. As a national organization under one name, they would be able to do this. While we still worried about whether or not they would be able to maintain all regions fully functional under one umbrella without a National Faculty Advisor, we hoped for the best.

In 2009, NBLHO finally joined the Latino Medical Student Association, known as LMSA-Northeast representing the Northeast region of the national organization. As such, it officially changed its name from NBLHO to LMSA-Northeast to reflect the cohesion of this new national network. This was a tremendous stepping stone for the northeast region and nationally given the existence of a significant populace of individuals committed to the advancement of Latinos in healthcare with a pointed emphasis on **recruitment, retention, and education**, to ensure accessible, culturally competent, and reflective medical care.

LMSA-NE 2009–2020

Since 2009, LMSA-Northeast has continued its mission and has expanded its membership to include nearly every osteopathic and allopathic medical school within the northeast corridor. Despite its growth and engagement, joining a national organization was not without its challenges. Each region within LMSA-National brought its own character and value with independent leadership structures and strategies to engage in its shared mission. Bridging that distinction and embracing change came with a simultaneous restructuring of how communication was executed, especially as it pertained to a national agenda and to joint rotating national conferences, which per region, transpired every 5 years.

Today, LMSA-NEs mission is to recruit Latinos into higher education, educate the public and one another about Latino health issues, advocate for increased Latino representation in health-related areas, and promote awareness about social, political and economic issues as they relate to Latino health. It also serves to create a support network for Latino students.

In 2022, immediate objectives of LMSA-NE were: [15]

- To recruit and admit Latin-American scholars who exhibit the potential to benefit their community through the health professions.
- Retaining our members in health professions programs by supporting academic and social support activities and by fostering close ties among members.
- Educating ourselves in areas of concern to our communities which may not be part of the health profession or allied health school curricula, ie: preventive and community medicine, politics of health care systems, mechanics of urban city primary care, family practice, etc.
- Orientation of our members towards actively accepting our principles of unity and aims of our organization.
- Community involvement for the purpose of strengthening working relationships with community groups and the overall aim of benefiting the community. A means of mutual education.
- Support and encourage prospective health professions school applicants throughout the admissions process.
- Writing and circulating our ideas and fostering the refinement and development of research skills among our members.
- Encourage the development of courses which better prepare our members to become high quality health care providers serving our community.
- To educate and sensitize the entire Medical Community to the specific needs and differences of the Latino regarding health and human well being.

Long term objectives have been: [15]

- Improve the health care delivery to Latino communities.
- Be advocates of the rights of Latino patients.
- Participate in the planning and implementation of research activities designed to identify the health care needs of our community.
- Networking with other organizations at the local and national levels to achieve common objectives.

Since the first chapter in 1972, BHO/BLHO/ NBLHO/LMSA NE has grown to have a chapter in 98% of accredited allopathic and osteopathic medical schools in the Northeast (Table 2.1) with student and faculty chapters and regional leaders (Table 2.2). The organization continues to sponsor yearly conventions (Table 2.3) which highlight regional issues and allow for dialogue between chapters. Between 2000 and 2023, conference titles reflected the desire for communication in English and Spanish and members to be unified, empowered, and overcome barriers for healthier communities (Table 2.3). The titles often called members to serve as leaders and facilitate change in the spheres of education, research and service. The same spheres that are listed in the mission of medical schools.

Jeans Miguel Santana, MD, Resident Physician Anesthetist, PGY-3, SUNY Downstate Medical Center (SUNY Downstate Medical School, 2012–2017) shares,

Table 2.1 List of States and School Chapters (stand alone or connected) in the LMSA Northeast Region (as of December 2022)

Maine: New England College of Osteopathic Medicine
New Hampshire: Geisel School of Medicine at Dartmouth
Massachusetts: Boston University School of Medicine, Harvard Medical School, Tufts University School of Medicine, University of Massachusetts Medical School
Rhode Island: Alpert Medical School—Brown University
Vermont: Larner College of Medicine at The University of Vermont
Connecticut: University of Connecticut School of Medicine, Yale School of Medicine, Frank H. Netter MD School of Medicine at Quinnipiac University
New York: Albany Medical School, Albert Einstein College of Medicine, Columbia University College of Physicians and Surgeons, CUNY School of Medicine, Hofstra Northwell School of Medicine, Icahn School of Medicine at Mount Sinai, New York Medical College, NYIT College of Osteopathic Medicine, NYU School of Medicine, Stony Brook University School of Medicine, SUNY Downstate College of Medicine, SUNY Upstate College of Medicine, SUNY at Buffalo Jacobs School of Medicine and Biomedical Sciences, Touro College of Osteopathic Medicine-Harlem, Touro College of Osteopathic Medicine-Middletown, University of Rochester School of Medicine & Dentistry, Weill Cornell School of Medicine
Pennsylvania: Drexel University College of Medicine, Geisinger Commonwealth School of Medicine, Penn State College of Medicine, Philadelphia College of Osteopathic Medicine, Temple University—Lewis Katz School of Medicine, Thomas Jefferson University—Sidney Kimmel Medical College, University of Pennsylvania—Perelman School of Medicine, University of Pittsburgh School of Medicine
New Jersey: Cooper Medical School of Rowan University, Rowan University School of Osteopathic Medicine, Rutgers—Robert Wood Johnson Medical School, Rutgers New Jersey Medical School, Rowan University School of Osteopathic Medicine
Maryland: Johns Hopkins School of Medicine, Uniformed Services University of the Health Sciences, University of Maryland School of Medicine
Washington D.C.: George Washington University School of Medicine, Georgetown University School of Medicine, Howard University College of Medicine

Table 2.2 Northeast Regional Leaders, 1994–2023

Year	Student Leader, Medical School
1994–1995	Belkis Pimentel, President, National Boricua/Latino Health Organization (NBLHO)
1995–1996	Romeo Morales, Boston University School of Medicine, President, NBLHO
1997–1998	Joseph Perez, Cornell University Medical College, President, NBLHO
1998–1999	Philip DeChavez, University of Pennsylvania School of Medicine, President, NBLHO; NBLHO Representative to NNLAMS Board
1999–2000	Edgar Figueroa, Cornell University Medical College President, NBLHO; NBLHO Representative to NNLAMS Board Added/restarted several chapters that academic year. Helped with drafting and ratifying first NNLAMS Constitution and led ratification in NBLHO constitution.
2000–2001	Catalina Vázquez, Albert Einstein College of Medicine Hector Vázquez, Mount Sinai School of Medicine NBLHO Co-Chairs and NNLAMS Board Representatives. First year Co-Chairs existed.
2001–2002	JosèAlberto Betances, Albert Einstein College of Medicine Lynn Hernandez, UMDNJ-New Jersey Medical School NBLHO Co-Chairs
2002–2003	Julissa Cruz, Albert Einstein College of Medicine Ana rodriguez, Temple University School Medicine NBLHO Co-Chairs
2003–2004	Lilia Reyes, UMDNJ-RWJ Medical School Edison Machado, Yale School of Medicine NBLHO Co-Chairs
2004–2005	Vashun A. Rodriguez, UMDNJ-RWJ Medical School Martine Aguiar, Temple University School of Medicine NBLHO Co-Chairs

(continued)

Table 2.2 (continued)

Year	Student Leader, Medical School
2005–2006	Esther Vivas, Albert Einstein College of Medicine Yirielis Sanguinetti, Temple University School of Medicine NBLHO Co-Chairs
2006–2007	Myrna Cortez-Perez, Temple University School of Medicine Raquel Murphy, UMDNJ-School of Osteopathic Medicine NBLHO Co-Chairs
2007–2008	Vennus Ballen, Mount Sinai School of Medicine Julian L. Castaneda, Temple University School of Medicine NBLHO Co-Chairs
2008–2009	Gezzer Ortega, Howard University College of Medicine Rajendra-Sawh Martinez, Yale School of Medicine NBLHO Co-Chairs
2009–2010	Frank Quintero, New York College of Medicine Felicia Rosario, Columbia College of Physicians and Surgeons NBLHO Co-Chairs
2010–2011	Christina M. Cruz, Columbia University College of Physicians and Surgeons Lisa Ochoa-Frongia, Mount Sinai School of Medicine NBLHO Co-Chairs
2011–2012	Amanda Lynn Hernandez, Yale School of Medicine Yelina Alvarez, New York University School of Medicine NBLHO Co-Chairs
2012–2013	Ismely Minaya, Mount Sinai School of Medicine David Martin, Columbia University College of Physicians and Surgeons NBLHO Co-Chairs
2013–2014	Amanda Lynn Hernandez, Yale School of Medicine Crystal Castaneda, Cornell School of Medicine NBLHO Co-Chairs
2014–2015	Jeffrey Uribe, Temple School of Medicine Diana Lopez, Harvard School of Medicine NBLHO Co-Chairs
2015–2016	Gricelda Gomez, Harvard School of Medicine Cindy Parra, Cornell School of Medicine NBLHO Co-Chairs
2016–2017	Jeans Santana, SUNY Downstate Medical School Seva G Khambadkone, John Hopkins School of Medicine NBLHO Co-Chairs
2017–2018	Adrianna Stanley, Geisel School of Medicine at Dartmouth Freddy Vazquez, Geisel School of Medicine at Dartmouth NBLHO Co-Chairs
2018–2019	Julia Su, Donald and Barbara Zucker School of Medicine at Hofstra/Northwell Iara Backes, Geisel School of Medicine at Dartmouth NBLHO Co-Chairs
2019–2020	Jessica Grenvik, Sidney Kimmel Medical College Mary-Catherine Skoulos, Cooper Medical School of Rowan University NBLHO Co-Chairs
2020–2021	Stacey Martinez, SUNY Upstate Medical University Luke Torre-Healy, Renaissance School of Medicine at Stony Brook NBLHO Co-Chairs
2021–2022	Bianca Ulloa Albert Einstein College of Medicine Juan Cerezo Temple University Lewis Katz School of Medicine NBLHO Co-Chairs
2022–2023	Jordan Juarez, Temple University Lewis Katz School of Medicine Claudia Torres, Icahn School of Medicine at Mount Sinai NBLHO Co-Chairs

Table 2.3 List of NE Regional Conference Titles and Host Institutions

• NBLHO, Latinos In The twenty-first Century: An Up And Coming Force, University Of Pennsylvania School Of Medicine, 1999
NBLHO, Closing the Gap: Health and Educational Challenges for Latinos in the New Millennium, UMDNJ—NJMS, 2000
Unknown
NBLHO, Changing Faces Latinos In Medicine, UMDNJ/Robert Wood Johnson, Piscataway, NJ, 2002
NBLHO National Conference, Albert Einstein College of Medicine, April 2003
NBLHO National Conference, NYIT College of Osteopathic Medicine, NY. April 2005
Advocating for Optimal Healthcare in Latino Communities, Jefferson Medical College, 2006
National Boricua Latino Health Conference, Opening Minds to Cultural Competency in Medicine and Health Policy, Johns Hopkins School Of Medicine, 2007
Excellence in Community Leadership, Mount Sinai School of Medicine, 2008
Improving Latino Healthcare Through Service, Education and Research, University of Pennsylvania College of Medicine, 2009
Cuidense Mi Gente! Promoting Wellness in Underserved Communities, Mount Sinai School of Medicine, 2011
Nuestro Futuro En Nuestras Manos: Empowering the Next Generation, Harvard, 2012
Soy Latino! Uniting the Leaders Among Us, Drexel College of Medicine, 2013
Abriendo La Puerta: Latin@S Promoting Unity, Education, & Rights Through Awareness!, Weill-Cornell Medical College, 2014
Creando Alianzas in Solidarity for Latino Health, Hopkins, 2015
Fortaleciendo Raices: Uniting Efforts in the Changing Face of Healthcare, Dartmouth, 2016
¡Aquí Estamos! Our Journey and The Climb to Greater Heights, Hofstra, 2017
Construyendo Puentes: Overcoming Barriers for a Healthier Community, Jefferson, 2018
Nuestros Vecinos, Nuestra Familia, Our Neighbors, Our Family, Suny Upstate, 2019
Juntos Tenemos Poder: Standing Together for Latino Healthcare, Albert Einstein, 2020
Siempre Unidos, Siempre Luchando: Empowering Our Communities Towards Health Equity and Justice, Icahn School of Medicine at Mount Sinai, 2021
Cincuenta Años De Comunidad: Fostering Service, Health Equity, And Leadership, Drexel University College of Medicine, Temple University Lewis Katz School of Medicine, Perelman School of Medicine, University of Pennsylvania, Jefferson, Thomas Jefferson University, Philadelphia, PA, 2022
Un Futuro Para Todos: Highlighting Latino Innovation, Service, and Leadership in Medicine, Johns Hopkins School of Medicine, 2023

I was born in Santiago, Dominican Republic and grew up in the Bronx. As an undergrad I met a LMSA member at a regional conference and I became hooked. When you look for what you need it's at LMSA—community, involvement, and leadership are intertwined—peers helped me appreciate this and it compelled me to become involved. I served as Northeast Co-Chair from 2015–2017 and helped to create a medical Spanish elective at Downstate to raised a greater consciousness of Hispanic culture and health

Julia Su (MD/PhD Student at Donald and Barbara Zucker School of Medicine at Hofstra/Northwell, 2017-present)

I joined my local LMSA chapter in medical school to learn Medical Spanish. Reminded by my grandparents' struggles, I wanted to become a physician that practices cultural humility. I wanted to understand other cultures and learn the language so I

could provide that comfort when I encounter my patients on their worst days. My medical school also happened to be hosting the National LMSA conference that year so after being selected as the Co-Chair of my LMSA chapter, I got involved with conference planning. Helping plan a conference that empowered medical students and working with incredibly passionate people drew me into LMSA. The organization's mission and values aligned with the kind of physician I wanted to become. There is no better way to learn about the problems and challenges affecting a specific population than from the population itself. By being present, attending LMSA events, befriending LMSA members, I heard about the issues that affect their community. From the atrocities of separation of families at the southern border to the DACA medical students facing uncertainty if they can stay in the country to finish their education, I learned a lot by being surrounded by the people these issues affected. At the 2017 LMSA National

Conference, I was elected as the LMSA-NE Co-Director Elect and led the Northeast region for two years.

The strong foundation of BHO, BLHO, and NBLHO has been attributed to building LMSA members as leaders, on-going mentorship, and maintaining their focus on community issues. For the organization's success it was necessary to engage first year medical students right away so they would be well-prepared to serve as chapter leaders by second year. The typical medical school schedule, with third years entering the clinical wards made the leadership hinge on first and second year students. Mentors who are senior administrators and know the culture and climate of the institution are invaluable and

therefore every chapter is required to have a faculty advisor. Lastly, promoting trainees' interests and maintaining their tie to the community has been the heart and soul of LMSA and often has helped trainees overcome the toughest academic times.

> And we had a saying that we passed on from year to year, which is that we don't want to become Harvardized. And that terminology kind of meant that we don't want you to just become a stereotypical Harvard academic—we want to maintain our community roots, our community involvement…. every year since we started over the 50 years— we've always had speakers at the conferences who are from the community, who are community activists, who are doing things for improving health in those that are more vulnerable [12]. Emilio Carrillo MD, MPH

Photos

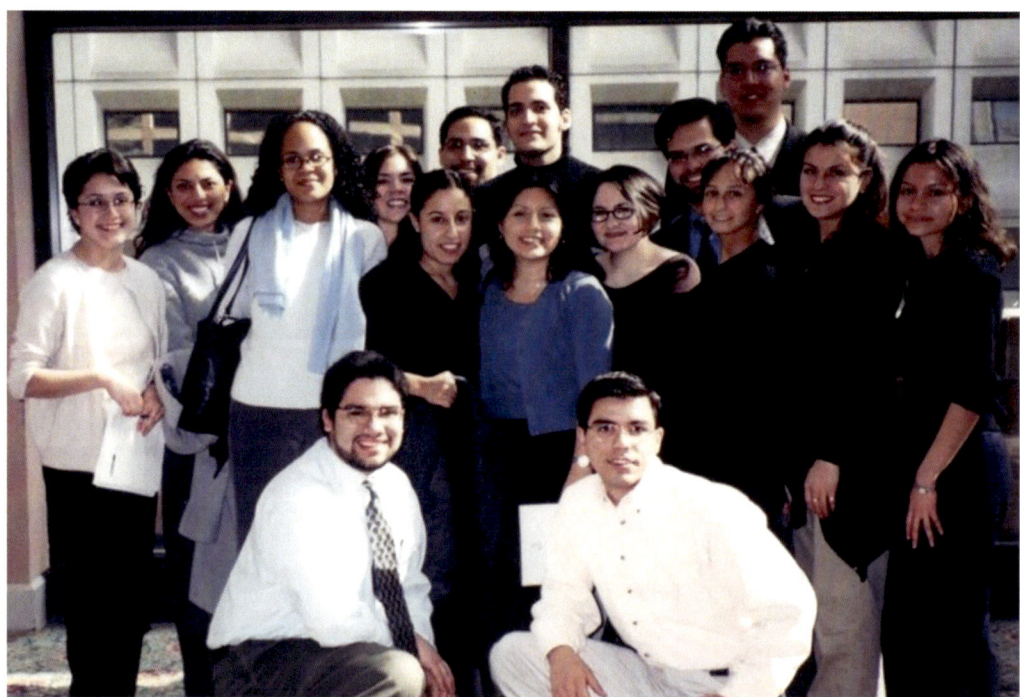

Above: NBLHO members attending the 4th Annual NHMA Conference (2000) in Washington, DC (©LMSA)

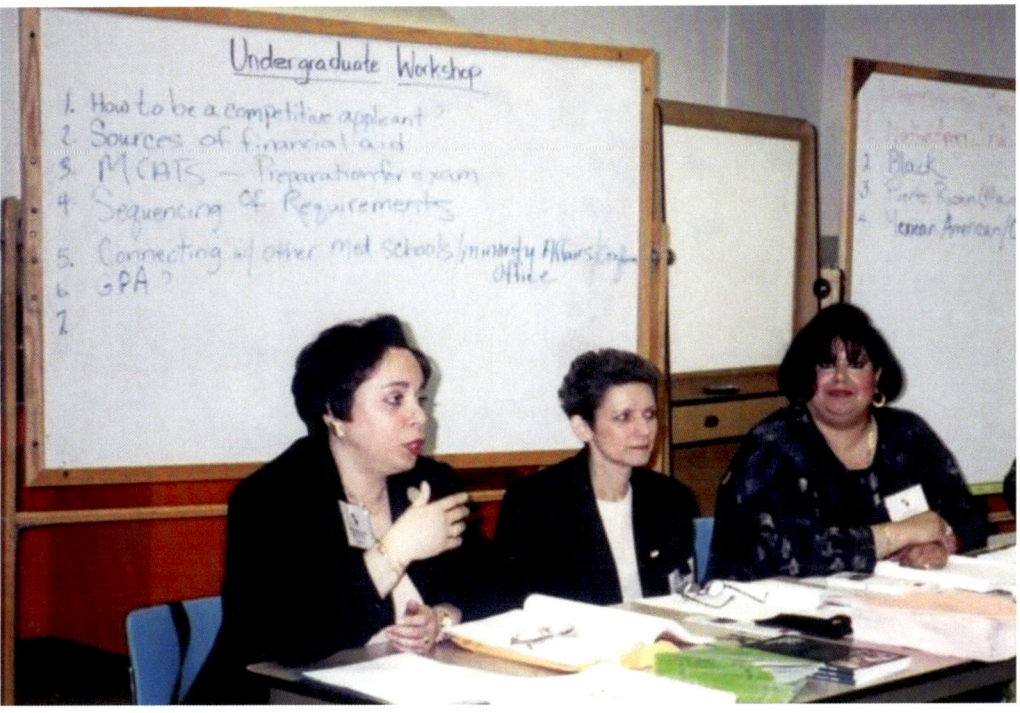

Photo above Three of the Comadres (Right to Left—Nilda Soto, Hilda Luiggi, Luz Torres) (©LMSA)

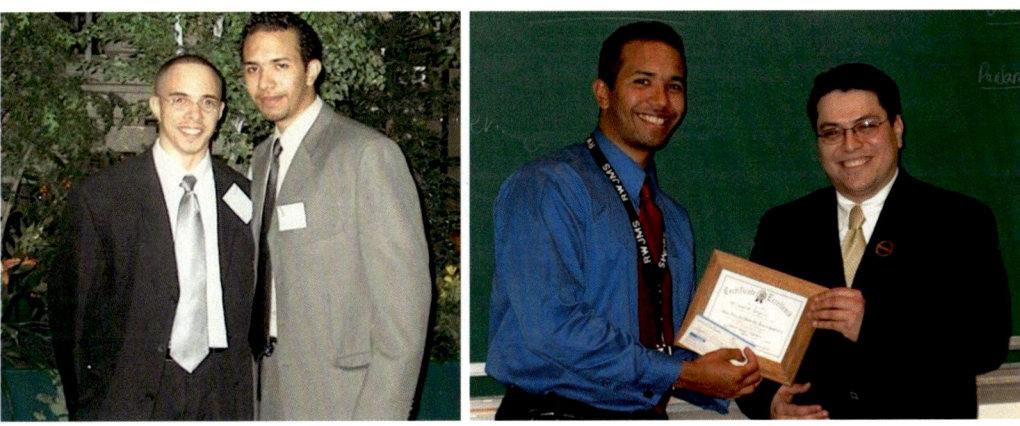

Photos above (Left): Jose Alberto Betances and Vashun Rodriguez 2002 NBLHO Conference, University of Medicine and Dentistry of New Jersey—Robert Wood JohnsonPhoto (Right): Vashun Rodriguez and Edison Machado, 2003 NBLHO Conference, Albert Einstein College of Medicine. (©LMSA)

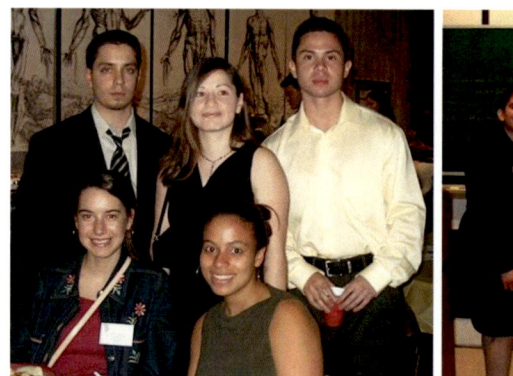 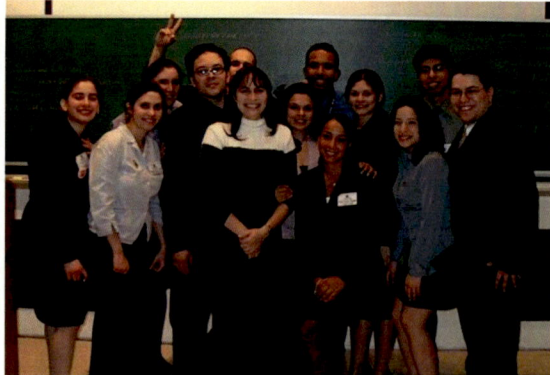

Photos above (Left): UMDNJ-RWJ NBLHO Board 2002Photo (Right): Albert Einstein College of Medicine. NBLHO Board 2003. (©LMSA)

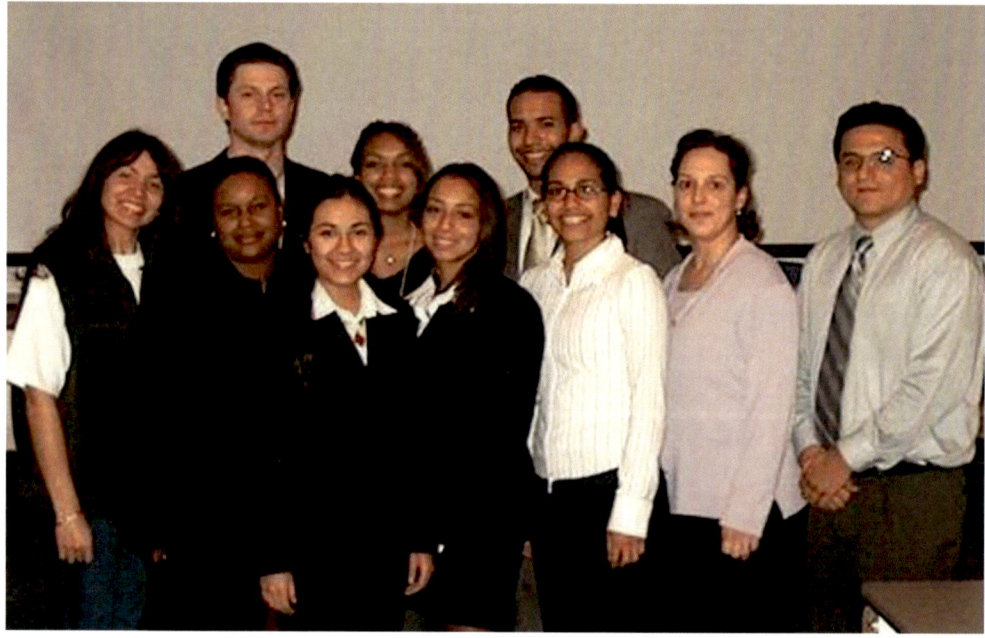

Photo above NBLHO Board, 2004 NYCOM. (©LMSA)

Personal Narratives
Thomas R. Ortiz, MD, FAAFP, Founder and Medical Director

Forest Hill Family Health Associates, PA in Newark, NJ, BHO Chapter President, NJ Medical School—Newark, NJ

When I went up to Harvard Medical School to be interviewed as a premed student for a spot in the class of 1981, I was fortunate in that, on that same day a meeting of the Boricua Health Organization, BHO, a new organization representing the needs of the Puerto Rican community,

was happening that evening and I was invited to attend. There was Emilio Carrillo, Juan Albino and Jaime Rivera walking the stage in a very classic Harvard Hall with all the trappings, talking about Latino lack of access to health care, working jobs, being abused, and not even offering insurance. I felt the enthusiasm in the room with the many Latino medical students from several Boston area medical schools. I felt a good understanding of the group's mission and high ideas. I was extremely impressed and vowed to bring this same movement, this same mission to the students and community in NJ. Just so happened that I got accepted into UMDNJ NJMS along with 4 other Boricuas in the class of 1981. Add that to the 2 in the class of 80 we amounted to 7 Latinos at NJMS that year. We all got together, and I introduced the idea of starting a BHO chapter here at NJMS after getting the go ahead from Emilio and BHO Boston.

I was very encouraged by the response to my fellow Latino students and I was tasked as the first NJMS BHO Chapter president. We knew we had to do several things, after adapting the BHO Constitution, then the first and foremost was getting more Boricuas into medical school, the second was to get the current medical staff, teachers, professors and hospital staff to join us in our mission and thirdly, we had to get more medical services, education and promotion out to our Latino community as well as sensitize the mainstream health care system to understand the culture and needs of the surrounding Latino community. Our task was to increase our representation in recruitment, retention and admission of medical students at NJMS while providing classes in medical Spanish, create a brown bag lunch series of sessions on the plight of the Latino patient in our health care system presented to the school populations of all students and faculty, and to outreach with resources to the community from whom we gained good support.

The newsletter" Curandero" was born, the brainchild of Ambrosio Romero, NJMS class of 82, a monthly newsletter that published articles and announcements on our movement and programs to achieve our mission. While doing all these as medical students, we realized that we could not do it by ourselves and we expected the institution to support us as well.

Since Aspira Inc. of NJ, led by Griesel Ubarry and later Maria Vizcarrondo, was always an integral part of developing student candidate in premed to be groomed for medical school in NJ, we therefore naturally closely aligned our missions and decided to call a meeting with UMDNJ President Stanley Bergen and all of his Deans in what became known as the "The Aspira Demands of 1977". In a coalition of medical students (BHO), Aspira officials and

community leaders, 10 demands were laid out on the table.

Among the demands was for the schools, both NJMS and RWJMS, would each hire a full-time recruiter/ counselor to support our recruitment and admission of Latinos and support the local activities planned out by BHO. This was accepted and the schools hired professions for these positions and they allowed BHO participation in the selection committee. This is how Mariano Vega, Jr., Luz Ortiz, Maxime Lisboa, Mercedes Rivera and others, all came to these institutions over the ensuing years as we gained strength and numbers, translating into institutional recognition and acceptance and increasing numbers of Latinos getting admitted into NJ medical schools.

Another demand was an assigned seat on the admissions committees, which was also adopted by the schools and over the next 4 years admissions began to climb.

By 1981, NJMS had over 10 Latinos admitted to the first-year class, a national 1-year record. The NJMS BHO Chapter that year also hosted the very first National BHO convention, a 2-day event that included students representing the east coast, 10 medical schools from Philadelphia, NYC and Boston, and a national mission statement and constitution was written.

BHO and its members were very instrumental in the inception and establishment of the Student Family Health Care Clinic at NJMS University Hospital, which was created by medical students to provide free medical care to those who would otherwise be left behind. Students had an opportunity to help the community with volunteer faculty and private practice physicians. This program has grown into an institutionalized NJMS student service program to this day, generously funded by charitable organizations to give students an early experience in patient care and the poor community an opportunity to get themselves checked out.

Since 1981, I have continued to help in mentoring students and supporting their efforts to maintain the momentum of the BHO movement. Now inclusive of all Latino or Spanish speaking students from all Latin American countries, thus the evolution of the name from BHO, to BLHO to its current name NJMS Latino Medical Student Association, LMSA.

The work that we did had an impact, unfortunately, for many reasons, medical school and achieving an MD remains a challenge for Latinos. Our original BHO mission is, sadly, still relevant even today.

Fidencio Saldaña, MD, MPH, Dean for Students

Harvard Medical School, LMSA Member, Harvard Medical School 1996–2001, Chapter President 1997–1998

As a prospective Harvard Medical student in 1996, I never could have imagined being where I am today. I applied to Harvard due to encouragement from faculty as well as peers from the Stanford chapter of Chicanos in Health Education, an organization that continues to provide prehealth support to Latinx undergraduates. I recall visiting Harvard Medical School (HMS) during the underrepresented minority revisit weekend. I was in awe that I would finally have the opportunity to become a physician. I came from a humble background. My parents were both immigrants from Mexico who only had the opportunity of an elementary school education. At the time, HMS appeared to be a daunting place—one where I did not necessarily belong. However, during that weekend, I was fortunate to meet a cadre of faculty and students from similar backgrounds to my own, who helped me put aside those feelings. They insisted that not only did I belong in medical school, there was a large population of patients who desperately needed me to be their physician.

My passion at the time was to become a physician that would help take care of underserved patients—specifically those of Spanish-speaking heritage. I wanted to be their linguistic and cultural interpreter to the world of medicine. I soon became the beneficiary of wonderful mentors who were crucial in allowing me to fulfill this dream. I vividly remember one of my first conversations with Dr. Alvin Poussaint, Director of the Office of Recruitment and Multicultural Affairs at HMS. He is unaware that he was the first person who made me believe that I could pursue a career in academic medicine. Dr.

Poussaint insisted that I could serve these patients on an individual as well as a collective level. He believed in both my capacity as a leader as well as my ability to have a broad impact on this population of patients.

At HMS, we had three LHS+ identified student organizations when I matriculated: the National Chicano Health Organization, Boricua Health Organization, and Latin American Health Organization. At the time, my colleagues and I formed the precursor to the HMS LMSA chapter—Medical Students de Las Americas or MeSLA. We recognized that as Latinx students we shared a common heritage and we would be stronger collectively speaking as one voice and being a source of support for one another.

There were two early formative experiences that had an incredible impact on me. The first was when one of my mentors, Ernesto Gonzalez, sponsored my trip to Washington D.C. to attend one of the first NHMA conferences, The second was taking a trip to Philadelphia to attend a Boricua Health Organization Conferences which led me to become more involved in the regional and national organization. These experiences allowed me to see that I did belong in the world of medicine. At these conferences, I was surrounded by students and physicians that looked like me and shared similar backgrounds and challenges. Every conference became a booster shot of energy and motivation that I would take back to Boston. Encouraged by one of my colleagues Fausto Mesa, past chair of the National Network of Latin American Medical Students (NNLAMS), I ran for and was elected to the national NNLAMS board and had the pleasure of attending the Garcia Leadership conference in Galveston, Tx.

Today I am part of the Harvard Medical School faculty. I am proud to say that the passion I felt as a prospective student has only grown with time. I am a clinical cardiologist and cardiac imager who serves Spanish-speaking Latino/a patients at the Brigham and Women's Hospital (BWH) as well as BWH affiliated community health centers. As I continue to build my practice, I am working to develop programs to improve the health of Latino/a patients beyond the clinic. I am humbled on a daily basis by the gratitude in patient's voices when I am able to communicate with them in their own language and culture while providing them with the highest quality in cardiovascular care. I enjoy being able to share this experience with the medical students and residents that join me in the clinic.

In addition to being a clinician, I have the privilege of serving as an educator both at the Brigham and Women's Hospital as well as Harvard Medical School. One of my most memorable moments in teaching happened the first day of one of my courses, when I looked out into the crowd and saw a Latino and an African American student. I felt a great sense of pride that I was able to serve as a role model, a fellow minority in an educational leadership position. I will continue to foster these educational roles and build on them into the future.

My third role was not initially part of a formal job description, but it is a role I take very seriously. It is that of mentor—to all fellows, residents, and students, not just underrepresented minorities. I am a strong believer that we all have something to offer those who are coming up behind us. Mentorship was incredibly important and I continued to work with the LMSA students throughout my training. I would not be where I am today were it not for the paths paved by those that came before me. It came as a surprise when I was awarded the excellence in mentoring award by the HMS underrepresented minority medical students in 2008. It is an incredible honor to know that you have affected the lives of a group of individuals in such a positive manner. I had the privilege of serving as Assistant Dean of Student Affairs and Assistant Director of the Office of Recruitment and Multicultural Affairs at HMS where I served as an advocate for recruitment and retention of underrepresented minority medical students. Four years ago I became Dean for Students at HMS. I have passed on my role as LMSA advisor but continue to serve as a regional advisor to LMSA.

As a successful minority physician, I believe it is my calling to use my talents as clinician, educator, and mentor to support the careers of the minority physicians of the future.

John Paul Sánchez MD, MPH, Full Professor with Tenure, Emergency Medicine, Inaugural Executive Diversity Officer (2000– 2022), University of New Mexico School of Medicine; Executive Associate Vice Chancellor, Office for Diversity, Equity and Inclusion, Health Sciences Center, University of New Mexico, LMSA Executive Director (2017-present years), Albert Einstein College of Medicine (2001–2006)

My parents were born in Puerto Rico, my mother in Moca and my father in Santa Isabel. Their parents brought them to New York City in the 1950s in pursuit of social support and economic opportunities. My parents met at a Salsa club and eventually married and gave birth to two sons, both born in the 1970s. Both parents worked for the NYC Board of Education as teachers of the English and Spanish languages. Myself and my brother Nelson Sanchez M.D. not only serve as physicians but have followed in their footsteps as educators. Growing up in the Bronx and witnessing the socioeconomic (e.g. Burning of the Bronx, decrepit buildings) and health disparities (e.g. asthma and HIV/AIDS) impacting Hispanic communities ignited a concurrent interest in medicine and public health. I was fortunate to have parents who supported educational attainment and nurtured career interests. This was critical in succeeding at schools (from elementary to medical school) where I was one of the few Hispanic identified students and often endured discrimination.

Like for many others my pursuit of medicine started in college as a pre-medical student. Unfortunately, being pre-med and associated coursework rarely addressed what it meant to be Hispanic. As such my academic performance during college suffered as I sought groups and experiences that aligned with my Hispanic upbringing and developed my knowledge and skills in understanding and addressing Hispanic community issues. NYU's Academic Achievement Program, led by Dr. Marcia Cantarella, was one of the few spaces, to be oneself and develop as a Hispanic professional. A second formative experience was participating in the Morehouse School of Medicine/Emory

Rollins School of Public/CDC Public Health Summer Fellowship Program, where I learned how to conduct health disparities research and met one of my most influential mentors, Dr. Kenneth Dominguez (medical epidemiologist extraordinaire).

Rebelling against the notion that "treatment" was the best approach to managing health, I opted to obtain an MPH in infectious disease epidemiology at the Yale School of Medicine to better understand prevention. I continued health disparity related service and research work through community based entities such as Alianza Domincana and the Hispanic AIDS Forum, culminating with a graduation thesis on "Culturally Sensitive HIV Programming for Latino Men Who Have Sex with Men?", and serving as a founding Board Member of the Bronx Lesbian and Gay health Resource Consortium (the first LGBT Center in the Bronx).

After several years working as an epidemiologist, and having attained practical experience in researching Hispanic health issues, I re-directed and commenced medical school in the Bronx at the Albert Einstein College of Medicine in 2006. During the Office of Minority Affairs Retreat, I first learned of NBLHO—and found a new family. NBLHO meetings served as an inviting space to have critical, open, safe, Hispanic centric discussions related to admissions (Why were there so few Hispanic medical students considering >40% of the Bronx was Hispanic identified?), student affairs and promotions (What else could be done to prevent the dismissal of friends RA and BS and so many Hispanic students?), medical education (Where are the Hispanic faculty and curricula content?), and diversity and inclusion (Are we offering a minority orientation retreat?). During medical school, I served as a member of LMSA, supporting social and educational events and as treasurer in year 2, but then took a step back to focus on academic challenges. My relationship with LMSA continued after medical school, as I assumed roles as Chair of the NHMA Council of Residents and as Founding Chair of NHMA Council of Young Physicians, making sure that LMSA members remained connected to a support system through NHMA. The

knowledge and skills acquired in supporting LMSA and NHMA members and constituents helped me to develop a leadership foundation to serve as an Inaugural Assistant and subsequent Associate Dean for Diversity and Inclusion at a state based medical school. In 2017, I was elected to serve as the Co-Executive Director of LMSA National Inc. and work towards giving back to a family that supported my completion of an MD and maintained my trajectory to addressing the health issues of LHS+ (Latina/o/x/e, Hispanic, or of Spanish Identified+) individuals.

Amanda Hernandez-Jones, MD, PhD, Assistant Professor, Department of Neurology University of Connecticut School of Medicine, LMSA NE Co-Chair (2010–2014), LMSA National President (2015–2016) Yale University School of Medicine 2009–2016

I am the proud child of two Puerto Ricans, both of whom spent the majority of their upbringing in the Bronx, NY. Growing up, I was taught not only to be proud of my heritage but to embrace the complexity, tradition, and diversity that came along with it. My parents met in the 1980s, my mother a bank teller and my father a contractor. At the time, neither of them had attended college or university but remained steadfast in their belief in the importance of education. I was born in the mid 1980s, my sister in the early 1990s, and we both spent our childhood being engrossed not only in rigorous academic practice but also in creative and open-minded spaces. Prior to my engagement in the life sciences, I was primarily focused on music as a singer and flautist. As such, the performing arts functioned as a brave and safe haven for me, especially as I navigated my frameshift into medicine and basic science research, an interest that was born out of what I witnessed in my community. Throughout my childhood and experience in New York City, I was overcome by the lack of cultural competency and bilingual providers. Apart from my intrigue for life sciences, I found myself committed to transforming these barriers and increasing accessibility to comprehensive care for my community.

At Columbia University, I set out on a premedical course that quickly shifted to include the neurosciences given my passion for cognition and neuronal circuitry. This interest led me to the laboratory, where for the first time I encountered the creativity of basic science research and instantly fell in love. Science afforded the capacity to be creative, think on your feet, and be bold in the approach to open ended questions and pursuit of knowledge. Initially I was torn between pursuing a medical degree and a degree in basic sciences, however, upon learning of dual-degree programs, I made the bold decision to pursue an MD/PhD. This path led me to ultimately spending 5 years at the bench during and following my undergraduate degree completing work pertaining to the neuroanatomical circuitry underlying the suprachiasmatic nucleus.

I matriculated at Yale University in 2009 to attend their medical scientist training program in pursuit of an MD/PhD. On arrival, my initial intent was to continue neuroanatomical investigations, however I found myself intrigued by autoimmunity and its intersection with neurosciences. This led me to study how dietary shifts in salt intake can alter regulatory mechanisms in multiple sclerosis and other autoimmune conditions. Much of these discoveries and curiosities dovetailed into my medical specialization as a neuromuscular neurologist wherein I am currently engrossed in research analyzing autoantibody and humoral responses in neurological inflammatory conditions.

Throughout my tenure in medical school, I was heavily engaged in communities of color starting with my local LMSA chapter which gave birth to engagement regionally and nationally with LMSA and also with the undergraduate community at Yale. In LMSA, I served as the northeast regional co-chair for 4 years from 2010 to 2014 prior to serving as LMSA National President from 2014 to 2015. At Yale University, this work was translated into the greater Yale College community and throughout this time I participated heavily in the Latinx Cultural Center, La Casa Cultural, initially as a graduate assistant and subsequently as a director. All in all, participating in academic spaces with a conscious focus on recruitment, retention, and mentorship for historically underrepresented communities added

substantial latitude to my medical training and provided invaluable leadership experiences.

Jeffrey Uribe, MD, LMSA NE Co-Chair (2014–2015), Temple University School of Medicine (2011–2015)

I was born and raised in New York City by parents who immigrated from Colombia. My father came to New York City in 1969 and my mother in 1984 and met each other through mutual friends. My mother began working when I was in high school after taking night classes to complete an associate degree, despite having a bachelor's degree in Colombia. My father worked as a taxi driver and then as a garment cutter. Early on, they understood the importance of education and they encouraged me to continue to study and not focus on working to help pay the bills which happens to many first-generation students.

My dream was to become a professional soccer player, but when I was asked by my middle school counselor what I envisioned as my future career, I could only answer "to become a doctor,", only because my mother came to my head with what she would frequently tell the family, "He is going to be a future doctor, my doctor!" This highlighted something very important to me from a very young age and that was the clear disparity in access to medical care in my community and the cultural barriers in medical care. This was evident in my frequent doctor visits. Soon enough, I took on that vision and with my parent's support, I entered a path that transformed my life and set my path into medicine. My middle school counselor enrolled me in a science pipeline program, a yearlong program during my freshman year at Columbia University (separate from my high school), where I had the opportunity to take college graduate classes. This introduced me to a different world, where I met other like-minded students and became immersed in the world of science. This experience was followed by another opportunity in another educational pipeline program during my junior year in high school, which involved learning medicine, SAT preparation and the opportunity of shadowing medical doctors. Sadly, but fortunately, it was here where for the first time in my life, I met Hispanic and Black medical doctors and role models. The mentors and volunteers from the medical school were members of the Black and Latinx Students Association (BALSA).

These experiences and encouragement from my mentors kept me on track as I applied to college and medical school. During medical school, I learned about the visible disparities that the Black and Hispanic communities faced. This encouraged me to become President of LMSA chapter at Temple University School of Medicine. I worked alongside Dr. Dela Cadena, who was the Assistant Dean for the Recruitment, Admission and Retention Office at Temple University School of Medicine. A very important lesson I learned is that we need more Latinos, not only in healthcare, but as administrators/Deans in very important positions including the admission committee. Dr. Dela Cadena strived to increase the number of underrepresented students at Temple, and it was here, where I felt most comfortable completing my medical degree. Working with other Latinx students as part of LMSA is where I learned that we as medical students can begin to make a difference in our communities. I was humbled to volunteer my time alongside Dr. Larson at Puentes de Salud, a non-profit healthcare clinic dedicated to serving the immigrant population in South Philadelphia. I continued leadership roles as Co-Chair of NE LMSA during medical school and as Chair of the NHMA Council of Residents during residency. I completed a fellowship in Emergency Medical Services (EMS) and as a medical director for an EMS system, so I can have a role in the intersection of healthcare, public health, and public safety and help educate and work on eliminating disparities. I will continue my role as LMSA chapter advisor, continue the fight to advance Hispanic health, and give back to the village that brought me to who and where I am today.

Julia Su (MD/PhD Student at Donald and Barbara Zucker School of Medicine at Hofstra/Northwell)

I am the daughter of two immigrants. My mother immigrated from China while my father immigrated from Taiwan. While my parents finished their graduate degrees, I was sent to China to live with my grandparents. After living in China for 4 years, I was reunited with my parents in California. Two years later, my grandparents immigrated to California and lived with me and my parents to help with childcare. Much of my passion for working with LMSA came from my formative experiences growing up and seeing the struggles my family had in navigating the health care system.

My grandfather is a two-time cancer survivor. He does not speak any English or drive so he was dependent on my parents to be translators and to provide transportation to all his appointments. To help, I would translate medical reports to my anxious grandpa, help with scheduling appointments, and drive them to their appointments. My family is lucky in that we had the social know-how and the resources to get my grandparents the care they needed, but what about the others who did not have family members that knew English, the education to understand and navigate the healthcare system, or had the means of transportation?

I joined my local LMSA chapter in medical school to learn Medical Spanish. Reminded by my grandparents' struggles, I wanted to become a physician that practices cultural humility. I wanted to understand other cultures and learn the language so I could provide that comfort when I encounter my patients on their worst days. My medical school also happened to be hosting the National LMSA conference that year so after being selected as the Co-Chair of my LMSA chapter, I got involved with conference planning. Helping plan a conference that empowered medical students and working with incredibly passionate people drew me into LMSA. The organization's mission and values aligned with the kind of physician I wanted to become. There is no better way to learn about the problems and challenges affecting a specific population than from the population itself. By being present, attending LMSA events, befriending LMSA members, I heard about the issues that affect their community. From the atrocities of separation of families at the southern border to the DACA medical students facing uncertainty if they can stay in the country to finish their education, I learned a lot by being surrounded by the people these issues affected.

At the 2017 LMSA National Conference, I was elected as the LMSA-NE Co-Director Elect and led the Northeast region for 2 years. My first year as Co-Director Elect was mainly focused on developing regional programming and learning what it takes to run LMSA-NE. It was not until I fully stepped into the Co-Director role that I learned about how LMSA-NE's fits in LMSA National and where it stands compared to other regions. Not all LMSA regions were created equal. We all face similar yet different challenges in terms of finances, history, and the support of faculty and student members. A more established region, with better infrastructure, was able to create a voter drive, and help Latinos register to vote on top of their regular four required quarterly meetings and annual conference where attendance from all chapters were required. While another region, due to lack of student leaders, was struggling to plan their own House of Delegates meeting and annual conference. Being able to sit at the National leadership table, I was able to learn the best practices from regions that were more advanced than ours and also assist regions that were newer than us by sharing our learned best practices. I also noticed that all Regional Directors including myself, always looked out for our region's interests first. At our monthly meetings, we took pride in the projects we led and our role as a board member on a national organization was secondary to our primary role as regional director.

When I asked Freddy Vazquez, the Co-Director before me, if he had any advice to give Iara and I as we took full reign of LMSA-NE, he said, "Buy into National." At that time, I did not understand what he meant, but as I took on the role as a voting Board of Directors member for LMSA National, I realized that my vote and my voice steered the direction of the organization. I would attend monthly National meetings and finally understood why the American government took so long to accomplish anything. If LMSA National wanted to release a statement or receive funding to do a project, all the Regional Directors would have to vote, and a simple majority would allow it to happen. However, if Regional Directors did not "buy in", there would be discussions and

no action would come about it. This can cause stagnation in the organization and frustrate student leaders so the most passionate and promising leaders would rather innovate and lead at the regional level than at the national level.

When LMSA-NE wanted to have a conference app, I did the market research and got funding approval within a month. Since it was a successful feature at our conference, I wanted to have all the LMSA regions to also have a conference app so we can all benefit from it. However, when I pitched this idea at the National meeting, I encountered resistance and the time it took from the initial pitch to final voting and adoption was five months. Once the regional leaders used the conference app themselves and saw how well-received by users. When reflecting on this experience, I realized that as Regional Directors, we have strong loyalties to the success of our region, and because there is a lack of in-person meetings at the National level, we may not always trust or cooperate as readily with people we have not met before or gotten to know well. When pitching an idea to LMSA National, one must always think about the people who vote i.e. the Regional Directors and recognize that each Regional Director will always be thinking, What's in it for me and my region? While this process may seem slow and tedious, it is also remarkably important because anything that is done by LMSA National is reflective of our organization and our values. There are real world consequences if we publish a statement that is harmful to our cause. While we always want positive attention to what our organization does in terms of our programming and our ability to empower Latinos to pursue medicine, we must always be cautious and on the alert for any negative attention that may harm our members and damage our organization.

After serving as the Co-Director for LMSA-NE, I became the first non-Latino identified President of LMSA National and it was controversial. Some people believed I deserved the position because they had personally worked with me before, and they knew that I would continue carrying out LMSA's mission and goals. Some believed that since the President is the face of the organization and I am not Latino, therefore, I should not be allowed to be in that position. After all, by not being Latino, how can I truly understand the struggles or culture if I did not experience it myself? Other arguments against my candidacy include: one of LMSA's objectives is "to provide leadership opportunities to Latinos"and by becoming President I am taking away one of those opportunities. The leaders in LMSA are role models for Latino pre-health students and many studies have shown the importance of seeing someone who looks like you, who had similar shared experiences, and who understands your culture to validate that you belong and can achieve the level of success. What does it mean and what is our organization stating by voting someone who is not Latino to represent their organization and their interests?

To me, being voted as President is an honor and privilege that others have entrusted me to carry out the mission of LMSA National. It is acknowledgement by the community that they recognize me for my allyship to their cause. If I failed my duty, I could be impeached. I was voted into power by the people and could also be removed from power by the people.

What is allyship? According to PeerNetBC [16], allyship "begins when a person of privilege seeks to support a marginalized individual or group. It is a practice of unlearning and relearning, and is a life-long process of building relationships based on trust, consistency, and accountability with marginalized individuals or groups. Allyship is not an identity, nor is it self-defined. Our work and our efforts must be recognized by the people we seek to ally ourselves with. Because of this, it is important to be considerate in how we frame and present the work that we do."

For me, my allyship began when I first joined LMSA to learn Medical Spanish. By getting involved in LMSA activities, I was able to practice critical allyship. LMSA allowed me to transform my motivation from the vague desire to help the less fortunate to concrete commitments like: "I learn from the expertise of, and work in solidarity with, historically marginalized groups to help me understand and take action on systems of inequality." [17] As the United States becomes more and more diverse, it is imperative for physicians to understand and help fix the health disparities. In order to achieve that, everyone should practice critical allyship because there is always some part of your identity that has more privilege than someone else, whether it be race, wealth, religion, sexual orientation, etc.

References

1. Massey D, Constant A. Latinos in the Northeastern United States": Trends and Patterns. https://www.researchgate.net/publication/316420751. Accessed 25 Mar 2020.
2. Tienda M, Mitchell F, editors. Hispanics and the Future of America. Committee on Transforming Our Common Destiny, National Research Council (US) Panel on Hispanics in the United States. Washington, DC: National Academies Press (US); 2006. ASPIRA of New York. https://aspirany.org/. Accessed 29 May 2020
3. Fernandez J. The young lords a radical history university. Chapel Hill: North Carolina Press; 2020.
4. Velasco-Mondragon E, Jimenez A, Palladino-Davis A, et al. Hispanic health in the USA: A scoping review of the literature. Public Health Rev. 2016;37:31.
5. Ana María García La operación. 1982, New York, NY: Distributed by the Cinema Guild, c2006.
6. Darder A. Colonized Wombs? Reproduction Rights and Puerto Rican Women. December 2006. http://publici.ucimc.org/2006/12/colonized-wombs-reproduction-rights-and-puerto-rican-women/. Accessed 29 May 2020.
7. Iris Ofelia López. Matters of Choice: Puerto Rican Women's Struggle for Reproductive Freedom. 2008. Published by: Rutgers University Press.
8. Bereknyei S, Foran S, Johnson K, Scott A, Miller T, Braddock C III. Stopping discrimination before it starts: the impact of civil rights laws on healthcare disparities - a medical school curriculum. MedEdPORTAL Publications. 2009;5:7740. https://doi.org/10.15766/mep_2374-8265.7740.
9. Iris Morales. ¡Palante Siempre Palante! http://archive.pov.org/palantesiemprepalante/. Accessed 30 May 2020.
10. Our History. LMSA Northeast. https://www.lmsane.org/our-history.html. Accessed 26 Dec 2022.
11. David J. Leonard and Carmen R. Lugo-Lugo Latino history and culture: an encyclopedia. New York: Routledge Publishing; 2015. p. 378.
12. Perspectives of Change. J. Emilio Carrillo, MD, MPH, 1976. https://perspectivesofchange.hms.harvard.edu/node/54. Accessed 26 Dec 2022.
13. In Memoriam: Luis Garden Acosta, Builder of Bridges. Published January 15, 2019. https://citylim-

its.org/2019/01/15/in-memoriam-luis-garden-acosta--builder-of-bridges/. Accessed 26 Dec 2022.

14. Carrillo EJ, Carrillo VA, Perez HR, et al. Defining and targeting health care access barriers. J Health Care Poor Underserved. 2011;22(2):562–75.

15. LMSA Northeast Purpose and Goals. https://www.lmsane.org/our-vision.html. Accessed 20 Dec 2022.

16. PeerNetBC. What is allyship? Why can't I be an ally? Chttp://www.peernetbc.com/what-is-allyship Posted on Nov 22, 2016. Accessed 30 May 2020.

17. Nixon SA. The coin model of privilege and critical allyship: implications for health. BMC Public Health. 2019;19:1637.

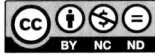

LHS+ Medical Student History and Heritage of the U.S. Southeast Region

Nicole McManus and Victor Cueto

Introduction

The southeast region of the Latino Medical Student Association (LMSA Southeast) encompasses a broad and large geographic area consisting of medical schools in the states of Alabama, Florida, Georgia, Kentucky, Mississippi, North Carolina, South Carolina, Tennessee, Virginia, and West Virginia, as well as the Commonwealth of Puerto Rico and the Caribbean islands. This represents a vast territory of approximately 440,000 square miles of land [1], with a diverse array of local and regional cultures, as well as, ethnicities and political views.

The largest populations of individuals identifying as Latino in this vast territory are largely concentrated in Puerto Rico and rural areas or around large metropolitan areas in the states of Virginia, Georgia, North Carolina, and Florida [1]. Notable areas in the region with large concentrations of Latino populations include Miami-Ft. Lauderdale, Tampa, Orlando, Jacksonville, Atlanta, and Raleigh-Durham [2].

The pioneers and founders of these populations in the region have represented the full spectrum of social, political, and economic classes. Some areas and populations owe their roots to factories and migrant farmworkers while others were founded by skilled laborers and highly educated professionals [1]. The Latin American nationalities and ethnicities represented in particular states and metropolitan areas largely reflect the history of U.S. immigration policies and Latin American geopolitical conflicts. As in other places in the United States, Latinos in the southeast have fled social and economic strife in their home countries, often seeking refuge from violence and political oppression. In turn, these brave men and women have brought an increasingly diverse array of Latin American cultures to the southeastern United States that has enriched the greater culture of the region.

The demographic history of Latinos in the region has paralleled the growth of LMSA Southeast. However, the increasing density of Latino populations in the southeast has not kept pace with the diversity of medical schools in the region. At a regional level, with the exception of Puerto Rico, Latinos continue to be severely underrepresented in medical education and are often dispersed in small numbers at individual medical schools throughout the country [3]. Accordingly, many medical schools in the southeast suffer from very small enrollments of Latino

N. McManus (✉)
Philadelphia College of Osteopathic Medicine, Philadelphia, PA, USA
e-mail: nicolemc@pcom.edu

V. Cueto
Department of Pediatrics and Internal Medicine, University of Miami, Miller School of Medicine, Miami, FL, USA

© The Author(s) 2024
J. P. Sánchez, D. Rodriguez (eds.), *Latino, Hispanic, or of Spanish Origin+ Identified Student Leaders in Medicine*, Sustainable Development Goals Series, https://doi.org/10.1007/978-3-031-35020-7_3

students, from which it was and continues to be difficult to create or sustain a thriving LMSA chapter. Even at some schools in the southeast with larger enrollments of Latinos, past leaders have noted challenges in organizing strong LMSA chapters, because some Latino students did not readily identify with their ethnic background or realize the potential benefits of involvement in LMSA. This has represented and continues to be a unique challenge to the growth of LMSA in the southeast region as compared to other regions where there has either been a larger, critical mass of Latino students, an inherently majority-minority population or a more robust history of Latino medical student organizations.

Historical Background

The story of LMSA Southeast and Latinos in the region is unquestionably tied to its geographic proximity to Latin America. Accordingly, its history is marked by the lasting impact of political upheaval, violence, economic disruption, and natural disasters in various Latin American countries and Puerto Rico. Presently, Latinos in the southeast identify with many different countries of origin. The most significant waves of migration and immigration to the region have been dominated by socioeconomic conditions and events in Cuba, Puerto Rico, Colombia, Venezuela, Argentina, El Salvador, Nicaragua, Honduras, Dominican Republic, and Mexico.

In telling the history of Latinos in the Southeast, the significance and contribution of the state of Florida and South Florida cannot be understated. The state of Florida has the third-largest Latino population in the country and the largest in the southeast [1]. In fact, there are more Latinos in Florida than in Puerto Rico. The early history of Latinos in Florida was largely shaped by the events and consequences of the Cuban Revolution. Undoubtedly, the overthrowing of Fulgencio Batista by Fidel Castro in 1959 and the resulting social, political, and economic upheaval that ensued for decades thereafter has impacted the demographics and politics of Florida for the last 60 years. Over the course of six decades, over

1.3 million Cubans have migrated to the United States in five major waves. It is on the backdrop of this history that South Florida's emergence as the "Gateway to the Americas" is predicated.

Before 1960, South Florida had a rather small Latino community. However, this changed dramatically with an influx of approximately 508,700 Cubans to the United States, in just over one decade from 1959 to 1973. A large majority of these political exiles and refugees settled in Miami and the surrounding communities, forever changing the character and culture of the city and surrounding South Florida region as well as the politics regarding immigration to the State of Florida. During the first wave of Cuban migration, over 14,000 children fled Cuba as part of a U.S. State Department project named Operation Peter Pan, from 1960 to 1962 [4]. These unaccompanied minors were airlifted to Miami, Florida. Upon arrival, they were placed in the care of Catholic Charities until they could be placed in foster homes or reunited with family members.

The 1960s was also an important decade of national immigration policy. In 1965, President Lyndon B. Johnson signed the Immigration and Nationality Act into law. This law abolished the immigration quota system and shifted the focus of immigration policy toward reuniting families. Additionally, this new policy also focused on bringing in skilled and educated workers, which allowed many physicians trained in other countries, including Latin America, a new pathway within the U.S. immigration process. One source has documented that at the time, approximately 388 physicians trained in Latin America immigrated to the United States, a tally that did not include Cuban physicians [4]. It is more difficult to quantify the number of Cuban doctors who immigrated during this time. However, based on the efforts of certain local institutions such as the University of Miami, which established an Office of International Medical Education, it is clear there was a significant number of Cuban physicians who also immigrated and sought to practice in the United States.

Over the past 60 years, a myriad of political events and natural disasters throughout both

Central America and South America have fueled immigration to the Southeast. Additionally, the politics, as well as the immigration and foreign policies of the United States, has also played a significant role. One such example is the history of Operation Condor (1968–1989), which was a U.S.-financed campaign involving several South American countries and dictatorships that punished political dissidents, social activists, trade unionists, and religious clergy [5]. Initially, Chile, Argentina, Bolivia, Brazil, Paraguay, and Uruguay were involved in this plan, and Peru, Colombia, and Venezuela joined later on as the project progressed. It is reported that thousands were raped, murdered, or "disappeared" in these countries and that this violence caused many to flee to the United States to escape authoritarian oppression [5].

The 1980s and 90 s were decades of a number of important immigration events. One notable event was the Mariel exodus and boatlift, a humanitarian crisis brought on by Fidel Castro's actions after approximately 10,000 Cubans flooded foreign embassies on the island, seeking political asylum. As a result, Castro proclaimed the port of Mariel open to anyone wishing to leave the country. The crisis lasted from April to October 1980, with approximately 125,000 Cubans leaving the island on boats and ultimately seeking political asylum in Florida [6]. However, a much larger influx of Latino immigrants during the 1980s resulted from civil wars in El Salvador, Guatemala, and Nicaragua. The violence and economic strife caused by these wars drove thousands of immigrants to seek refuge in the United States. In a single decade from 1980 to 1990, the population of Central Americans in the United States tripled, with many taking residences in the Southeastern states, chiefly Florida and Virginia. Later in 1994, the Cuban balsero crisis brought approximately 30,900 Cubans to the U.S. and punctuated years of countless lives lost at sea while attempting to cross the ocean in homemade rafts. As a result, the Clinton administration negotiated with the Castro regime and established new policies including the "wet foot - dry foot" policy for those apprehended by border patrol or Coast Guard agents, in addition to a yearly legal immigration lottery system organized by the U.S. State Department.

Another contributing factor to immigration has been the destruction, displacement, and economic turmoil caused by natural disasters such as hurricanes. Although hurricanes are a common occurrence for the Caribbean islands, Central America, and the coastal southeastern United States, the damage caused by large and powerful hurricanes often causes individuals to abandon their homes and relocate. One such storm was Hurricane Mitch in 1998, which devastated the countries of Nicaragua and Honduras, resulting in a large number of refugees, a number of which took up residence in Florida. Similarly, Hurricane Maria in 2017 devastated Puerto Rico, causing over 400,000 individuals to move out of the island, with the largest amount, 43%, relocating to Florida [7].

As one might imagine, the events, conditions, and circumstances prompting immigration as well as the process itself do not come without significant health repercussions. Post-traumatic stress disorder related to the immigration process was not uncommon [8]. Individuals who have experienced trauma may also exhibit distrust of medical providers and other officials [5]. Other significant related health concerns include substance use and its many medical complications [6, 8]. Lastly, many immigrants face economic hardship once arriving in the United States [6], a contributing factor to the development of health disparities.

An additional source of stress and fuel for health disparities is the labyrinth of immigration policies that govern legal status in the United States. These policies often divide and discriminate against Latinos based on national origin and the circumstances underlying their immigration. The consequences of these policies have resulted in divided families and communities labeled by their "status" and afforded different access to full participation in society depending on whether they are legal permanent residents, undocumented, refugees, asylum seekers, or temporary protected status [9].

Overall, the southeast has experienced consistent and rapid growth of the Latino community.

This history of immigration and the events surrounding them are the context in which the students of the LMSA were raised and planted the seeds for Latinos in medicine. In one way or another, every member of the LMSA community has been affected by immigration and immigration policies, be it directly, within their own family, or in the communities that they serve.

Putting the Pieces Together: The Early Years (1987–2010)

The precursor to LMSA-Southeast was the National Network of Latino American Medical Students (NNLAMS) whose origins date to a national meeting of regional medical student leaders in Chicago in 1987 but was later formally organized in 1999. In 2003, national records indicate that the southeast region adopted the NNLAMS name. However, details of the role of leaders from the southeast during this time have been lost to time, but it is loosely known from oral history that there were active student groups in the region at the time and possibly a number of decades earlier. Under NNLAMS, regional groups acted collaboratively, yet functioned largely independently with limited communication and structure. As such, many of the details of the organizational and regional activities during these early years have also been lost to history. Nonetheless, it is known that a number of individual medical student organizations at several medical schools, who identified as either Hispanic or Latino, were active and functional in the region, and that a number of these organizations predated the creation of either NNLAMS or LMSA. For example, two schools in Florida, the University of Miami and the University of Florida had chapters that went by the name of the Hispanic American Medical Student Association (HAMSA). Conversely, the local chapter at the University of South Florida utilized the name Latino American Medical Student Association (LAMSA), and later the Hispanic Medical Student Association (HMSA). Some institutions had different names altogether, whose focus was beyond that of students, such as Edward Via

College of Medicine in Virginia, which preferred the name Hispanic Community Medical Outreach (HCMO). There were also groups outside of the United States, such as at Ross University in Dominica, who used the name Organization of Latin American Students (OLAS). "For whatever reason, it was hard getting the students to buy into the LMSA agenda, and they chose to be called the Association of Latino Medical Students (ALMS)," Dr. Jose Rodriguez, former Chapter Advisor at Florida State University explained. "FSU's chapter was still going by 'ALMS' at their campus by the time I moved [in 2016]."

Furthermore, Dr. Rodriguez recounted the motivation behind starting ALMS at that time. "Initially, the group was part of SNMA (Student National Medical Association), but they felt that organization wasn't fully meeting their needs." This sentiment was a common theme of the formation of many chapters of LMSA (and similar groups) in the Southeast region.

The success of the group at FSU was especially notable as the medical school was new, yet still had sufficient interest to support the new organization. Dr. Rodriguez remained the chapter advisor throughout his time working at FSU. During that period, he notes the university also benefited from starting an LMSA chapter, both in terms of recruiting Latino students and being recognized at a national level as FSU was ranked as one of the Top 10 medical schools for Latinos for 6 years.

During this same time period, a separate organized medicine movement outside of medical schools began forming at the professional level, organized by Latino physician leaders on a regional and national stage. Dr. Onelia Lage, a chapter advisor of the student group at the University of Miami, recalls attending the southern regional conference call of the National Hispanic Medical Association (NHMA) in 1994. Dr. Lage noted, "It's about creating opportunities...The way I see it, I push so that others behind me can have it easier and have more room to grow professionally in academia." NHMA would later serve to support NNLAMS' first national conference in 2006 under a joint collaboration with NHMA.

As the region began to take on a stronger regional structure, facilitating face-to-face meetings and improving collaboration on a national level became a greater priority. Most notably, in 2005 the southeast region hosted the Garcia Leadership Seminar (GLAS) at Duke University School of Medicine. GLAS was an important annual event that brought together Latino student leaders from across the nation. This was the first time that a major national event was hosted in the southeast region. Duke University was chosen as the host for the event because it had ample resources and was at the time the home institution of Dr. Omar Rashid, former National Coordinator and then-current Southeast Regional Co-director.

However, this time period was not without its challenges. In the spring of 2006, there were reported interpersonal conflicts which resulted in the schism of leadership, resulting in the following 2006–2007 academic year being a lost year of leadership in the Southeast region. As far as it is known, there is no record of a regional executive board on file and no formal regional activities noted. It is likely that local chapters were able to carry on their activities without major impact, but the guiding regional infrastructure was not active. This was followed by a figurative rebirth of the region in 2007, facilitated by the NNLAMS conference in San Antonio, TX. At that meeting, there were approximately 4 students from medical schools representing the southeast region. These students had either been aware of NNLAMS through their undergraduate institutions or had friends from other regions who informed them of the existence of NNLAMS. Two of these students, Aisha Rivera and Mario Nieto, were appointed by the NNLAMS leadership to serve as ad-hoc chairs for the Southeast, and they began rebuilding the region. Dr. Homan-Sandoval notes the constitution at that time stated that representatives must be elected by members of their own region, yet there no other members from the Southeast region present to elect them, thus this rule was exempted in order to appoint the new regional leadership. Dr. Aisha Rivera recalls the meeting as follows:

"I went to the meeting held in San Antonio and that's where I met other folks involved around the country involved with the organization." Dr. Rivera noted. "They were so excited to see that there were medical students in the Southeast who were interested in NNLAMS (or I should say LMSA) and we were there, so it was like 'there's no one else here, so you're representing the southeast!'"

Soon thereafter the region would return to growth. In 2009, the Southeast hosted its inaugural regional conference at the University of South Florida on February 27–28, 2009. As conference chair and Southeast Co-Director, Annellys Hernandez was instrumental in organizing the first two regional conferences. Despite being a landmark project for the Southeast region, Dr. Annellys Hernandez recalls her experience as a student planning the first Southeast regional conference was not as stressful as one might imagine and was well supported. "We teamed up with our local AHEC [Area Health Education Consortium] to host the conference. They provided monetary support and mentorship, even helping us develop the logo and posters used to promote the event."

Another significant project embarked on by the Southeast region was an annual medical mission trip to the Dominican Republic, organized by a chapter at the University of South Florida. Dr. Annellys Hernandez recounted that several students from other chapters in the region would join in on this effort, which not only provided a great service opportunity for members but also helped support the clinic by augmenting the time each year during which services could be delivered.

Joining Forces: Continued Growth (2010–2014)

As the region continued to grow, it became more involved with national activities. The region once again hosted GLAS, the 12th Annual Garcia Leadership & Advocacy Seminar on August 12–13, 2011 at Duke University. Topics discussed included managing student debt, occupational risks among farmworkers, and leadership in the public sector. At this time, there was concern about cultural organizations losing their vote in the Medical Student Section of the American Medical Association House of Delegates. At the 2010 Minority Health Summit, leaders of these student groups discussed supporting each other by attending each other's conferences, forming alliances, and being more collaborative as they shared similar goals and missions. This show of solidarity also helped fortify the pipeline of diversity in medicine as well as address the inter-sectionality of latinidad.

This period in the history of the Southeast region was one focused on increasing the visibility of the region on a national level as well as strengthening the region internally. Over the next few years, the region was presented with both many opportunities and successes as well as challenges. Miguel Gosalbez, then a medical student at the University of Miami Miller School of Medicine, notes that several organizational issues within the southeast region took some time to resolve during his tenure as regional Co-Director from 2011 to 2013.

> When I initially became president, we weren't fully aware how many chapters we had or how many were active. It was a little disorganized initially, so one of the things we wanted to try while I was there was reaching out to the different chapters, making sure people were involved, and trying to get at least one long-term contact at each one.

During this time in 2012, Dr. Gosalbez was also instrumental in the creation of the LMSA Premedical Latino Undergraduate Society (PLUS) both regionally and nationally. The aim of this effort was to help build a continuum and pipeline of students that unified premedical students, graduate students, and medical student LMSA members. Under this banner, several institutions began forming undergraduate LMSA groups and served as a bridge between the undergraduate experience and medical school. As a student, Dr. Gosalbez was a strong advocate of the program on behalf of the Southeast, and sought allies among members of the LMSA national leadership. He was united in this effort by then Yale MD-PhD student, national leader, and northeast regional co-chair leader, Amanda Lynn Hernandez. Together they championed these efforts at the national level and LMSA

PLUS would go on to replace the former program named Premedical Association of Latino Students (PALS). Fittingly, Dr. Gosalbez, who helped coin the term of LMSA PLUS, later served as an LMSA PLUS chapter physician advisor at the University of Florida.

By 2013, the Southeast region continued to have strong leadership and served as host for the 8th annual LMSA National Conference. The event was held as a joint national and regional conference at the University of Miami on March 15–17, 2013. This was the first national conference ever held in the Southeast region. Dr. Elizabeth Homan-Sandoval, who at the time was completing her psychiatry residency at the University of Miami-Jackson Memorial was instrumental in advising the regional leadership and helping to organize the conference. Dr. Homan-Sandoval's experience as an LMSA alumna and former national leader from the Midwest was a tremendous asset to the burgeoning and rebuilding Southeast region.

In four years from 2010 to 2014, the region experienced strong growth and leadership. After three very well-attended conferences in Miami and one in North Carolina, the executive board focused on continuing to build a strong foundation upon which the Southeast region could continue to grow and flourish. Regional leaders from the time reported they had accumulated a sizable nest egg to provide financial stability for the region. "It was not entirely under our control, but our goal was that when things fall apart when you lose some interest if there's a year med students are too busy—at least there's something to fall back on," explained former Co-Director Dr. Beth Batchelor.

The physician advisor of the region from 2014–2016, Dr. Victor Cueto, also notes the success and strength of the region during this time. "The Southeast leadership truly did a phenomenal job of growing and shepherding the region. As a student leader just a couple of years earlier in the Northeast, I had witnessed my peers in the Southeast such as Annellys Hernandez, Noemi LeFranc, Miguel Gosalbez lay the groundwork that later blossomed under the leadership of Beth Batchelor, Felix Chinea and others. Having grown up in South Florida, I was especially proud to see the region flourish and show LMSA what it has to offer."

Un Pasito Pa'lante, Un Pasito Pa'tras (2015–2020)

The success of the preceding years had positioned for continued growth and resilience. Chapter membership was strong throughout the region and new chapters in Puerto Rico had been successfully established. This growth set the stage for an ambitious plan to host the 7th Annual LMSA Southeast Regional Conference in Puerto Rico, at San Juan Bautista School of Medicine in March 2015. This was especially noteworthy as it was the first time that a regional conference or any LMSA conference was held outside the contiguous United States.

The main goal of hosting the conference in Puerto Rico was to acknowledge the contribution that Puerto Rican medical schools provide to overall diversity in medicine, as well as increase awareness of Puerto Rican medical students as US graduates. Unfortunately, students from Puerto Rico have been discriminated against and perceived as others, among both peers and residency program directors, who often mistake medical students studying in Puerto Rico for International Medical Graduates (IMGs). Dr. Amnha Zambrano (née Elustra) reported that the conference was very effective in raising awareness of the role of students in Puerto Rico, "Only about 5% of physicians in the US identify as Latino, and of those, half are from or have trained in Puerto Rico. Without Puerto Rican med schools, there would only be 2%. It was important to have the conference in Puerto Rico to say 'we're here'" she explained.

The conference was truly a rousing success with regard to visibility and programming. It was very well attended by those on the island of Puerto Rico and those from the mainland. Schools from all over the United States sent students and representatives to the conference. Additionally, the American Association of Medical Colleges (AAMC) also had representatives and leaders in attendance. Even a number of LMSA alumni from various regions attended and participated as speakers. However, the cost of hosting the conference placed a large financial strain on the region. The cost of hosting the conference at a hotel rather than a medical school or other educational institution was a particularly significant expense.

Dr. Cueto recalls that "The students did an amazing job of planning the conference. I remember that Estevan and Amnha were the champions and cheerleaders of the whole effort and they put together a really strong team. The conference was absolutely wonderful all around, the programming was engaging, the venue was beautiful, the students were great hosts, and there were even faculty and alumni in attendance. It was only after the conference that we realized how it had turned out to be really financially tough on the region."

The subsequent years of 2016 and 2017 were not as strong for the region. In 2017, the number of positions on the regional executive board was reduced from 11 to 7. Marvin Valencia and Lauren Silva, Co-Directors of the Southeast region at that time, cited difficulty filling board positions and decreased participation as the impetus for this change.

In 2019, an effort to increase member engagement resulted in a virtual rather than in-person House of Delegates meeting, which was hosted on September 18, 2019. Over 11 chapters were in attendance. Major business included reviewing requirements for the year, as well as discussing the resolutions to be voted upon at the upcoming Policy Summit in Washington D.C. The concept of a virtual assembly was ultimately successful as it helped overcome two of the main challenges to participation in the region: geographic distance and financial limitations for travel. This new concept has been built on a history of openness and collaboration among student leaders in the region. For instance, Dr. Beth Batchelor noted that during her tenure as a Southeast Co-Director, monthly conference calls hosted by the regional board were open to all LMSA chapter presidents to attend; she stated this helped increase transparency and involvement throughout the region.

During the 2019 academic year, Dr. Elizabeth Homan-Sandoval gained approval from the LMSA national board, Southeast regional board, and the LMSA Physician Faculty Advisory Council to establish a regional Physician Faculty Advisory Council in the Southeast using a parallel framework as the National Faculty Physician Advisory Council. Several physicians in the Southeast region banded together to form the Southeast Faculty Physician Advisory Council, composed of 5 physicians LMSA alumni either working in the Southeast or trained in the region previously. The members of the inaugural board included Dr. Lorena Bonilla, Dr. Claudia Alvarez, Dr. Franklyn Cabrero-Rocha, Dr. Giselle Dutcher, Dr. Elizabeth Batchelor, and Dr. Elizabeth Homan-Sandoval. The main goals of the LMSA Southeast FPAC include increasing continuity within the region, providing opportunities for LMSA alumni to engage with current students, and providing mentorship. As the journey through medical school and matching into residency programs has become more challenging, the Regional FPAC provided hope for additional stability in the region. Additionally, it has become more common for recent alumni to be invited back to regional and national LMSA conferences as speakers and exhibitors, leading to increased interaction with more individuals with institutional memory.

The advisory council had been successful in helping support the region, evidenced by the well-attended conference at Jackson Memorial Health and the election of a full incoming Southeast regional board. Dr. Franklyn Cabrero-Rocha felt it had been rewarding to be part of the Southeast FPACand "though there are definitely times where I might be busy there are several physicians on the advisory council and we all work together to help out." A precursor to this established advisory board, was the contributions of several individual advisors and alumni, such as Dr. Elizabeth Homan-Sandoval, Dr. Victor Cueto, and Dr. John Paul Sanchez.

Hacia el Futuro: Great Promise (2022 and Beyond)

The rhythm of the southeast region has been an ebb and flow of success and struggle. Several decisions have been made and then reverted over time. The tenor of the region's growth and the path forward has imbued the composition of the regional student leadership and history of conferences. The locations of conferences and the medical schools represented by the regional student leaders have reflected both the major areas of LHS+ populations in the Southeast as well as the states where LHS+ populations continue to grow. Although 7 of the 11 conferences to date have been held in Florida, with 5 conferences hosted in Miami (Table 3.1), the region has more recently expanded its reach to Georgia, Virginia, North Carolina, and Puerto Rico (Table 3.2). The regional leadership (Table 3.3) has also reflected the growth of chapters in these states and territories. The conference themes also tell the story of the evolution of the region as a whole. The first conference theme—"Sembrando Raíces: A Focus on Latino Health"—illustrates the effort to develop an organizational presence as LMSA Southeast began to take hold. Over time, the conference themes became more specific and discrete, while between 2016 and 2022, the themes have focused on elements of growth, unity and progress. The future of the region will inevitably grow through an ongoing ebb and flow, yet there is hope and evidence that the tide of progress will continue to rise in the Southeast region.

Table 3.1 Regional conference title, date, and host

1. University of South Florida
"Sembrando Raíces: A Focus on Latino Health"
February 27–28, 2009

2. Florida State University
"Healthcare Reform: The Impact on Latino Communities"
February 5–6, 2010

3. University of Miami
"Abriendo Puertas: Empowering Future Medical Leaders to Have Ethical Care of Every Patient"
January 14–16, 2011

4. University of Miami
"Pa'Lante Juntos: Aligning to Discover Health Solutions for Our Communities"
February 17–19, 2012

5. University of Miami
"Tomando Accion (Taking Action): Ensuring Health Equity for All."
March 15–17, 2013

6. University of North Carolina SOM
"Hablamos Espanol: Understanding the Diversity Behind One Language"
February 7–9, 2014

7. San Juan Bautista SOM
"But You Don't Look Latino/a…"
February 27–March 1, 2015

8. Virginia Commonwealth University
"Sigue Pa'lante"
January 29–31, 2016

9. Philadelphia College of Osteopathic Medicine—Georgia Campus
"Unidos por un Futuro: Together We All Rise"
February 3–5, 2017

10. Miami Dade College
"Siempre Unidos: Celebrating Diversity & Bridging the Gap
April 13–15, 2018

11. Jackson Memorial Hospital,
"Siempre Unidos: Advancing Through Advocacy and Activism"
February 29, 2020

12. Mercer University School of Medicine (Virtual),
"El Futuro Depende Del Presente"
February 25–27, 2022

13. Nova Southeastern University Dr. Kiran C. Patel College of Allopathic Medicine
"Raices Fuertes, Futuros Seguros"
March 3–4, 2023

Table 3.2 List of States and School Chapters (stand alone or connected) in the LMSA Southeast Region (as of December 2022)

Alabama: Alabama College of Osteopathic Medicine, Edward Via College of Osteopathic Medicine, University of Alabama School of Medicine, University of South Alabama College of Medicine.

Florida: Florida International University Herbert Wertheim College of Medicine, Florida State University College of Medicine, Nova Southeastern University, University of Central Florida, University of Florida College of Medicine, University of Miami Miller School of Medicine, University of South Florida Morsani College of Medicine, Charles E. Schmidt College of Medicine at Florida Atlantic University, Nova Southeastern University KPCOM, LECOM Brandeton.

Georgia: Emory University School of Medicine, Medical College of Georgia, Mercer University School of Medicine - Columbus, Mercer University School of Medicine - Macon, Mercer University School of Medicine - Savannah, Morehouse School of Medicine, Philadelphia College of Osteopathic Medicine - North GA Campus, Philadelphia College of Osteopathic Medicine - South GA Campus.

Kentucky: University of Kentucky, University of Louisville, University of Pikevile.

Mississippi: University of Mississipi Medical Center, William Carey University College of Osteopathic Medicine.

North Carolina: Duke University School of Medicine, East Carolina University Brody School of Medicine, University of North Carolina School of Medicine, Wake Forest School of Medicine.

South Carolina: Medical University of South Carolina, University of South Carolina School of Medicine Greenville, University of South Carolina School of Medicine Columbia, Edward Via College of Osteopathic Medicine Spartanburg.

Tennessee: Lincoln Memorial University - DeBusk College of Osteopathic Medicine, Vanderbilt University School of Medicine, East Tenessee State University, Meharry Medical College, University of Tennessee Health Science Center College of Medicine.

Virginia: Eastern Virginia Medical School, University of Virginia School of Medicine, Virginia Commonwealth University School of Medicine, Virginia Tech Carilon School of Medicine, Edward Via College of Osteopathic Medicine Blacksburg, Liberty University College of Osteopathic Medicine.

West Virginia: Marshall University, University of West Virginia, West Virginia School fo Osteopathic Medicine.

Puerto Rico & The Caribbean: American University of the Caribbean School of Medicine, Ponce Health Sciences University, Ross University School of Medicine, San Juan Bautista School of Medicine, School of Medicine University of Puerto Rico, Universidad Central del Caribe School of Medicine.

Table 3.3 List of Southeast Co-Director(s)

2022–2023	Christopher Vazquez, University of Miami SOM
	Darisel Ventura Rodriguez, Nova Southeastern University Dr. Kiran C. Patel College of Allopathic Medicine
2021–2022	Roxana Gonzalez, Mercer University School of Medicine
	Emily Rabinovich, University of Virginia School of Medicine
2020–2021	Olga Chamberlain, University of Miami SOM
	Yanelys Fernandez, University of Miami SOM
2019–2020	Roxana Navarro, University of Miami SOM
	Victoria Fernandez, University of Miami SOM
2018–2019	Nicole McManus, Philadelphia College of Osteopathic Medicine—Georgia
	Roxana Navarro, University of Miami SOM
2016–2018	Marvin Valencia, Lincoln Memorial University DeBusk
	School of Osteopathic Medicine
	Lauren Silva, Virginia Commonwealth University
2015–2016	Maria Fernanda Perry, Edward Via College of Osteopathic Medicine
	Marvin Valencia, Lincoln Memorial University DeBusk School of Osteopathic Medicine
2014–2015	Adrian Diaz, Virginia Commonwealth University SOM
	Estevan Torrez, San Juan Bautista SOM
2013–2014	Felix Chinea, Duke University SOM
	Elizabeth Batchelor, University of Miami Miller SOM
2012–2013	Miguel Gosalbez, University of Miami Miller SOM
	Felix Chinea, Duke University SOM
2011–2012	Noemi LeFranc Matta, Florida State University
	Miguel Gosalbez, University of Miami Miller SOM
2010–2011	Annellys Hernandez, University of South Florida SOM
	Enrique Huerta, Vanderbilt University
2009–2010	Aisha Rivera, University of Virginia SOM
	Annellys Hernandez, University of South Florida Morsani SOM
2008–2009	Jason Castellanos, Vanderbilt University SOM
	Irving Zamora, University of Florida
2007–2008	Mario Edmundo Nieto, Vanderbilt University SOM
	Aisha Rivera, University of Virginia SOM
2005–2006	Omar Rashid, Duke University SOM
	Ali Rashid, University of South Florida Morsani SOM

References

1. Pew Research Center. Demographic and Economic Profiles of Hispanics by State and County, 2014. www.pewresearch.org/hispanic/states
2. Constant, AF, Massey DM. Latinos in the southeastern United States: trends and patterns. Office of Population Research, Princeton University; 2019 Oct.
3. Diversity in Medicine: Facts and Figures 2019 https://www.aamc.org/data-reports/workforce/data/table-7-us-medical-schools-200-or-more-hispanic-or-latino-graduates-alone-or-combination-2009-2010
4. Anderson M. Pedro Pan: A children's exodus from Cuba. Smithsonian Insider, 2017 July 11. www.insider.si.edu/2017/07/pedro-pan-childrens-exodus-cuba/. Accessed 25 Feb 2020.

5. West KM. Foreign Interns and Residents in the United States. J Med Educ. 1965;40:1110–29.
6. Hollander NC. Psychoanalysts bearing witness. In: Gherovici P, Christian C, editors. Psychoanalysis in the Barrios. New York: Routledge; 2019. p. 38–53.
7. Hinojosa J, Meléndez E. Puerto Rican exodus: One year since Hurricane Maria. Center for Puerto Rican Studies; 2018.
8. Portes A, Stepick A, Truelove C Three years later: The adaptation process of 1980 (Mariel) Cuban and Haitian Refugees in South Florida. Population and Policy Review, Summer 1986.
9. Cislo AM, Spence NJ, Gayman MD. The mental health and psychosocial adjustment of Cuban immigrants in South Florida. Soc Sci Med. 2010;71(6):1173–81.

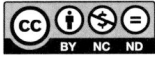

LHS+ Medical Student History and Heritage of the U.S. Midwest Region

Emma B. Olivera, Jorge Girotti, and Monica Vela

"Oral history provides a useful tool for beginning to fill significant gaps in our knowledge about the history of [Latina/o] experiences, but it should also prompt us to collect and preserve important documents in publicly accessible archival repositories."

—Delgadillo & Weaver, 2017, p. 249.

Migration and Immigration of Latinos to the Midwest

Since the mid-nineteenth century, several push and pull factors have contributed to the migration of Latinos to the Midwest region of the United States (U.S.). All Midwestern states—including Illinois, Indiana, Iowa, Kansas, Michigan, Minnesota, Missouri, Nebraska, North Dakota, Ohio, South Dakota, and Wisconsin—saw increases in the Latino population during this time period. Many forces driving immigrants to the Midwest were related to these individuals' desire to achieve the ever-elusive "American Dream," with economic opportunities prompting Latino laborers to establish initially transitory residence in the region.

For migrant laborers in the 1880s, the Midwest region served as a source of seasonal work, not a place for permanent settlement [1]. Jobs in the agriculture, railroad, meatpacking, stockyard, and manufacturing industries attracted primarily unaccompanied males of Mexican descent; these individuals would move to and within the U.S. Midwest according to seasonal harvests or project availability and would return to Texas, California, or Mexico after their work was complete. With these expectations, Midwest-based employers directly sought out these males, often offering wages too low to support workers' families in order to depress expenses. Moreover, established residents of Midwestern communities often welcomed this strategy, as many feared that, if migrants were offered equitable salaries, they might settle permanently into their communities and affect access to employment [1]. These employment practices contributed to a generally transitory community of Latino workers in the Midwest through the turn of the twentieth century.

War in the 1910s saw a disruption of this pattern of temporary residence. Mexican immigration to the United States increased as individuals sought greater salaries, stability, and safety in the wake of the Mexican Revolution. Alongside this, World War I depressed European migration to the Midwest, creating an immense workforce void. Under pressure from the agricultural sector to

E. B. Olivera (✉)
College of Medicine - Rockford General Pediatrics, Advocate Children's Hospital, Advocate-Aurora Health, University of Illinois, Rockford, IL, USA
e-mail: eolive2@uic.edu

J. Girotti · M. Vela
Hispanic Center of Excellence, University of Illinois College of Medicine, Chicago, IL, USA

© The Author(s) 2024
J. P. Sánchez, D. Rodriguez (eds.), *Latino, Hispanic, or of Spanish Origin+ Identified Student Leaders in Medicine*, Sustainable Development Goals Series, https://doi.org/10.1007/978-3-031-35020-7_4

address labor shortages, the U.S. Congress implemented the Immigration Act of 1917, allowing Mexican immigrants to enter the United States under a temporary guest-worker contract program. Agricultural employers in the Midwest began to replace their European immigrant workers with ethnic Mexican laborers. This trend accelerated after quota laws in the 1920s reduced the number of legal immigrants allowed from Southern and Eastern Europe [1]. Employers thus started to entice married men with families and, for the first time, hire entire families. This strategy proved successful, and migrants established a more permanent presence in the region. While ninety percent of the Mexican-origin population during the 1930s in the United States resided in five southwestern states, 7% made their home in the Midwest [2]. As cities like Chicago, Detroit, and Minneapolis attracted migrants to the industrial industry, laborers moved from rural to urban areas during times when work slowed in the fields.

World War II created more opportunities for Latinos, as many Americans left to join the military. This led to further expansion of rural laborers into urban settings as they found higher-paying and more stable employment. The war also reduced European agricultural production, leading to an increased demand for U.S. harvests. To address this demand, the U.S. and Mexico established a formal guest-worker agreement, the Mexican Farm Labor Program (Bracero Program), that supplied contract male guest workers to fill the voids in the agriculture and railroad industries [3]. The economic success brought on by the Bracero Program led to a continued agreement even after the war. Another agreement was made with Mexico in 1951 to address labor shortages caused by the Korean War.

The evolving sociopolitical climate of the mid-twentieth century, coupled with corresponding changes in U.S. immigration policy, led to a diverse expansion of the Latino diaspora within the U.S. Midwest. As part of Operation Bootstrap (Manos a la Obra), Puerto Rican contract laborers joined Mexicans in the Midwest. To both control the island's "overpopulation" and facilitate Puerto Rico's industrialization, the Puerto Rican government sent male agricultural laborers and female domestic servants to the mainland United States [4]. Prior to the 1940s, mainland Puerto Rican communities were concentrated primarily in the U.S. Northeast region. Migration of Puerto Rican workers following World War II led many such individuals to establish themselves in various Midwestern cities, including Chicago, Illinois; Milwaukee, Wisconsin; and Gary, Indiana. Notably, Operation Bootstrap failed at increasing employment in Puerto Rico and ultimately led to more poverty on the island, displacement, and migration to the mainland United States [1]. Due to the Jones-Shafroth Act, which granted Puerto Ricans statutory U.S. citizenship in 1917, Puerto Rican laborers could not be deported once their work contracts expired, or even if they abandoned their contract before completion—unlike laborers recruited from Mexico [4]. This permanent status contributed to the establishment of stable Puerto Rican communities throughout the U.S. Midwest. Moreover, immigration laws implemented in the latter half of the twentieth century "significantly transformed the Latina/o population in the Midwest" by facilitating migration from several other Latin American countries. By the 1970s, half of all immigrants to the United States were from Latin America [1]. The number of political and economic refugees from Central and South America, as well as Cuba, the Dominican Republic, and other Caribbean nations, surged in the late 1960s through the 1980s.

The growth of this diverse Latino population considerably changed the demographics and culture of the U.S. Midwest. In 2003, data released by the U.S. Census Bureau showed Latinos had become the nation's largest racial or ethnic minority group [2]. 2021 Census data demonstrate that Hispanics/Latinos comprised 18.9% of the nation's population. and Illinois is ranked tenth among states with the highest proportion of Latinos [5].

Education of Latinos in the Midwest

As more Latinos began to call the Midwest home, their children entered the education system. As many immigrant parents did not speak proficient

English and the majority of teachers and administrators were not proficient in Spanish, immigrant parents were less able than their Anglo counterparts to advocate for their children. Ineffective communication between parents and teachers/administrators was one major factor limiting the number of students that experienced academic success [1, 6]. Parents who were monolingual Spanish were labeled as "uninterested" and "uncaring" because they were not as engaged with teachers in conferences or at extracurricular activities. However, Colvin and co-authors dispelled this idea and discovered that parents were frustrated with the typical communication models between parents and schools [1]. Adding to the challenges facing Latino families and their children's education, Spanish-speaking children were often separated from English-speaking peers and placed into mobiles outside of the main educational structure [7]. Districts engaging in this practice delivered disparate education to non-English speakers in comparison to English speakers. As educators have more recently identified the benefits of bilingual education on children's brain development, the physical division of the learning environment on the basis of language deprived all groups of children from potential educational and social benefits [8]. Moreover, such educational practices forced Latino children to forgo Spanish, learn English, and fall behind in their learning until mastery of the English language was attained.

Notably, while children across the Latino diaspora faced the challenges described above, individual subgroups encountered unique obstacles to their educational and social advancement. Unlike Mexican and Mexican American groups who were dispersed throughout the Chicagoland area, Puerto Ricans established themselves in distinct barrios (neighborhoods) in Chicago's Northwest side [4]. In the 1950s and 1960s, these barrios experienced a "lack of service workers who spoke Spanish and respected sociocultural differences; high infant mortality rates and incidence of preventable diseases; increasing unemployment due to industrial restructuring; police brutality; inadequate educational opportunities; and high incidence of fires induced by white

supremacists to drive residents in the area out of the area." [9]

In response to the verbal and physical abuse Puerto Ricans endured, several community organizations arose to promote and safeguard the education of Latino youth. Among these was the Young Lords Organization, which emerged in the Lincoln Park neighborhood of Chicago and expanded nationally through the late twentieth century [4, 10]. Initially labeled a street gang, the Young Lords became a youth organization: they helped denounce police brutality, advocate for living wages, and demand community control of institutions and land. They developed daycare programs, demanded low-cost housing, and challenged urban renewal efforts that displaced Puerto Ricans in efforts to gentrify the area. Continued unrest prompted the emergence of the ASPIRA Network in Chicago; first founded in New York, ASPIRA established a presence in Chicago in 1968 after the "Division Street Riots" catalyzed efforts to address the growing social and educational needs of youth in the city's Puerto Rican community [11]. ASPIRA's mission was to promote the self-determination of Latinos and other underserved youth, through education, leadership development, and cultural awareness. To accomplish this, ASPIRA began operating student clubs and a youth development center geared at providing academic enrichment and career counseling for Latino students. These and other initiatives of the post-Civil Rights era reduced high school dropout rates and promoted the retention of Latino students throughout the U.S. Midwest. In 2020, Latino children—99% of whom are US-born or naturalized citizens—represented nearly one in four public school students in Illinois. While many of the issues fought by the Young Lords, ASPIRA, and others persisted through the turn of the twenty-first century, Latinos have gone on to comprise the largest proportion (46%) of students in Chicago Public Schools as of this chapter's writing [12].

As the share of Latino students in primary and secondary education grew, a concomitant increase in the number of Midwestern Latino college students followed. For example, the number of Latino students between the ages of eighteen to twenty-four attending college in Illinois increased to over 2.1 million students in 2011 [13]. At the time of writing, Latinos represent the largest non-white racial or ethnic group enrolled at U.S. college campuses [14]. As such, university administrators have a unique opportunity to add curricular elements reflective of their students' ethnic backgrounds and to create programs geared at improving graduation rates for all students [1]. The Illinois State Legislature established a blueprint for such a program upon creating the Urban Health Program at the University of Illinois in 1978 [15]. Introduced in response to health inequities disproportionately affecting African-American, Native American, and Latino communities in Illinois, this program began to assist not only in the acceptance and retention of Latino students in the University of Illinois College of Medicine (UICOM), but also in the creation of a space in which students could support and mentor each other. The establishment of the Hispanic Center of Excellence at the University of Illinois Chicago (UIC HCOE) built upon the successes of the Urban Health Program. To address the severe shortage of Latinos in medicine, UIC HCOE developed an educational pipeline program to support students as they progress from high school to the level of medical school faculty. In the period from 1991 to 2006, UIC HCOE and its counterparts across the U.S. received federal funding to support their shared mission. When federal financial support for all COEs was cut in 2006, UIC maintained its commitment to its HCOE, allowing the latter to continue combating the underrepresentation of Latinos in the medical profession.

Origin of the Latino Midwest Medical Student Association (LMMSA)

The point is not to pay back kindness but to pass it on.
—Julia Alvarez, Dominican American author and poet

The support provided by UIC HCOE and similar programs proved critical for Latino students to not only enter medical school, but also to network with their counterparts throughout Chicagoland and beyond. In the early 1980s, a small number of universities in the U.S. Midwest began to focus on supporting the development and/or enhancement of student organizations that brought together Latinos/as interested in medicine and other health professions. From such efforts, two organizations in Chicago emerged and became very important for the aspirations of Latino premedical students: the Latin American Student Association – Pre-Health Committee at Loyola University; and the Health-Oriented Latino Association (HOLA) at UIC. Some of the students that entered the UIC College of Medicine in the fall of 1982 had been involved in these premedical organizations. Jorge Girotti, PhD, former Director of the UIC HCOE, reflects that the students "felt that Latinos in medicine did not have a voice that addressed the issues of Latino communities. They looked at other areas of the country to see if any organizations were already doing that work, and found them on the East and West Coasts."

These ambitious students established La Raza Medical Student Association at UIC in 1983. Often referred to as "La RaMA," the UIC chapter chose this name based on a medical student organization in California, which had a mission that spoke most directly to their interests. The Spanish phrase "la raza" was thought to "instill a sense of ethnic and cultural pride extending to all Latin American people." [11] In the late 1980s, the UIC La RaMA students met with their counterparts at other schools in Chicago and surrounding Midwestern states. This included students from the University of Michigan, who had founded their institution's Latin American & Native American Medical Association in 1985. Students during this time period met during medical conferences and remained in contact through telephone meetings. They would share with one another what meetings they were likely to attend and seek funding from their institutions for travel costs. Over time, these in-person and virtual encounters fomented a desire to connect disparate institution-based medical student groups together under a larger regional umbrella.

This Midwest regional organization came to fruition with the formal establishment of the Latino Midwest Medical Student Association (LMMSA) in Chicago in 1990. That same year, LMMSA held its first regional conference, uniting approximately twenty students primarily from UIC College of Medicine and the University of Michigan Medical School (Table 4.1). Juan J. Guerra, MD, who attended the UIC College of Medicine in 1990, reflects that the "individuals he trusted the most were the medical students in the Midwest that were like" him. "This trust," Dr. Guerra recounts, "was critical in helping me get through the challenging times of exams and the stress that comes with graduate school." He recalls the time when an administrator at the College of Medicine addressed his class and stated that a large number of the class would fail their medical exams. Discussions like these were a driving force to rely on peers for support rather than faculty members. Many medical students had similar stories from their institutions and

Table 4.1 List of States and School Chapters (stand alone or connected) in the LMSA Midwest Region (as of December 2022)

Illinois: Midwestern University Chicago College of Osteopathic Medicine, University of Illinois at Urbana-Champaign Carle Illinois College of Medicine, Windsor University School of Medicine, Chicago Medical School of Rosalind Franklin University of Medicine and Science, Loyola University Chicago Stritch School of Medicine, Rush Medical College, Southern Illinois University School of Medicine, University of Illinois College of Medicine - Chicago, University of Illinois College of Medicine - Peoria, University of Illinois College of Medicine - Rockford, Northwestern University Feinberg School of Medicine, University of Chicago Pritzker School of Medicine

Indiana: Indiana University School of Medicine - Fort Wayne, Indiana University School of Medicine - Gary, Indiana University School of Medicine - Lafayette, Indiana University School of Medicine - Muncie, Indiana University School of Medicine - South Bend, Indiana University School of Medicine - Terre Haute, Marian University College of Osteopathic Medicine, Indiana University School of Medicine - Evansville, Indiana University School of Medicine - Indianapolis

Iowa: Des Moines University College of Osteopathic Medicine, University of Iowa Roy J. and Lucille A. Carver College of Medicine

Kansas: University of Kansas School of Medicine - Salina, University of Kansas School of Medicine - Wichita, University of Kansas School of Medicine - Kansas City

Michigan: Michigan State University College of Osteopathic Medicine - Clinton Township, Michigan State University College of Osteopathic Medicine - Detroit, Michigan State University College of Osteopathic Medicine - East Lansing, Western Michigan University Homer Stryker M.D. School of Medicine, Central Michigan University College of Medicine, Michigan State University College of Human Medicine - East Lansing, Michigan State University College of Human Medicine - Grand Rapids, Oakland University William Beaumont School of Medicine, University of Michigan Medical School, Wayne State University School of Medicine

Minnesota: Mayo Clinic College of Medicine, University of Minnesota Medical School - Duluth, University of Minnesota Medical School - Twin Cities

Missouri: A. T. Still University Kirksville College of Osteopathic Medicine, Kansas City University of Medicine and Biosciences College of Osteopathic Medicine - Joplin, Kansas City University of Medicine and Biosciences College of Osteopathic Medicine - Kansas City, University of Missouri - Columbia School of Medicine, Saint Louis University School of Medicine, Washington University School of Medicine, University of Missouri – Kansas City School of Medicine

Nebraska: Creighton University School of Medicine, University of Nebraska College of Medicine

North Dakota: University of North Dakota School of Medicine and Health Sciences

Ohio: Cleveland Clinic Lerner College of Medicine, Ohio University Heritage College of Osteopathic Medicine - Athens, Ohio University Heritage College of Osteopathic Medicine - Cleveland, Ohio University Heritage College of Osteopathic Medicine - Dublin, Northeast Ohio Medical University College of Medicine (NEOMED), Boonshoft School of Medicine at Wright State University, Case Western Reserve University School of Medicine, The Ohio State University College of Medicine, University of Cincinnati College of Medicine, University of Toledo College of Medicine

Oklahoma: Oklahoma State University Center for Health Sciences College of Osteopathic Medicine, University of Oklahoma College of Medicine, University of Oklahoma School of Community Medicine

South Dakota: Sanford School of Medicine of the University of South Dakota

Wisconsin: Medical College of Wisconsin - Green Bay, Medical College of Wisconsin - Wausau, Medical College of Wisconsin - Milwaukee, University of Wisconsin School of Medicine and Public Health - Madison could relate to one another. The shared experiences of Latino medical trainees fostered a growing sense of interconnectedness across universities in the U.S. Midwest and, eventually, across the nation.

Transition to NNLAMS Midwest

In 1999, at its tenth regional conference, LMMSA members and leaders (Table 4.2) welcomed medical student representatives from the National Boricua Latino Health Organization (NBLHO), LMMSA's counterpart in the U.S. Northeast. Founded as the Boricua Health Organization (BHO) in 1972, NBLHO had established numerous chapters of Latino medical students at Northeastern medical schools. In traveling to the Medical College of Wisconsin in Milwaukee, NBLHO leaders Philip DeChavez, MD, MPH; Edgar Figueroa, MD; and others sought to persuade LMMSA members to join a burgeoning national consortium called the National Network of Latin American Medical Students (NNLAMS). As a medical student at the University of Pennsylvania, Dr. DeChavez served as NBLHO President and strongly advocated for the unification of Latino medical students into one national organization. LMMSA co-presidents Marcelo Venegas, MD, from UIC, and Sandra Torrente, MD, from the University of Missouri-Kansas City, appeared open to the idea of joining NNLAMS and agreed to discuss the prospect further. Dr. Figueroa recalls the Midwest and Northeast groups celebrated this moment of progress by going salsa dancing shortly after the conference ended. The two groups bonded and kept in touch until attending the 2000 National Conference of the recently established National Hispanic Medical Association (NHMA). There, LMMSA formalized an agreement to join the nascent NNLAMS consortium later that year.

As LMMSA developed national connections, its regional identity, infrastructure, and programming continued to expand. Midwest leaders developed a logo showcasing the caduceus staff in front of a globe highlighting the map of North and South America, with flames from the sun in the background. The organization formally assumed the name NNLAMS Midwest, as the national consortium obtained federal recognition as an established non-profit organization under Internal Revenue Code Section 501(c)(3). NNLAMS Midwest established two annual meetings for the academic year: the House of Delegates meeting and the Annual Regional Conference. The House of Delegates meeting allowed for the regional board to have direct contact with chapter leaders and review strategies for regional development. The Annual Regional Conference (Table 4.3) continued to facilitate networking between medical students across the U.S. Midwest, while providing career development opportunities and education on health disparities facing Midwestern Latino communities. Moreover, regional conference workshops included panels of physician leaders and medical admissions faculty providing advice on building a successful path into medicine. By connecting medical students to faculty and professionals committed to supporting the next generation of Latino physicians, NNLAMS Midwest began to address the gap identified earlier by Dr. Guerra and others. This provision of potential mentors, advisors, and role models represented a core element of NNLAMS programming, both regionally and nationally, and remains apparent in modern-day efforts of NNLAMS's successor, the Latino Medical Student Association (LMSA).

At the local level, NNLAMS Midwest supported its institutional chapters as the latter focused on hosting health fairs, volunteering at various medical centers, and providing mentorship to undergraduate students. Trina Helderman, MD, was a medical student at Indiana University (IU) School of Medicine and NNLAMS Midwest regional president from 2003 to 2004. She founded a chapter at her institution known as the Society of Latinos (SOL) in response to the large Spanish-speaking community they served. Locally, students advocated for these patients and provided Medical Spanish courses for classmates. She remembers, "At the time, there were a lot of Spanish-speaking patients and very insufficient interpreters or bilingual providers and a lack of translated materials." The SOL Chapter hosted

Table 4.2 Previous LMMSA, NNLAMS Midwest, and LMSA Midwest Co-Presidents and Co-Directors

Year	Midwest president	Chapter
1999–2000	Marcelo Venegas Sandra Torrente	University of Illinois COM at Chicago University of Missouri-Kansas City SOM
2002–2003	Esmeralda Llanas	Rush Medical College at Rush University
2003–2004	Trina Helderman	Indiana University SOM
2004–2005	Rebeca Sandoval Lourdes (Luly) Gomez	University of Illinois COM at Chicago Loyola University Stritch SOM
2005–2006	Rebeca Sandoval Lourdes (Luly) Gomez	University of Illinois COM at Chicago Loyola University Stritch SOM
2006–2007	Emiliano Sol Higuera Mayra Mendoza	University of Wisconsin SOM University of Illinois COM at Chicago
2007–2008	Jared Terronez Gina Waight	University of Illinois COM at Chicago University of Michigan Medical School
2008–2009	Daisy Cortes Matthew Carazo	University of Illinois COM at Chicago University of Illinois COM at Chicago
2009–2010	Elizabeth Homan Sandoval Raymond Morales	University of Illinois COM at Chicago University of Illinois COM at Urbana
2010–2011	Mayra Cruz-Ithier Anthony Acosta	University of Illinois COM at Chicago University of Illinois COM at Chicago
2011–2012	Emma B. Olivera Stacey Pereira	University of Illinois COM at Rockford Rush University Medical College
2012–2013	Stacey Pereira Luis Rivera	Rush Medical College at Rush University University of Illinois COM at Chicago
2013–2014	Thalia Torres Alex Cortez	University of Illinois COM at Chicago University of Cincinnati COM
2014–2015	Alex Cortez Ana Mauro	University of Cincinnati COM University of Illinois COM at Chicago
2015–2016	Ana Mauro Valeria Valbuena	University of Illinois COM at Chicago University of Illinois COM at Chicago
2016–2017	Valeria Valbuena Grace Keeney-Bonthrone	University of Illinois COM at Chicago University of Michigan Medical School
2017–2018	Jose Grajales-Reyes Alexandra Alejos	Washington University of St. Louis University of Michigan Medical School
2018–2019	Jose Grajales-Reyes Donald Rodriguez	Washington University of St. Louis University of Chicago Pritzker SOM
2019–2020	Donald Rodriguez Gracia Vargas	University of Chicago Pritzker SOM University of Michigan Medical School
2020–2021	Gracia Vargas Christian Hernandez	University of Michigan Medical School Medical College of Wisconsin
2021–2022	Jesús Acevedo Cintrón Jennifer Chinchilla Perez	Washington University of St. Louis Michigan State University College of Human Medicine (MSU COM)
2022–2023	Larissa de Souza Kimberly Flores	Case Western Reserve University SOM MSU COM

lunch talks on topics specific to Latino health and formed a peer support group much like that offered by the regional conferences. Many SOL members participated in various outreach clinics and helped develop the IU Student Outreach Clinic which functions to this day.

The spring of 2006 was also a historical time for medical student activism in the Midwest and the nation. In cities both large and small, hundreds to thousands of people took to the streets to protest H.R.4437, a congressional bill that would have classified undocumented immigrants as fel-

Table 4.3 Regional Conference History

2003 (13): Medicina: Hoy y Mañana – Prevenir – Educar – Curar
•Advocate Illinois Masonic Medical Center
2005 (15): Liderazgo y Tradición: Preparing for the Changing Face of Medicine
•Loyola University Stritch SOM
2006 (16): Derribando Fronteras: Beyond the Boundaries of Traditional Medical Practice
•Advocate Illinois Masonic Medical Center
2007 (17): Salud sin Barerras: Healthcare for All
•University of Michigan Medical School
2008 (18): Devuelve: Honoring our Communities Through Service and Advocacy
•Northwestern University Feinberg SOM
2009 (19): The New Faces of Medicine
•Medical College of Wisconsin
2010 (20): Breaking Barriers: Rompiendo las Barreras
•University of Chicago Pritzker SOM
First Independent LMSA National Conference: A United Voice[a]
•University of Illinois at Chicago
2011 (21): Adelante con Salud
•Rush University Medical College
2012 (22): Academic Medicine: Educating Tomorrow's Doctors
•Instituto Health Sciences Career Academy
2013 (23): The 23rd Annual Latino Medical Student Association Midwest Regional Conference
•Loyola University Stritch SOM
2014 (24): Advancing the Front Line: Latino Physicians Across All Specialties
•Northwestern University Feinberg SOM
2015 (25): Llegamos, Seguimos: Celebrating a Decade of Progress[a]
•Case Western Reserve University SOM
•Cleveland Clinic Lerner COM
2016 (26): Quienes Somos? Creating Your Identity as Future Health Leaders
•University of Cincinnati COM
2017 (27): Creating Comunidad Through Mentorship and Research
•University of Michigan Medical School
2018 (28): El Querer es Poder: Empowering Latinx Physicians in Uncertain Times
•Loyola University Stritch SOM
2019 (29): Unicos, Unidos, y Orgullosos: Celebrating Diversity in Medicine
•University of Chicago Pritzker SOM
2020 (30): Unidos por Medicina y Más: A Multidisciplinary Approach to Latinx Health[a]
•Washington University in St. Louis SOM
2021 (31): Unity in Community / Unidad en Comunidad
•Virtual
2022 (32): Health Leaders of Tomorrow: Continuando la Lucha por la Equidad
•Northwestern University Feinberg SOM
2023 (33): Sin Fronteras: Celebrating Latinx Excellence & Pioneering Tomorrow's Leaders in Medicine
•College of Human Medicine, Michigan State University

[a]Denotes: National Conference in conjunction with Regional Conference

ons. Across the nation, these mega-marches drew an estimated total of 3.5 to 5 million participants [16]. The March 10th demonstrations in Chicago saw more than 100,000 people march for immigrant rights. On May 1, over 400,000 Chicagoans marched from Union Park to Grant Park, the largest such demonstration in the city's history. Among these participants were Latino medical students from LaRaMA and surrounding chapters in Chicago, including former NNLAMS Midwest regional president, Jared Terronez, MD. Dr. Terronez shared that the students in attendance "all felt the calling to bring some form of awareness for immigrant rights at that time.

We wanted it made clear that we, as Latino/a medical students, were the future of medicine and that we were going to advocate for our underserved patient population. Our white coats [worn at the event] were a visual representation of our place in society that could not be ignored, both metaphorically and visually."

The heightened socio-political awareness of immigrant communities and their struggles drove Latino student leaders to propose a "national day of action." This effort was championed by Daniel Turner-Lloveras, MD, then a medical student at the University of Chicago with roots in California. He nostalgically recollects learning from his father about César Estrada Chavez, the prominent Latino American civil rights activist, and traveling seven hours as a young boy to attend Chavez' funeral procession. Dr. Turner-Lloveras still remembers waking up with 50,000 people camped out across the fields around him. "I will never forget that. It made a great impression on me. A year later, I entered an essay competition in Sacramento, California, and tried to continue to spread the word about [Mr. Chavez] in college and medical school." Dr. Turner-Lloveras attended Chicago's May 2006 rally, where then-UIC medical student Christina Chavez-Johnson, MD, delivered a powerful speech in support of immigrant rights. Coincidentally, the two had met many years prior to medical school at the funeral of Mr. Chavez, Dr. Chavez-Johsnon's tio (uncle). Shortly after the march, Dr. Turner-Lloveras approached Dr. Chavez-Johnson to pitch and flesh out the day of service idea. Dr. Chavez-Johnson recollects she was excited about the idea, and both leaders presented the proposal together to the NNLAMS national executive board with "a PowerPoint and a smile." In March 2007, NNLAMS passed a resolution to establish the "National Latino Healthcare Day" and became a part of "honoring and supporting Chavez' legacy to educate, inspire, and empower the community." The Friday closest to Mr. Chavez's birthday, March 31, was designated as the day on which all NNLAMS chapters nationally would act in solidarity by performing a community service activity, thereby honoring the legacy of Cesar Chavez. The Midwest region chose to honor this day of action with a service event following each regional conference thereafter.

Rebranding as LMSA Midwest

As regional and national programming expanded and became more intertwined, a growing push for unification led to the adoption of a new organizational name in 2010: the Latino Medical Student Association (LMSA). As national leaders discussed changing the organization's name from NNLAMS to LMSA (the name used by the NNLAMS region representing the West), the Midwest favored this change as it reflected the latter's previous regional title and allowed for easy branding of one unified, national student body. As the new LMSA Midwest, the region temporarily shared the LMSA West logo until artwork for the entire organization was finalized. Moreover, at the UIC Forum in 2010, LMSA Midwest co-hosted the national organization's first standalone national conference, independent from external organizations. The event also marked the adoption of the name LMSA National, bringing the community together to celebrate a shared title and identity. Notably, this milestone was commemorated through an event separate from the LMSA Midwest regional conference held only weeks prior at the University of Chicago Pritzker School of Medicine. Elizabeth Homan Sandoval, MD, MPH, LMSA Midwest co-president at the time, recalls how exciting it was to host two conferences in the Midwest: one for the region and another for the national organization. "However, the workload for two conferences was intense. Ever since then, the National Conference has been held in conjunction with the regional conference instead of separate [events]." This practice has only recently ended, with LMSA National slated to host a separate National Conference in the fall of 2023. Dr. Homan Sandoval recollects how well attended the conference was and how profusely advisors and alumni expressed their admiration. With signature events, such as a welcome reception at the renowned National Museum of Mexican Art,

LMSA "set the bar high that year for all future national conferences."

Between 2010 and 2020, LMSA Midwest began to increasingly stress Latino physician involvement in academia. Through mentorship and fellowship, students worked together on research publications. Starting in 2011, Midwest regional conferences incorporated Research Poster Presentations. Students from across the region traveled to present their scholarly work and a panel of Latino academic physicians assisted in judging. This allowed for alumni to strengthen their commitment to the regional organization and its student body.

As part of this growing emphasis on Latino scholarship, in early 2011, LMSA Midwest leaders raised the issue of the importance of language concordant care to the quality of health care being delivered to Spanish-speaking populations. Students were quick to point out that a dearth of Spanish-speaking physicians may be contributing to health and health care disparities among Latino/a patient populations. As LMSA Midwest co-president and a medical student at UICOM – Urbana, Raymond Morales, MD, PhD, MS, suggested that LMSA conduct a regional survey of medical Spanish components within medical school curricula. This project was pursued with the goal of establishing a call to action and an LMSA policy statement regarding this issue. "Our study was part of a movement to improve the care of Spanish-speaking populations starting with provider representation and linguistic and cultural competency in medical school," states Lauren Rodriguez, MD. "This study occurred at a time of significant student advocacy at my institution [University of Michigan] for the first longitudinal, institutionalized medical Spanish curricula, which was advanced in tandem with a new Global Health & Inequities Path of Excellence. By leveraging our administration's interest in global health and inequities, we were able to gain participation in the study and support for our goal of a more sustainable medical Spanish program." Monica Vela, MD, faculty mentor for the Midwest region, urged the leadership to consider a national survey and pursue a publication that would allow educators to raise

the level of urgency regarding the issue of medical Spanish. LMSA convened a committee to study the issue of medical Spanish curricula and over the next month conducted a series of focus groups among medical students to better inform the survey development. The committee found few studies on medical Spanish courses in the extant literature. LMSA leaders from the Midwest, including Dr. Morales, Dr. Rodriguez, and Lydia Mendoza, MD, published the "National Survey of Medical Spanish Curriculum in U.S. Medical Schools" under the mentorship of Dr. Vela. The article was initially rejected due to a poor response rate on the survey—less than 45 percent of schools completed the survey. To address this, Dr. Vela used her contacts in the AAMC's Group on Diversity and Inclusion, and LMSA leadership encouraged each of their chapters to contact their school leadership to complete the study. Marshaling the social capital of LMSA furthered the survey completion rate. The study was ultimately published in the Journal of Internal Medicine in 2015 with a national survey completion rate of over 80%. This was the first study to describe the expanding state of medical Spanish curricula in schools of medicine across the U.S. and the need for standardized testing to ensure the cultural and language proficiency of students and faculty working with non-English language preference patients. This article is repeatedly cited as the landmark article regarding medical Spanish curricula and has served as an impetus for more scholarship in this area [17]. Dr. Vela believes "the process demonstrated the importance of alumni commitment to LMSA, the sociopolitical power of the LMSA student leadership, and the importance of representation of minority-led scholarship regarding Latino/a issues."

These goals of mentoring and developing future physician faculty members permeated the 22nd Midwest Regional Conference, titled "Academic Medicine: Educating Tomorrow's Doctors" and held in 2012 at the Instituto Health Sciences Career Academy (IHSCA), a public charter high school in Chicago. IHSCA provides an education focused on "preparing urban youth to succeed in competitive colleges and universities, obtain job-readiness certification for entry-level positions with higher wages in health care, and gain new awareness of and seek out a healthier lifestyle [18]. Then co-presidents Emma B. Olivera, MD, and Stacey Pereira, MD, sought to strengthen pipeline efforts with high school students. "It was important for us to show these young minority students that the possibilities were endless and, more importantly, they were attainable," remarks Dr. Olivera. During this conference, high school students attended workshops geared specifically towards them, including overviews of anatomy/physiology, career development sessions, and even an exercise and fitness workshop. The high school students also acted as volunteers in organizing the day's events. While the 2012 event represents the only instance in which a regional conference was held at a high school institution, LMSA Midwest has included programming for local high school and undergraduate premedical students at each major event since then.

Also in 2012, LMSA Midwest mentorship efforts more greatly intersected with policy and advocacy in the wake of inaction by the U.S. Congress regarding immigration reform. President Barack Obama spoke on the failure of Congress to pass the "DREAM Act," which would have provided a path to citizenship for certain immigrants brought to the country undocumented as children. President Obama stated that, in the absence of congressional action, the Department of Homeland Security would institute a temporary program to defer deportation for "eligible individuals who do not present a risk to national security or public safety." [19] Referred to as the Deferred Action for Childhood Arrivals program (DACA), this program allowed eligible individuals to obtain work authorization and attend school. In the spring of 2012, Loyola Stritch School of Medicine became the first medical school in the nation to amend its admissions policy to welcome applications from "DREAMers" who had DACA status. Mark G. Kuczewski, PhD, HEC-C, Director of the Neiswanger Institute of Bioethics & Health Policy at Loyola University, had attended LMSA Midwest Conferences since the early 2000s. He

recalled receiving an email from a colleague in California regarding a student who was labeled as "the best student his colleague ever had," but also happened to be undocumented. This propelled him on a journey to research the possibility of accepting such a student. When DACA was announced, Dr. Kuczewski "knew exactly what this meant." It meant that these students had the possibility to attend Loyola Stritch. The medical school, encouraged by the Dean, used social media and networking to get the word out. Alongside LMSA, another organization called Pre-Health Dreamers served as a primary channel for Loyola to use to inform undergraduate students that it was now possible to enter medical school. Dr. Kuczewski claims the DACA students at the School of Medicine "changed the face of the medical school." He believes the increased diversity of the student body drove students to learn about and become more involved in social justice causes, such as those surrounding immigration. They accepted their first DACA student in the Fall of 2013 and, as of 2020, nearly half of all undocumented U.S. medical students were enrolled at Stritch School of Medicine.

Among these students was former LMSA Midwest leader Ivonne Beltran Lara, MD. Her path to medicine was not easy, but was one of dedication and perseverance. Born in Colombia, Dr. Beltran Lara immigrated to New York at the age of six with her family, and later settled in Georgia. She "always wanted to be a doctor" since she was a young girl. Her grandmother was a nurse and instilled a love for medicine in her at an early age. Dr. Beltran Lara signed up for college as a pre-medical student; however, she could not attend for very long as the costs of tuition were too great a burden for her and her family. When the DACA program was announced, she was given the opportunity to resume her studies, all the while working full time. While she was not accepted her first time applying to medical school, this led her to seek out organizations like Pre-Health Dreamers and LMSA for guidance and mentorship. With the aid of organizations like this, she found "the light at the end of a dark tunnel" and successfully entered medical school the following year. This experience led her to realize the important role mentorship plays in one's successful path in medicine. She has taken this lesson into both her past role as chapter president, forming a mentorship program at her school with a grant offered by LMSA Midwest, and her role as 2020–2021 LMSA Midwest Mentorship Chair, working to promote the advancement of her peers across the region.

As LMSA students continued to support each other through growing initiatives, national and regional infrastructure evolved to match. In 2012, the LMSA Midwest regional organization obtained recognition as a 501(c)(3) non-profit. Thalia Torres, MD, was the Regional Treasurer at the time and worked diligently with a non-profit organization called Odysseus to complete the task. The executive board at this time also established a chapter development grant where monies would be given to a chapter with a project consistent with the organization's core principles and would be sustainable beyond the funding period. The intent was to allow smaller chapters to thrive and develop community or institutional projects they might not have accomplished without financial support. In 2014, the LMSA National Board of Directors reviewed the positions within the regional and national organizations. The following year the following changes were formalized. At that time it was decided that the Regional Co-Presidents would now be identified as Regional Co-Directors. The Regional Co-Directors form part of the voting body and Board of Directors within the national organization. Within the regional organization, the board members were also re-named. The regional organization restructured the following elected positions: Chief Financial Officer, Chief Development Officer, Chief Information Officer, Public Relations Chair, Policy and Academic Affairs Chair, Mentorship Chair, Community Affairs Chair, Regional Conference Chair, and Webmaster. To this day, LMSA Midwest officers holding these positions collaborate closely with their LMSA National counterparts via the latter's Internal and External Affairs Committees (recently renamed to Operations, Programming, and Communications branches of LMSA National).

Community service, advocacy, research, and mentorship have been the longstanding principal threads that have propelled the Midwest region forward in helping end disparities in medicine. At least through 2020, the Midwest Region has continued to provide funding at various levels for students in the Midwest medical schools. These include funding for leaders of several chapters to attend regional and national meetings, academic scholarships for premedical and medical students, and seed grants to support community-engaged projects. Beyond financial contributions, the regional organization connects with medical societies, such as the National Hispanic Medical Association (NHMA) and the Medical Organization for Leadership Advancement (MOLA) to gain access to mentors, research support, and collaboration in policy forums. Christian Hernandez, MD, alumnus of the Medical College of Wisconsin and past LMSA Midwest co-president stated, "2020 posed unique challenges for various medical societies, including the LMSA Midwest region amid the COVID-19 pandemic. The region explored strategies to host regional meetings remotely." Moreover, the leadership believed that the need to connect virtually due to COVID-19 could be optimized strategically to increase overall engagement with LMSA chapters across the Midwest without having distance or travel costs serve as barriers to participating in regional gatherings.

Conclusion

Since its inception as LMMSA, and through its transitions to NNLAMS Midwest and now LMSA Midwest, the region has continued to promote its core values of unity, service, and advocacy on behalf of its students and its communities. Whether through in-person or remote programs, LMSA Midwest has rallied its chapters across twelve states to continue pushing for the eradication of health disparities and the establishment of a diverse, equitable, and inclusive field of medicine. Like the rays of the sun represented in its first logo design (Table 4.4), the future is bright

Table 4.4   Conference Program Artwork (All artwork property of LMSA) (©LMSA)

2005	2006	2009
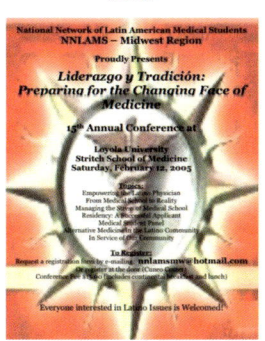	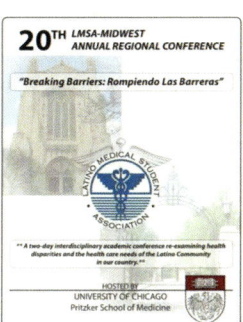	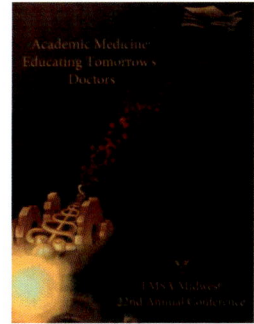

2010	2011	2012
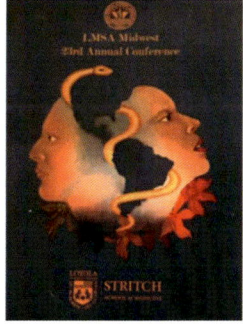	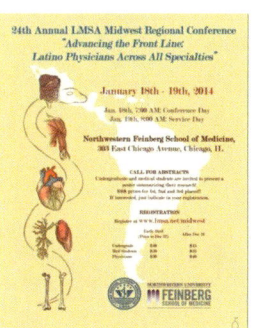	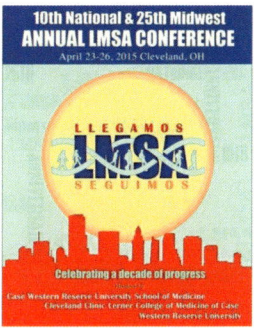

2013	2014	2015

2016	2017	2018

Table 4.4 (continued)

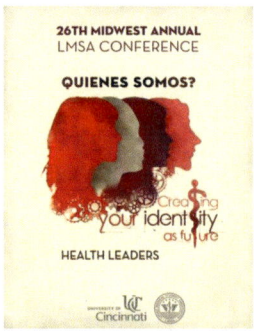

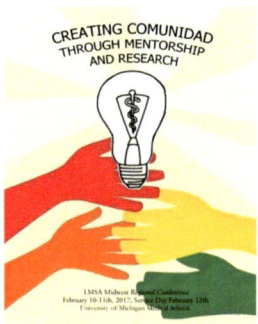

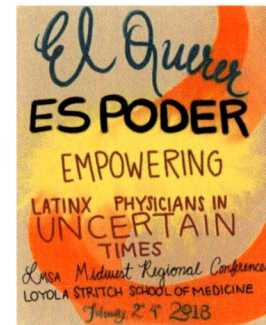

2019   2020   2021

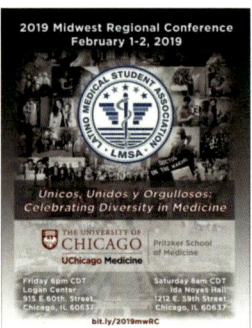

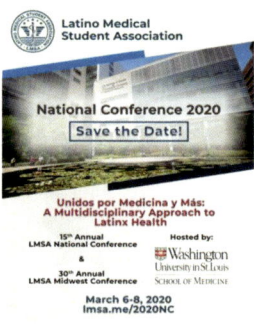

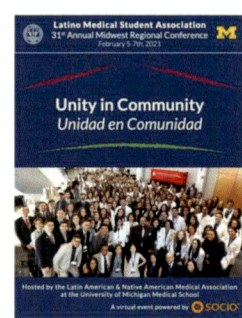

2022

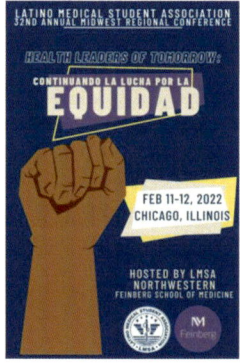

for LMSA Midwest, with more organizational support, growth, and unity ahead.

Personal Narratives:

Evelyn Figueroa, MD

University of Illinois at Chicago (UIC) LaRAMA President (1996–1997)

I am from the north side of Chicago, born to parents born in Puerto Rico (PR). Presently, my father is retired and lives with my stepmother, Mary, in Vega Alta, PR. My mother Lucille and her domestic partner Ray (together x 3.5 decades) live near where I live in Logan Square.

I have always loved science and human interaction. As a child, I verbalized interest in all sorts of scientific careers. Throughout high school, I was active in the Chicago Public Schools science fair and acquired an amazing science fair sponsor, Mr. Rosenbaum, a biology teacher. Mr. Rosenbaum and other teachers really encouraged me; they advised me to apply to medical school.

I never knew a doctor growing up (we only went for fee-for-service urgent issues or physicals). Their support affected me and helped me think of a career completely outside of my world. Because of my science teachers, I focused on medicine and never looked back.

UIC College of Medicine and its structure offered many more opportunities than my undergraduate institution, Northeastern Illinois University (NEIU). At NEIU, I focused on work, volunteering, and studying; I don't recall hearing about leadership opportunities. Through student-centered organizations like LaRaMA and Chicago Medical Student Council, I was able to develop as a leader. I served in three positions for LaRaMA: treasurer ('95–'96), president ('96–'97), and M4 representative ('98–'99). LaRaMA, like LMSA, worked to connect with the greater UIC community and during my presidential year, I coordinated over 100 medical volunteers for Alivio Medical Center's Fiesta del Sol event. In addition, the UIC HCOE helped connect us to the regional and national networks of Latino students through NNLAMS and NHMA. The learning and networking at these larger events showed me Underrepresented Minorities (URM) in leadership positions, which was very important for my journey.

My biggest career goal was to be recognized as a leader, not as a Latinx leader. Since tokenism is a huge threat to any minority's success, I have also joined mainstream organizations in order to promote diversity and inclusion. At the UIC Department of Family Medicine, I feel that I reached that; I recall during my nine-year maternity director role realizing that I was being counted upon as a leader due to my knowledge, not due to my heritage. This addressed my internal imposter phenomenon and, perhaps, the implicit bias of others. My 10 years in residency administration gave me the power to recruit, hire, and support young minorities in Family Medicine. I have been active in the Society of Teachers in Family Medicine (STFM) since 2008. I chaired a collaborative for 3 years, was a co-primary investigator for a minority mentorship grant, served on the Board of Directors for 3 years, and now am on the Foundation's board. During this time, we

(respectfully) challenged the status quo of URM promotions at STFM and the leadership responded fully to our suggestions.

My community work dating back to LaRaMA is currently the focus of my career – I am now a community activist. Our family founded a non-profit, the Pilsen Social Health Initiative, and I direct the organization. I am able to incorporate my perspectives as a minority woman in medicine into the community work that I do. LaRaMA was the first organization that helped me realize my voice and gave me the structure to create impact. In August 2019, I reached the full professor rank – I am the first URM in the history of our department to achieve this milestone. My journey thus far has had many ups and downs, unexpected twists, and some heartache – but persistence, resilience, organization, and patience are common strategies I use to persevere. I feel really good about my contributions and the opportunities ahead.

Jimena Alvarez Soto, MD
LMSA National Secretary (2009–2010), LMSA National Scholarship Co-Chair (2010–2011)

My Latino buddies in M1 year of medical school talked about LMSA as "the" organization to join, and the encouragement coupled with unfamiliar and intimidating concepts like advocacy, representation, community, minority leadership. Even the thought of conferences, regional or national, proved to be foreign to me. Yet, my let's-go-for-it spirit made the short drive from Rockford, IL, to Milwaukee, WI, and brought me to my first live introduction to NNLAMS (now known as LMSA) at the 2008 Midwest Regional Conference. The auditorium was full of medical students from all medical school years within the region, along with faculty physicians, discussing topics like creating awareness, finding ways to make healthcare more available to the Latino community, and ways to facilitate the medical school experience for Latino medical students. Before the end of the meeting, I had "mind-scanned" my upbringing in Peru and some of my new life experiences in the U.S., and I had decided that LMSA was an organization I was meant to be part of.

I was born in Lima, Peru, to a pair of supportive parents who, among many lessons, instilled in me the values of service, humility, and dedication. They taught me que si se puede pensar en metas grandes y justas porque mis sueños son alcanzables si trabajo duro para lograrlos. I still wonder if they were the biggest influence in my life to pursue a medical career. What I do know is that ever since I can remember, I wanted to be a doctor and that everyone I knew growing up gave me nothing but encouragement towards this goal.

International college students have narrow chances of entering a U.S. medical school, and I had been warned about that. I moved to the U.S. at 16 years old after high school graduation, holding an F-1 student visa, but my family only continued giving their encouragement from across the continent. I found very similar support from my extended family and friends in the U.S once they learned about my goal. My pre-med counselor at Brigham Young University seemed intimidating to say the least when I first heard him speak. Plus, I was one of the very few Latino pre-med students sitting in the room. Regardless, after I met with the counselor, it turned out that he became one of my biggest advocates to make my way to medical school. Then came what I like to call a miracle: my long-awaited green card was issued a couple of months before the time I was due to apply to medical school. Life seemed good between the support and blessings I had received. Only once did I get negative feedback about my goal to attend medical school, but I listened, humbly gave thanks, and kept moving forward. Looking back, I am thankful for the polarizing feedback because it was that lack of support that would later make the value of LMSA become more evident to me.

The LMSA National Conference in 2009 was my next opportunity to engage. I served as the LMSA National Secretary, communicating with the national board and taking minutes during the board meeting teleconferences. A great way to serve and learn about the different components of the organization! One day, I thought to contribute by creating something that students could directly benefit from. The project took lots—and I mean lots—of hours of brainstorming, phone calls, sending emails, finding donors, and creating awareness, but ultimately, this is how the LMSA National Scholarship for U.S. Medical Students was created. It was directed to Latino medical students or medical students from any background who demonstrated interest in the Latino community. We raised funds for our first scholarship award, and although the amount was not comparable to the medical school tuition total, everything counts and it was a contribution that in the future could potentially grow and continue helping students—it still is.

LMSA influenced my personal life by creating a platform to meet peers who have become leaders in their medical communities and to make incredible and long-lasting friendships. Academically, LMSA provided opportunities to meet in person with a variety of OBGYN programs and their program representatives in the friendly setting of the LMSA conferences. Unlike today, when we have video posts on social media and webinars at our fingertips to learn about the residency application process, LMSA was making the effort to help orient its students in their path, but live! These live interactions with different residency program leaders increased my understanding and expectations of the residency application process and residency programs. Professionally, the networking opportunities were so vast within the organization and during conferences, that I have to admit, it helped me overcome any fears related to networking, which comes in handy in any profession. My experiences in LMSA also became a topic of conversation during residency interviews. In sum, the perfect boot camp!

Participating in LMSA took extracurricular time and commitment that I had to set aside from academic time, but with the logistical organization and support provided by the organization, it was very worth the experience. Not only did the LMSA Regional Conference break the ice between me and so many intimidating concepts I was meant to unavoidably face in the long run, but it also increased my awareness of disparities based on socioeconomic status and cultural background within the U.S. medical student community. This made me look back at my strong village of support but also the instances when I felt like a minority and unsupported by discouraging feedback. It became my goal to be a part of a boat that rowed toward creating opportunities and facilitating the path for minorities in medicine, and what a better way than working with an organization that was directly involved in this purpose y poder alentar a estudiantes y mostrar que al final, si se puede!

Emma B. Olivera, MD, Assistant Clinical Professor of Pediatrics

UICOM Rockford, LMSA Midwest Regional President (2011–2012), National Coordinator (2012–2013)

I was born in a Northwest neighborhood of Chicago, Illinois. My mother immigrated as a political refugee from Matanzas, Cuba, to Chicago, Illinois, at the age of eight. My father immigrated to Chicago from Tarija, Bolivia, during a time of political unrest in his homeland in his mid-twenties. I am a prime example of the Inter-Latinidad which permeates throughout the Chicagoland area. I identify myself as Latina, but foremost as an American-Bolivian-Cuban woman, as all these cultures form who I am today.

My pediatrician, Enrique Lujan, MD, was from Bolivia and became a strong role model in my formative years. Dr. Lujan would call me colega, or colleague, when I was only 4 years old. My family instilled a strong value of an education and the importance of learning both English and Spanish. As my interest in medicine grew, much of my high school and early college years were spent volunteering at a local medical center. I saw a great need for Spanish-speaking physicians right away and knew I could make a difference in the care of my community.

During my undergraduate education at the University of Illinois at Chicago (UIC), I found a flyer for the Health Oriented Latino Association (HOLA) and immediately knew that I had to join. HOLA provided me with the additional support of peers to reach my goals as a pre-medical student and introduced me to the Hispanic Center of Excellence. It is during this time period I learned of both the National Hispanic Medical Association (NHMA) and the National Network

of Latin American Medical Students (NNLAMS) and attended the first NNLAMS Midwest regional conference in 2005. I was offered a travel grant by NHMA in 2006 and coincidentally attended the first NNLAMS conference as an undergraduate student. As I did not have a family in the healthcare field, these organizations provided me with much-needed mentorship in achieving success in applying to medical school. The medical students at the time were very inviting and encouraged me to participate in regional and national activities. The individuals I met helped me stay laser-focused on my chosen path, as I had received advice from my undergraduate counselor against applying to medical school.

In 2008, Ruben Font, MD, offered me the role of Webmaster for the NNLAMS national organization. I had always been artistically inclined growing up and learned graphic and web design as a hobby during my early years in college. While working together, I remember he referred to me as "the chosen one." It is through his encouragement that I became Webmaster of the Midwest region shortly thereafter and helped organize conferences as a pre-med. During this time, I was also a part of the NNLAMS National "Name Change Committee," which worked to unify the organization under the name of the Latino Medical Student Association (LMSA). I graduated with a Bachelor's degree in Biological Sciences and Latin American and Latino Studies and I was accepted to the UIC College of Medicine - Rockford after completing a post-baccalaureate program with the UIC Urban Health Program. I attribute a large part of my confidence in applying to medical school to this much-needed mentorship and to the support of my family. In medical school, I held leadership positions at my local chapter, including LMSA chapter President for my first 2 years. I organized local educational events, and community service events, and established a mentorship pipeline program with pre-medical students. I continued to hold LMSA national and regional positions, including National and Midwest regional Webmaster and National Secretary, all the while helping with the organization of annual conferences. As I had worked on the unification process of LMSA, I was also a part of the organization's Branding Committee for the new logo design. I later was elected as the Midwest Regional Co-President in 2011, during which time I also was elected as National Coordinator-Elect. As a regional co-president, I was dedicated to increasing the strength of smaller chapters and fortifying a pipeline for high school students. Our leadership team was able to establish 501(c)(3) nonprofit status for the region, chapter development grants, and scholarships. In 2012, I had the honor of acting as National Coordinator, now known as the National President. My vision as National Coordinator was to create stronger partnerships with other health organizations, such as the NHMA, Student National Medical Association (SNMA), and National Association of Hispanic-Serving Health Professions Schools (HSHPS), and facilitate the growth of regional development. My participation in these projects afforded me the opportunity to network with medical and academic professionals around the nation, which was useful when applying to pediatric residency.

In residency at the Children's Hospital of Michigan (Detroit, Michigan) I continued to work closely with the underserved community. I was nominated as Class Representative and was also my class representative on the Liaison Committee for Graduate Medical Education (LCGME). My program director recommended me for the position of chapter representative to the American Academy of Pediatrics (AAP) Section on Medical Students, Residents, and Fellowship Trainees (SOMSRFT). It seemed natural when I attended the AAP National Conference and Exhibition I was elected AAP SOMSRFT Region V Communications Director. It also seemed inherent that I would translate my passion in medical school and LMSA to advocacy as a physician. Along with AAP membership, I met with congress members in Lansing, MI to discuss harmful laws affecting our youth with regard to e-cigarettes. I later gave a workshop on advocacy to premedical and medical students at the 2015 LMSA National Conference held in conjunction with LMSA Midwest.

LMSA has undeniably shaped who I am as a Latina physician. It has instilled in me a passion for service, advocacy, and mentorship. I use these lessons every day in my role as a board-certified pediatrician, all while continuing to serve the underserved community and provide mentorship through my participation with NHMA and local medical school programs.

References

1. Valerio-Jiménez O, Vaquera-Vásquez S, Fox C. The Latina/o Midwest Reader. Urbana, IL: University of Illinois Press; 2017.
2. Facts on Latinos of Mexican origin in the U.S. Pew Research Center's Hispanic Trends Project. https://www.pewresearch.org/hispanic/fact-sheet/u-s-hispanics-facts-on-mexican-origin-latinos/. Published 2020. Accessed 19 May 2020.
3. Mandeel EW. The Bracero Program 1942-1964. Am Int J Contemp Res. 2014;4(1):171–84.
4. Pérez G. The near northwest side story: Migration, displacement, and Puerto Rican families. Berkeley: Univ of California Press; 2004.
5. United States Census Bureau. https://www.census.gov/quickfacts/fact/table/US/PST045221 Quick Facts. United States. Accessed on 15 July 2022.
6. García J. Conóceme en Iowa, cited in Teresa A. García, "Mexican Room: Public Schooling and Children of Mexican Railroad Workers in Fort Madison, Iowa, 1923–1930" (Ph.D. diss., University of Iowa, 2008), 51.
7. Gonzalez GG. Chicano education in the era of segregation (No. 7). Austin: University of North Texas Press; 2013.
8. Baker C. Foundations of bilingual education and bilingualism. Bristol: Multilingual Matters; 2017.
9. Ramos-Zayas AY. National performances: the politics of class, race, and space in Puerto Rican Chicago. Berkeley: University of Chicago Press; 2003.
10. Jeffries J. From gang-bangers to urban revolutionaries: the Young Lords of Chicago. J Illinois State Hist Soc (1998-). 2003;96(3):288–304.
11. Rivera-Perez, Christian, "ASPIRA Inc. of Illinois: a tale of educational success?" (2007). Capstone Projects – Politics and Government 14.
12. Demographics. Chicago Public Schools. (n.d.). Retrieved January 30, 2023, from https://www.cps.edu/about/district-data/demographics/
13. III. Hispanic College Enrollments. Pew Research Center's Hispanic Trends Project. https://www.pewresearch.org/hispanic/2012/08/20/iii-hispanic-college-enrollments/. Published 2012.
14. Hanson M. College Enrollment & Student Demographic Statistics; 2022, July 26. EducationData.

org. Retrieved January 30, 2023, from https://educa-tiondata.org/college-enrollment-statistics

15. About | Urban Health Program | University of Illinois Chicago; n.d. Retrieved January 30, 2023, from https://uhp.uic.edu/about/.

16. Pallares A, Flores-González N. Imarcha! Latino Chicago and the immigrants rights movement. Urbana: University of Illinois Press; 2010.

17. Morales R, Rodriguez L, Singh A, Stratta E, Mendoza L, Valerio MA, Vela M. National survey of medical Spanish curriculum in U.S. medical schools. J Gen Intern Med. 2015;30(10):1434–9. https://doi.org/10.1007/s11606-015-3309-3.

18. Our Mission; n.d. ihsca.org. Retrieved January 30, 2023, from https://www.ihsca.org/apps/pages/index.jsp?uREC_ID=371586&type=d&pREC_ID=835555

19. Remarks by the President on Immigration. (2012, June 15). Whitehouse.gov; The White House. https://obamawhitehouse.archives.gov/the-press-office/2012/06/15/remarks-president-immigration

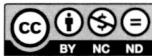

Victor H. Rodríguez, Valerie Romero-Leggott, and Eric Molina

Tiempo Pasado con Pena Recordado: Effects of Health Disparities in Latino Communities in the Southwest Region

In the famous words of Jorge Agustín Nicolás Ruiz de Santayana y Borrás, better known by his English name as George Santayana, "Those who cannot remember the past are condemned to repeat it." This statement continues to be true throughout the history of our country, seeing similar effects of health disparities in the Latino community as well as the sociopolitical climate that Latinos and Latino medical students face in the Southwest region. The LMSA Southwest region comprises Arkansas, Colorado, Louisiana, New Mexico, Oklahoma, and Texas. In interviewing Latino physicians for this chapter, we found many similarities in their sentiments about health disparities. Systems that perpetuate health

disparities have negatively impacted the health of our Latino communities; addressing these health disparities served as a driver for some Latinos to go into medicine. However, without support, we, as a community, are doomed to continue this cyclical effect of health disparities.

Since the annexation of the southwest regions' constitutive states in the late 1800s, disparities have been documented in the health of the then newest Americans. Initial public health surveys by Dr. John Hunter Pope noted that South Texas needed "drastic improvements in housing stock, basic primary care, and working conditions" to protect the Mexican people from future epidemics that could impact the rest of the country [1]. Unfortunately, despite the recommendations to improve the health of its new citizens, Latinos continued to face similar issues early in the twentieth century. John Mckiernan-González comments, "social class and political powerlessness limited [Mexicans'] access to clean water, decent housing, food, and sanitation services," and notes the impact these factors had on healthcare such as infant mortality rates that were, "three times higher for Latinos than for Anglos," during this time [1]. Due to the lack of support of its new government, the Latino community began to mobilize and help improve its health situation. Latinos began to pool their money together to create sociedades mutualistas to address deaths, injuries, and illnesses; with one of the largest

V. H. Rodríguez (✉)
Tulane University School of Medicine,
New Orleans, LA, USA
e-mail: vrodriguez@tulane.edu

V. Romero-Leggott
UNM SOM Combined BA/MD Program,
Albuquerque, NM, USA

E. Molina
Interventional Radiology Residency – Integrated,
Massachusetts General Hospital – Mass General
Brigham, Boston, MA, USA

© The Author(s) 2024
J. P. Sánchez, D. Rodriguez (eds.), *Latino, Hispanic, or of Spanish Origin+ Identified Student Leaders in Medicine*, Sustainable Development Goals Series, https://doi.org/10.1007/978-3-031-35020-7_5

being the Alianza Hispano Americana, co-founded by Dr. Mariano Samaniego, which spanned far north to Colorado and down to South Texas, to address deaths, injuries, and illnesses [1].

From the time of the Mexican Revolution to the Great Depression, infectious diseases began to considerably impact those in the border communities. Additionally, local community members added racist ideology to these diseases, demanding "the United States Public Health Service differentiate healthy Mexican border-crossers [from] anyone who looked like a 'dirty and lousy immigrant" instead of improving the local health system [1]. The El Paso community blamed working-class immigrants for being carriers of tuberculosis (TB), smallpox, and typhus. Immigrants were sent for "inspections, fumigation of their bodies and their property, and unwanted vaccinations," setting an unwelcoming tone for Latinos interacting with medicine in America [1].

The unwelcoming tone continued during the Great Depression, where the idea of citizenship and public charge played an important role. During this era, the government used public funds to "move approximately half a million ethnic Mexicans to Mexico, regardless of citizenship." Moreover, those that had "received public assistance through medical clinics or relief offices [while in the U.S.] were likely to be considered a public charge," and would be denied return to the U.S.; adding a dimension of healthcare issues that Latinos would face alongside immigration [1]. Racial re-categorization served as an additional barrier for Latinos in receiving equitable care. In the 1930s dysentery and infant mortality rates were high in Latino dense neighborhoods of San Antonio, but TB rates were the highest reported in the nation [1]. Data from the Texas Department of Health showed "Latinos were dying of TB at five times the rate of their white neighbors and twice the rate of their African American neighbors." [1] To help address the issue, Texas health officials changed, "the racial category for Mexicans from 'white' to 'colored,'" which was met with outrage by the

community as this did not address the underlying societal issues [1].

Post-World War II, in the mid-1940s, the U.S. began to implement progressive initiatives in medical education to help fill needs in the country. The country increased the construction of new medical schools and pushed for desegregation of medical schools, in an effort to increase the number of available Latino doctors [1]. Nevertheless, desegregation did not eliminate continued racial discrimination in the country. Dr. Héctor Pérez García, later mentioned in this chapter, was described as being denied residency in his home state. Working with the Veteran's Administration hospital in Corpus Christi, Texas, he saw how race impacted the treatment of veterans of color – veterans were left in the halls waiting while there were vacant beds in the white wards. However, with his white coat, he was able to advocate and demand that "the hospital treat Mexican veterans like white patients." [1]

Although the Civil Rights Movement brought racism and discrimination to the national forefront during the sixties, the advent of the sexual exploration showed there was still more work to be done in terms of health disparities. It was not until 1978 that Thomas McKeown first described the concept of social determinants of health, where he discussed the idea that the health of an individual had both biological and socioeconomic components [2]. Dr. Hector Chapa, an OBGYN faculty member at Texas A&M University College of Medicine, recalls his time as a medical student at the University of Texas Southwestern in the mid-1990s and saw the impact of social determinants of health in the Latino community he served.

Social determinants of health were present, the concept was there, but it wasn't described. In medical school, I worked in Dallas county with a large indigent community. HIV/AIDS was still a death sentence at the time. These patients would come in with PCP, Meningitis, or Crypto and die. The patient demographics I saw would be skewed. A lot were undocumented and didn't have access to these services. People were critically ill at the time. Diseases were characterized by ethnicities. There were illness presentations then, as there are now too, like diabetes, that disproportionately affected Hispanics. I noticed that these high-risk populations were always designated/grouped together not by disease processes or diagnoses, but by ethnicities. I grew up in Laredo, Texas. Not until I went to college, I learned other people had more than me growing up. In medical school, I learned that certain races and ethnicities were disproportionately affected by certain diseases and diagnoses [3].

The nineties brought its own set of health issues to the Texas-Mexico Border. This was a time of increased urbanization brought on by the maquiladora or assembly plants, a boom led on by foreign industries that wanted to make use of the low wages and operating costs in Mexico [4]. With the demand for low-income housing brought on by the increase in population rates for the region, landowners took advantage of the abundant supply of idle agricultural fields to sell plots of land for people to build their homes [4, 5]. The new homes in these lots are what spurred the growth of the colonias in South Texas. Due to lax development regulation, people bought these pieces of unincorporated land, sacrificing access to portable water, sewers, utility services, and paved roads, which led to the creation of health issues such as waterborne illnesses among others [4, 5]. Access to ambulances, firefighters, police, or other city infrastructure became an issue in these communities because the "responsibility for colonias [became] complex due to the considerable ambiguity surrounding government and service provider jurisdictions." [5] Moreover, the access to healthcare was limited to those living in colonias, as few hospitals were able to care for low-income individuals, referring patients to hospitals miles away [5].

Apart from the issues brought on by urban and colonia development, maquiladoras proved to cause issues among its workers. Maquiladoras exposed its workers to "poor ventilation, few rest periods, excessive noise levels, unsafe machinery, … and exposure to toxic chemicals and carcinogens." [6] These working environments led to health conditions such as depression, pulmonary issues, eye problems, dermatitis, and hand injuries, among many other devastating ailments [6]. Unfortunately, these health issues fell short of the femicides that made national and global news. Women made up about two-thirds of workers in the maquiladoras, and were thought to play the role of "the 'liberation' of women from the household and their dependency role." [4] Unfortunately, growing rates of murdered women and failure of "the state to provide murdered women—and their families—rights and justice", challenged women's newfound freedom [7].

Dr. Chapa has noticed that over time, health issues in the Latino community have improved [4]. Medical schools continue to create initiatives to diversify medicine and train physicians to address health disparities in the country. However, some issues that the Latino community faced in the past, including but not limited to overt Latino discrimination, sexism, and immigration, has continued to play a prevalent role today. Dr. Chapa stated, "While improving, it remains critical for us to look back at history and continue to reassess issues not addressed so that we can play an active role in improving the health equity of our underserved Latino communities."

Ni De Aquí, Ni De Allá: The Ever Changing Border of the South and Its Role in Identity

The sentiment of not belonging is a common thread amongst medical students, particularly those from underrepresented backgrounds. Latino medical students face impostor syndrome as they step into the classroom, feeling different from their peers, whether it be because of differences in ethnicity, race, gender, or socioeconomic status (amongst some of the feelings) [8]. Furthermore, some reflect on the idea of feeling like outsiders since they were young. The concept of ni de aquí, ni de allá, highlights the struggle that bicultural students face when both groups they belong to challenge their identity. The concept is most interesting in the Southwest region, where many Latinos stress the idea that the border crossed them not the other way around.

The Southwest has faced several political and geographic transformations in comparison to other parts of the country. The U.S.-Mexico border evolved considerably throughout the years with the colonization by the Spanish and French, later having established countries such as Mexico and Texas, and having its border finalized by the Treaty of Guadalupe Hidalgo after the Mexican-American War in 1848 [9]. This long history of Spanish and Mexican rule in the region thus forms identity issues that differ from those found in other regions of the country such as the Northeast. Moreover, Louisiana, unlike other parts of our Southwest region, was controlled by Spain for 4 years, but "the culture and society of Louisiana remained French," due to its long history of French control [9].

Post-Treaty of Guadalupe Hidalgo, many "former Mexicans suddenly became U.S. citizens" becoming the new Latinos in the nation, with "86% of the nation's new Latinos [living] in New Mexico, which remained the only dense concentration of Latinos in U.S. territory for many years." [9] This sudden change in identity has had lasting impacts on not only those that continue to live there but also new immigrants that enter. Dr. Mary Headley Treviño de Edgerton was one of the first few Latina physicians recorded in history to have gone through discrimination of belonging and being accepted in the country. Despite being one of the "first Tejanos to attend medical school in Texas … at the University of Texas—Medical Branch in Galveston… [and] graduating at the top of her class and receiving the highest grade in the state medical exam in 1909," there was not a county medical association that would allow her to practice other than her home county of Starr, on the Texas-Mexico border [1]. Although Dr. Headley Treviño de Edgerton struggled to find a job in the U.S., her story was not unique during this time. Between 1890 and 1920, "the [number] of Latino doctors trained in American medical institutions fell," as did physicians from other underrepresented groups in that time [1].

Wartime brought more Mexicans to the U.S. during both World War I and II with the introduction of programs like the Braceros program to offset labor populations that went off to war [9]. Postwar time would follow cycles of discrimination where American workers felt as though Mexicans were taking away their jobs. The sentiment was followed by xenophobic rhetoric in favor of restricting immigration [10]. These emotions bled into the educational system that children of immigrant workers would enter. Muñoz notes how the American educational system encouraged students to assimilate into the American way, showing students the "'virtues of American democracy,' [and] that Mexican culture was a major factor in the "backwardness" of Mexican Americans." [10]

Dr. Héctor Pérez García was a physician that grew up in South Texas during these times, attending a segregated Mexican school. Similar to Dr. Headley Treviño de Edgerton, through his hard work he graduated cum laude from the University of Texas Medical Branch—Galveston in 1940; however, "every hospital in Texas rejected him because he was 'Mexican.'" [1] He returned to South Texas in 1946 after he acquired a residency in Omaha, Nebraska and after volunteering for the Army Medical Corps in World War II, he secured a job in the Veteran's Administration hospital in Corpus Christi, the only hospital that provided him visiting privileges [1].

These discriminatory attitudes persisted for many decades. Dr. Carlos Campos, a family physician in New Braunfels, TX, remembered the impact of Latino discrimination in his journey into medicine. Dr. Campos recalls growing up in a segregated town, which inspired him to go into medicine so that he could go back to his hometown and help those neglected in his community. Dr. Campos graduated from Baylor College of Medicine in 1981. During his time, not only did he experience rejection from segregation in New Braunfels, but he still vividly recalls being unwanted by a Mexican patient, a person of a similar background he hoped to serve.

> As a third-year medical student, I rotated at Kelsey Seybold. I had a patient, a Mexican lady, from Mexico City. When I went in to introduce myself, she said, 'I didn't come to Houston to see a Mexican doctor. I came to see a white doctor.' I still remember my attending, who later went in to talk to the patient and told her, 'If you don't want to see my medical student, you can grab your stuff and leave. He is part of my medical team and will see you as well.' After that, the patient grabbed her bag and left [11].

A few years later, Dr. Carrie Byington, a graduate of Baylor College of Medicine in 1989 and current Executive Vice President and Head of the University of California Health, recollects similar sentiments of not belonging as a medical student.

> As a woman and Latina, the first time I saw LMSA was as faculty at the University of Utah. I appreciated how much advice people had for pre-meds. I could have used all those things. I always felt alone. When applying to medical school, I didn't have anyone to go to. It was a lonely process, anxiety-provoking. I couldn't judge how to get in. I couldn't imagine how interviews would go. It was all a surprise. Felt lucky I got in and made the best of it [12].

As noted by Dr. Byington, being Latina and the first to go to medical school, or for that matter, college, poses another dimension worth considering. Dr. Maria del Carmen Espinoza, a graduate of the University of Texas Health Science Center at Houston in 1995 and currently a private practice pediatrician, discusses her experience wanting to go to medical school.

> When I was young, even though I always wanted to be a doctor, I was the only girl in my family. I came from a family that had never had anybody go to college… When I told my dad I wanted to go away for school [college], he asked 'Why don't you just stay here and become a secretary?' [13]

Being the first in your family to pursue higher education comes at a cost. Not only is it unknown to the student, but it is also new territory to family members. Discouragement may not necessarily stem from disparagement of a student's skills, but rather from fear of the unknown. The Latino community has roots in communal traditions. Sometimes Dr. Espinoza found it difficult to explain why she would be absent from so many family functions.

> They didn't understand that I was constantly studying, pretty much 24/7. It was a challenge with the family events. I would have to say 'I can't go. I can't go to this because I have to study.' [13]

Despite Latinos becoming the largest non-white minority group in the country, Latinos continue to be marginalized and underrepresented in medicine. According to AAMC data from 2019 to 2020, 7.6% of matriculants in Texas identified as Latino or Hispanic, whereas 39.6% of the Texas population identifies as Latino or Hispanic [14, 15]. Additionally, even though the number of medical school matriculants from underrepresented groups has increased by 30% nationally from 1997 to 2007, there has been an unfortunate 16% decrease in URM matriculants due to the overall increase in the first-year medical school slots [16].

Medical schools have learned to appreciate the value of diversity in the physician workforce and have attempted to address the low rates by creating pipeline programs. For example, Baylor College of Medicine and the University of Texas – Pan American, now formally known as the University of Texas Rio Grande Valley (UTRGV), created a BS to MD partnership initiative in 1994 to increase access to medical education for residents in South Texas. By 2008, the program produced 134 medical school matriculants, with 82% identifying as underrepresented racial and ethnic minorities and 79% identifying as Latino [17]. They also produced 65 MDs to date, 55 of which were Latino [17]. Dr. Monica Verduzco-Gutierrez, a graduate of Baylor College of Medicine in 2005 and Department Chair of Physical Medicine and Rehabilitation at UT Health San Antonio, was part of a similar pipeline program. Dr. Verduzco-Gutierrez notes her experience in the program and its importance in diversifying the physician workforce.

> There were always barriers to getting into medicine. Coming from one of the most impoverished areas in the US, the Rio Grande Valley, I didn't have the best high school education. College was hard for Latinos with a lot of competition. Plus, there we were not rich, so it was hard to access the MCAT courses. I have many Latino friends from undergrad who wanted to be physicians, but lack of privilege, systemic Hispanic discrimination, and poverty basically blocked them. I was in a pipeline program and was very grateful for that. Most of the Latino (and other URM) students in my medical school class were from pipeline programs. And for the most part, we may have had our struggles, but we made it out as outstanding physicians [18].

Being a Latino medical student poses identity struggles through the lack of shared experiences with peers or mentorship from individuals of the same background. Moreover, growing up in a country where one's nationality is put into question, the medical school classroom intensifies the feeling of not belonging. Fortunately, organizations such as LMSA, have helped to create a space of shared experiences that allows for students to thrive.

En Búsqueda De La Igualdad: Texas Student Chicano Movements for Educational Equity

The 1960s was a time for revolution and organization to create change against discriminatory actions against minority populations. In particular, the Chicano movements inspired many youths to take action into their hands. During this time, textbooks had omitted contributions of Mexican Americans, and teachers reprimanded students for speaking Spanish [19, 20]. School officials encouraged Latino students to "pursue manual labor jobs, learn a trade, or join the military" if they were male and consider lives as homemakers if they were female instead of encouraging them to go to college like their Anglo peers [17]. Students were chastised at higher rates than their white classmates for similar issues such as the length of skirts or sideburns [14]. These unfair treatments were absurd, as Mexican-American students made up about ninety percent of the student population [17].

Latino parents recognized the discrimination in schools and many did not hesitate to give their children a better chance at education. Dr. Rodolfo Molina, a Baylor College of Medicine graduate from 1976 and current rheumatologist at a private practice, recollects his memories of when his family moved in search of better schools.

> My dad moved our family to Corpus Christi because he didn't feel like Robstown, Texas was an appropriate place for his kids to grow up or have opportunities. I lived in a part of Corpus that was mostly Latino with some African Americans - almost no 'Anglo' people. In Junior high, my dad moved us to the 'white' side of town so that we could go to better schools. I felt like an outsider in the mostly white classrooms. I credit this move with helping meet one of my best friends, and helping me get into college. I was second in my family to go to college. My sister, just 2 years older was the first [21].

Unfortunately, not all students were as lucky to have the ability to change districts or cities. Students eventually mobilized and pressured school officials to set up meetings to address their grievances. Sadly, administrators and board members refused to listen to student demands [17]. Chicano students' frustration thus fueled their ambition to take action into their own hands. Similar to the Los Angeles Walkouts, many cities throughout the country were inspired to voice their concerns about the American education system. For example, two high schools in South Texas, Edcouch-Elsa High School and Crystal City High School had walkouts in 1968 and 1969, respectively [17, 20]. Despite their efforts, both walkouts resulted in different endings.

The Edcouch-Elsa High School students received advice and support from the Mexican American Youth Association (MAYO), a San Antonio Chicano student group. MAYO's preferred tactic was the walkouts, in order "to drastically lower a school's average daily attendance and thereby reduce its educational funding" as a method to force the schools to give in to student demands [17]. After the first day, the principal warned students they would receive a "three-day suspension and be subject to action by the school board" as a way to stir up fear and break up the walkouts [17]. On the second day of student protests the school principal called sheriffs to arrest students [17]. The protests escalated and eventually the school board opened meetings with students involved in the walkouts.

R.P. (Bob) Sánchez, an attorney from nearby McAllen, worked with the Edcouch-Elsa High School, supporting their cause. In an interview with The Monitor, the local newspaper in McAllen, he said:

> Our forefathers gave us some civil rights which the poor, downtrodden Mexican American students are just now waking up to and thank God they are.

Despite his support, the school board did not meet students' request and expelled vital participants of the walkouts [17].

The story ended on a lighter note in the Crystal City walkouts a year later. Students went to their school board requesting fair treatment but found it challenging to make meetings to meet with the board. Texas senators got involved and took students to Washington D.C. to talk with "officials in the Civil Rights Division of the Department of Justice and the Department of Health, Education, and Welfare [and discussed] the serious situation in Texas." [20] Through their struggle, school officials met student demands in 1970 [20].

These student movements continued throughout the nation, inspiring each other to bring about change in the educational system of Latinos. In 1969, all national groups, such as MAYO, came together to create the Movimiento Estudiantil Chicano de Aztlán, also known as MEChA [9]. Without the valiant efforts of these student groups in the late sixties, our educational system would not be where it is today. Although the effort to increase Latino representation in higher education continues, and more importantly to the theme of the book Latino physicians, we look back at these Chicano movements to resume their work for educational equity.

La Llamada A La Acción: The Formation of LMSA Southwest

With the Chicano Movement's push for equity in education, the rates of students pursuing higher education increased. In interviewing physicians, few people recall knowing of organized Latino medical student groups in the 1980s in the Southwest region. However, this makes sense with the slow increase in Latinos in professional careers. Initial groups were geared to URM medical students, such as the Student National Medical Association (SNMA), which Dr. Hector Chapa participated in and which allowed him to be in a more encouraging and inclusive environment that provided mentorship [3]. Similarly, in New Mexico, Dr. Patrick Rendon, a graduate of the University of New Mexico (UNM) School of Medicine in 2009 and now an Associate Professor, was part of the Association for the Advancement of Minorities in Medicine because there were no organized Latino groups [22].

As Latino populations began growing and seeing the need to address Latino student specific-issues, organizations began to emerge. Dr. René Salazar, former Assistant Dean for Diversity at

Dell Medical School, mentioned his involvement in the Texas Association of Latin American Medical Students. Dr. Salazar attended the University of Texas Health Science Center at San Antonio, graduating in 1999. He mentioned some of the issues students faced during this time were the lack of close-knit mentorship groups from people that looked like them as well as class retention [23].

These Latino student groups allowed learners to have a safe space to grow and motivate each other through the struggles of medical school. Many students were motivated to come back as faculty in medical schools and to provide mentorship to students and lead diversity efforts at their institutions. Dr. Valerie Romero-Leggott, a graduate of UNM School of Medicine in 1992 and current Vice President for Diversity, Equity & Inclusion for the UNM Health Sciences Center, notes the importance of these affinity groups.

> Although an organization like LMSA or SNMA did not exist while I was in medical school, I have a true appreciation for how important these organizations are in supporting students. They are a place to celebrate identity, culture, language, and belonging. You look for that. You yearn to feel a sense of community and belonging. It doesn't matter where you're from, these similarities bring you together. Mentors are another critically important part of medical student success, actually life success. We have all been the beneficiaries of mentors; many of whom did not have opportunities but made sure that we did [24].

Over time, students realized that these Latino student groups were all on the same mission. Dr. Anthony Oliva, a graduate of the University of Colorado School of Medicine in 2009 and now Assistant Professor of Anesthesiology played a vital role in the unification of all these Hispanic chapters across the nation. Attending the National Hispanic Medical Association (NHMA) conference in 2001 inspired him to take action in uniting Latino medical students across the nation.

> I attended the NHMA conference my first year of medical school. I didn't know about the Latino student group that existed throughout the country, for example, ULAMS [the United Latin American Medical Students] in Texas, the Chicano Medical Student Association, and the Boricua Health Organization in the Northeast. I solicited to become an officer right away, and with the help of

the national president at the time, Omar Rashid, and Dr. Elena Rios, President & CEO of NHMA, we worked in unifying the regions into the National Network of Latino American Medical Students (NNLAMS). Later I became president-elect and worked on having a unified nomenclature for all Latino student organizations to adopt. We wanted to work on the NMA [National Medical Association] and the SNMA model with NHMA, but we ended up adopting LMSA as the name [25].

With his hard work and other Latino medical students across the nation, NNLAMS held its first conference in conjunction with NHMA in 2006 [26]. NHMA and NNLAMS held conferences for a few years. However, in 2009, the NNLAMS Executive Board of Directors unanimously voted in favor of an independent National Conference as well as the common name of the Latino Medical Student Association [27].

Dr. Oliva helped to bring the Southwest region into the spotlight with his national presence, precipitating its start in 2007. Unfortunately, despite the unification of LMSA as a national organization, the Southwest region of LMSA historically suffered from a lack of communication and high officer turnover, among other factors [28]. The lack of strong leadership in the Southwest triggered the region to be fragmented and lose communication with the national organization shortly after the 2007 National Conference [28]. Although the population of the Southwest at the time was roughly a quarter Latino, many of the medical schools in the region did not know about LMSA [28]. Surviving chapters had motivated students that kept their individual LMSA entities afloat. Over time, the number of chapters increased and they eventually reached out to the national organization [28].

Dr. Ray Morales played a vital role in bringing back LMSA to the region in 2011. He contacted LMSA chapters at the major medical schools in the Southwest region leading efforts to hold face-to-face House of Delegate meetings to reconnect the region and centralize communication [28]. Dr. Ray Morales met with chapter leaders on November 5, 2011, at the University of Texas Southwestern [28]. With his help, the LMSA SW Regional Board drafted a constitution and reconnected the region to the national LMSA network, and most importantly, the students from various medical schools across the Southwest region [28].

In 2012, several Southwest regional officers (Table 5.1) attended the National LMSA Conference in Boston and the Garcia Leadership

Table 5.1 List of Southwest Co-Directors

2012–2013
- José Cruz, University of North Texas Health Science Center Texas College of Osteopathic Medicine
- Roger Romero, University of Texas Southwestern School of Medicine

2013–2014
- Giselle Dutcher, Baylor College of Medicine
- Humberto Mendoza, University of Texas Medical Branch

2014–2015
- Eric Molina, Baylor College of Medicine
- Marisa Castillo, University of North Texas Health Science Center Texas College of Osteopathic Medicine

2015–2016
- Eric Molina, Baylor College of Medicine
- Marisa Castillo, University of North Texas Health Science Center Texas College of Osteopathic Medicine

2016–2017
- Javier Santiago, Baylor College of Medicine
- Melissa Montoya-Vasquez, University of North Texas Health Science Center Texas College of Osteopathic Medicine

2017–2018
- Denise Mendez-Romero, University of Texas Southwestern School of Medicine
- Sonia Parra, Baylor College of Medicine

2018–2019
- Christian Aquino, Long School of Medicine at at UTHealth San Antonio
- Saul Perez, The University of Texas Southwestern Medical School

2019–2020
- Isabel López-García, The University of Texas Southwestern Medical School
- Christian Aquino, Long School of Medicine at at UTHealth San Antonio

2020–2021
- Munir H. Buhaya, McGovern Medical School at UTHealth Houston
- Victor H. Rodríguez, Texas A&M University College of Medicine

2021–2022
- Andrea Hernandez, UTHealth Houston McGovern Medical School
- Laura Garcia, Texas College of Osteopathic Medicine

2022–2023
- Luis Valdez, McGovern Medical School at UT Health
- Sierra Sossamon, Louisiana State University Health New Orleans

& Advocacy Seminar (GLAS), coming back inspired and with a vision for the future of the Southwest region [28]. GLAS was a leadership seminar created to commemorate Dr. Héctor Pérez García's work in civil and educational rights of Mexican-Americans, being appointed into Commission on Civil Rights in 1968 and the the first Mexican-American to serve as an ambassador to the United Nations in 1987 [29]. Attending these meetings served as essential learning experiences to help LMSA Southwest organize its first national conference in 2012 [28].

LMSA Southwest held its first regional conference on October 13, 2012 (Table 5.2), with the help of the Doctors Hospital at Renaissance [28]. The theme was Salud En La Frontera: Inspiring Future Leaders Through Mentorship and Education. The conference topic helped to reflect, "the culmination of many months of hard work from the conference organizers and the potential for growth in our region." [28] Through hard work, the first conference attracted over 75 medical students from various medical schools in the region and 30 undergraduates from the University of Texas – Pan American [28].

As the region gained momentum, the Southwest region hosted its first National Conference on April 2014, co-hosted by The University of Texas Health Science Houston, now known as McGovern Medical School, and

Baylor College of Medicine [28]. This conference helped to demonstrate the infrastructure the Southwest Regional Board predecessors established for Latino medical students in the region to the national organization.

Slowly, LMSA Southwest began expanding outside its Texas borders, adding chapters from Louisiana in 2016 and 2017 (Table 5.3). Motivated by the previous conference, Davis Mas, chapter president at the time and three-time Regional Chief Development Officer, from Louisiana State University Health Sciences Center (LSUHSC) New Orleans pushed his institution to host the sixth regional conference in 2018. He and other students believed it was an ideal location due to the city's "plethora of diverse ethnicities and identities along with a top-class hospital" [30]. This conference was monumental for the region holding its first conference outside of Texas, as well as having to move the conference from LSUHSC to the University Medical Center within a few days' notice due to inclement weather [30]. Despite this setback, the conference was successful at attracting 60 medical students along with pre-medical students [30].

The conference also highlighted a year of growth for the Southwest region, expanding chapters to two states, Arkansas and New Mexico. Similar to LSUHSC New Orleans, R. J. Parkinson, a medical student at the New York

Table 5.2 list of regional conference title and host schools and institutions between 2012 and 2023

- Salud En La Frontera: Inspiring Future Leaders Through Mentorship and Education, Doctors Hospital at Renaissance, 2012
- 2013?
- Creciendo Juntos: Improving Health Care For and By Latinos (National), Baylor College of Medicine and UT Health Science Center Houston, 2014
- Saber es Poder, University of North Texas Health Science Center Texas College of Osteopathic Medicine, 2015
- Cuidando La Salud, UT Health Science Center San Antonio, 2016
- Prevenir es Vivir, UT Health Science Center Houston, 2017
- Derribando barreras: Empowering the Community through Health, Louisiana State University Health Sciences Center New Orleans, 2018
- Todos Tenemos Valor (National), Texas Tech University Health Sciences Center School of Medicine, 2019
- Identidad Latina: Soy más que…, UTRGV School of Medicine, 2020
- El Lider Dentro de Mi: Advancing Latinx Leadership in Medicine, Texas A&M University College of Medicine, 2021
- Es Tiempo De Cambiar: The Importance of Diversity in Medicine, Tulane University School of Medicine, 2022
- El Futuro es Nuestro: Embracing our Roots to Build a Better Future in Medicine, Texas College of Osteopathic Medicine, 2023

Table 5.3 List of States and School Chapters (stand alone or connected) in the LMSA Southwest Region (as of December 2022)

Arkansas: New York Institute of Technology College of Osteopathic Medicine at Arkansas State University (ind. 2018), University of Arkansas
Colorado: University of Colorado School of Medicine (ind. 2019)
Louisiana: Louisiana State University Health Sciences Center New Orleans (ind. 2017), Louisiana State University Health Shreveport (ind. 2016), Tulane University School of Medicine, VCOM at Monroe, UQ Ochsner (Louisiana)
New Mexico: University of New Mexico School of Medicine (ind. 2018), Burrell COM
Oklahoma: OSU College of Osteopathic Medicine
Texas: Baylor College of Medicine (ind. 2012), Dell Medical School (ind. 2019), Long School of Medicine at UT Health San Antonio (ind. 2012), McGovern Medical School at UTHealth Houston (ind. 2012), Paul L. Foster School of Medicine, Texas A&M University College of Medicine (ind. 2014), Texas A&M University LMSA Plus (ind. 2020), Texas Christian University and University of North Texas Health Science Center School of Medicine (ind. 2020), Texas Tech University Health Sciences Center School of Medicine, Texas Tech University LMSA Plus (ind. 2019), University of the Incarnate Word School of Osteopathic Medicine (ind. 2020), The University of Texas Medical Branch at Galveston (ind. 2012), The University of Texas Southwestern Medical School (ind. 2012), University of Texas Rio Grande Valley School of Medicine (ind. 2017), University of Texas Rio Grande LMSA Plus (ind. 2019), University of North Texas Health Science Center Texas College of Osteopathic Medicine (ind. 2012)

Institute of Technology (NYTI) College of Osteopathic Medicine at Arkansas State University, was inspired by attending an LMSA Southwest regional conference to create a chapter.

> Our school was pretty new. We had students from Texas, Florida, and Southern California. The reason why we started our LMSA chapters was that we wanted a club where we could talk in Spanish and celebrate the Latino culture. Majority of our Spanish-speaking populations are migratory farm workers in northeast Arkansas. I have seen patients that only spoke Spanish, probably one of the few that could at school. I've encountered patients whose eyes light up when they see someone that could speak their language. Although I'm not Latino, having someone that shares or understands your culture helped the patient encounter [31].

His chapter elected him chapter president for his exceptional leadership and strong advocacy for Latino communities, inducting the chapter into the Southwest region in 2018.

In 2019, LMSA Southwest had the opportunity to host once again the National LMSA Conference at Texas Tech University Health Sciences Center School of Medicine in Lubbock, Texas. The conference was a resounding success with over 350 attendees from across the country [32]. Apart from its successful attendance, the Southwest region continued to grow its outreach to more states in the region, inducting the University of Colorado School of Medicine. Additionally, LMSA Southwest began to inspire and work with undergraduates to help increase mentorship with the addition of two LMSA PLUS chapters, one at UTRGV and the other at Texas Tech University.

Despite LMSA Southwest's flourishing momentum, the lack of communication and the announcement of officer turnover, shook the region at the end of 2019 and start of 2020, repeating errors from the region's early start. However, through extraordinary leadership from Dr. Christian Aquino and Isabel López-García, the Southwest Regional Board was able to hold its eighth annual regional conference at UTRGV School of Medicine. The conference was titled "Identidad Latina: Soy más que…" which explored the intersectionality of Latino identity. The speakers and workshops "allowed participants to challenge the stereotypes that may be associated with Latinos in the medical field." [33]

The LMSA Southwest region has built community partnerships for health fairs, scholarships, and research symposia and continues working to engage all students about health in our underserved communities and professional development. The culmination of hard work from many individuals has helped the Southwest increase in the number of members as well as increase connections between various institutions. Despite its short organized presence in comparison to other LMSA regions, the Southwest region has left a lasting impact in its chapters and LHS+ medical students through a shared space of experience and encouragement to become leaders in medicine.

References

1. Mckiernan-Gonzalez J. "American Science, American Medicine, and American Latinos" in American Latinos and the Making of the United States. Edited by Stephen Pitti. Washington, DC: National Park Service/ Organization of American Historians / Government Printing Office; 2013. http://www.nps.gov/history/heritageinitiatives/latino/latinothemestudy/.
2. McKeown T. Determinants of health. Life. 1978;60(40):3.
3. Chapa H. Faculty at Texas A&M University College of Medicine. Phone interview. 6 Apr 2020.
4. Williams DM, Homedes N. The impact of the maquiladoras on health and health policy along the US-Mexico border. J Public Health Policy. 2001;22(3):320–37.
5. Ward PM. Colonias and public policy in Texas and Mexico: Urbanization by stealth. Austin: University of Texas Press; 2010.
6. Guendelman S, Silberg MJ. The health consequences of maquiladora work: women on the US-Mexican border. Am J Public Health. 1993;83(1):37–44.
7. Córdoba MST. Transnational narratives, cultural production, and representations: blurred subjects in Juárez, México. Global Mexican Cultural Productions. New York: Palgrave Macmillan; 2011. p. 75–94.
8. Brooks R. "Study: Impostor syndrome causes mental distress in minority students." USA Today (2017).
9. Constant AF, Massey DS. Latinos in the Southern United States: Trends and Patterns. Office of Population Research, Princeton University; 2019.
10. Muñoz Jr, Carlos, and Power Identity. "The Chicano Movement." Mexican American History and the Struggle for Equality. New York: Rosa Luxemburg Stiftung; 2013.
11. Carlos Campos. Phone interview. 3 Apr 2020.
12. Byington C. Executive Vice President and head of the University of California Health. Phone interview. 7 Apr 2020.
13. Espinoza, Maria del Carmen. Phone interview. 21 Apr 2020.
14. Table A-11: Matriculants to U.S. Medical Schools by Race/Ethnicity and State of Legal Residence, 2019–2020. Association of American Medical Colleges, 15 Nov. 2019, https://www.aamc.org/system/files/2019-11/2019_FACTS_Table_A-11.pdf
15. "U.S. Census Bureau QuickFacts: Texas." Census Bureau QuickFacts, www.census.gov/quickfacts/fact/table/TX/POP010210.
16. Talamantes E, et al. Closing the gap – making medical school admissions more equitable. N Engl J Med. 2019;380(9):803–5. https://doi.org/10.1056/NEJMp1808582.
17. Thomson WA, et al. A baccalaureate–MD program for students from medically underserved communities: 15-year outcomes. Acad Med. 2010;85(4):668–74.
18. Verduzco-Gutierrez M. Department Chair of Physical Medicine and Rehabilitation at UT Health San Antonio. Email interview. 27 Apr 2020.
19. Barrera B. The 1968 Edcouch-Elsa High School walkout: Chicano student activism in a south Texas community. Aztlán J Chicano Stud. 2004;29(2):93–122.
20. Barrios G. Walkout in crystal city. Teaching Tolerance. 2009;35:41–3.
21. Molina R. Phone interview. 21 Apr 2020.
22. Rendon P. Associate Professor at the University of New Mexico. Email interview. 8 Apr 2020.
23. Salazar R. Assistant Dean for Diversity at Dell Medical School. Email interview. 4 Apr 2020.
24. Romero-Leggott V. Vice Chancellor for Diversity, Equity & Inclusion for the University of New Mexico Health Sciences Center. Phone interview. 29 Apr 2020.
25. Oliva A. Assistant Professor of Anesthesiology at the University of Colorado School of Medicine. Phone interview. 28 Apr 2020.
26. "1st Annual National Conference National Network of Latin American Medical Students." The National Latino Student Medical Association, 23 Mar. 2020, lmsa.net/files/nnlamsconference06.pdf.
27. "Conference History." The National Latino Student Medical Association, 2020, national.lmsa.net/conference-history.html.
28. "Latino Medical Student Association Annual Journal Volume 4." Edited by Felipe Camero et al., The National Latino Student Medical Association, 2014, national.lmsa.net/uploads/1/2/7/2/127219773/lmsa-journal-2014-double-page-view-final-version.pdf.
29. "Dr Hector P Garcia." The National Latino Student Medical Association, 2014, https://lmsa.net/events/glas/bio.
30. Mas D. "LSUHSC Hosts Latino Medical Student Association Regional Conference" The Pulse: The LSUHSC School of Medicine Electronic News, 28 Mar. 2018, https://lsuhscpulse.wordpress.

com/2018/03/20/lsuhsc-hosts-latino-medical-student-association-regional-conference/

31. Parkinson RJ. Phone interview. 23 Apr 2020.
32. Cisneros S, Skousen A. "TTUHSC Hosts National Latino Medical Students Association Conference." TTUHSC Hosts National Latino Medical Students Association Conference: TTUHSC Daily Dose, 5 Apr. 2019., https://dailydose.ttuhsc.edu/2019/april/LMSA.aspx.

33. Trejo D. "Latino Medical Student Conference at UTRGV Discusses Themes of Identity for Young Medical Professionals." The Newsroom - Latino Medical Student Conference at UTRGV Discusses Themes of Identity for Young Medical Professionals, 6 Apr. 2020., http://www.utrgv.edu/newsroom/2020/02/17-latino-medical-student-conference-at-utrgv-discusses-themes-of-identity-for-young-medical-professionals.htm.

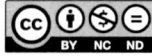

LHS+ Medical Student History and Heritage of the U.S. West Region

Minerva A. Romero Arenas and Alvaro Galvis

"True wealth is not measured in money or status or power. It is measured in the legacy we leave behind for those we love and those we inspire."

—Cesar Chavez

El Movimiento: The Chicano Civil Rights Movement

In the 1960s, in parallel with the Civil Rights Movement of African-American communities, Hispanic Americans of various backgrounds organized to advocate around their own struggle for civil equality and fairness. Among Mexican Americans in the Southwest United States (U.S.), this struggle came to be known as the Chicano Civil Rights Movement [1]. The Chicano movement in California was known as El Movimiento (the Movement) and encompassed a variety of issues, including restoration of land grants; protection of farm workers' rights; and equality in education, voting, and political rights. The dire needs for migrant farmworkers were also brought to light through the United Farm Workers Union (UFW), established in 1962 and led by revolutionaries like Dolores Huerta and Cesar E. Chavez. These needs included a minimum wage for migrant farmworkers, birthright citizenship for their children, and health protections, such as reducing the use of harmful pesticides and initiating unemployment and healthcare benefits [2]. In Arizona, the Mexican American Student Organization, which would later take the name Movimiento Estudiantil Chicano de Aztlán (MEChA), organized a sit-in at the President's Office of Arizona State University to protest treatment of the Chicano community within the institution and its surrounds [3].

Around the same time, Executive Order 19025 issued by U.S. President John F. Kennedy—commonly referred to as Affirmative Action—opened doors to higher education for many Chicano students. Undergraduate students started to enter college in larger numbers and began to form various organizations. At the pre-medical level, these organizations included Chicanos for Creative Medicine, C.H.I.S.P.A., Stanford Chicano Pre-Medical Society, Los Curanderos, Chicanos for Community Medicine (CCM), and Chicanos for Health Education (CHE), among others [4, 5]. These students who later entered medical schools would subsequently form the corresponding medical student organizations, and later, the professional physician societies. Thus, the organiza-

M. A. Romero Arenas (✉)
New York Presbyterian Brooklyn Methodist Hospital, Weill Cornell Medicine, New York City, NY, USA
e-mail: mar9462@med.cornell.edu

A. Galvis
Department of Pediatrics, Division of Pediatric Infectious Diseases, Loma Linda University Children's Health, Loma Linda, CA, USA

© The Author(s) 2024
J. P. Sánchez, D. Rodriguez (eds.), *Latino, Hispanic, or of Spanish Origin+ Identified Student Leaders in Medicine*, Sustainable Development Goals Series, DOI https://doi.org/10.1007/978-3-031-35020-7_6

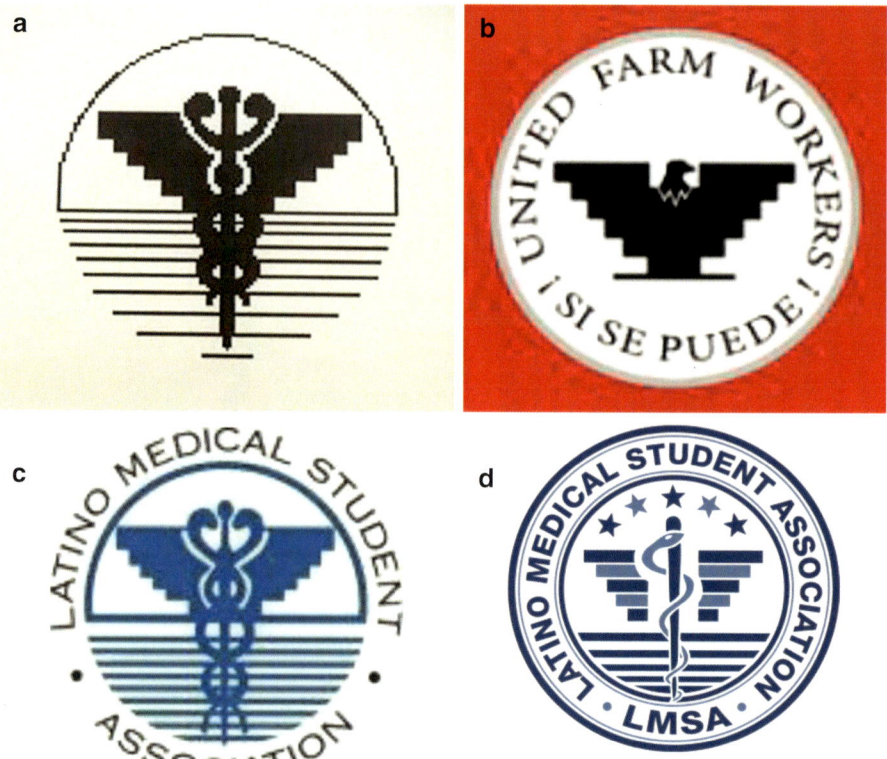

Fig. 6.1 LMSA Logo Influence and Evolution (©LMSA). (**a**) The original LMSA (West) logo was designed by a medical student at UCI. It took inspiration from the United Farm Workers logo (**b**). (**c**) The LMSA (West) region logo was updated in 2005 with the organization name added around the graphic. It was then adopted by LMSA National (2009–2011) as homage to the West region during the process of national unification. (**d**) The LMSA National logo was redesigned in 2011. The Staff of Aesculapius replaced the Caduceus, five stars were added to represent each region, and the eagle wings surrounding the medical caduceus remained as a homage to the roots of the West Region's logo

tions and leaders that would eventually give rise to today's Latino Medical Student Association (LMSA) developed during the Chicano Movement.

The influence of El Movimiento, specifically that of the farm workers' movement, can be seen in the original logo of LMSA (Fig. 6.1a). The logo drew inspiration from the UFW logo (Fig. 6.1b) in the eagle wings surrounding the medical staff. The original logo was designed by a medical student at the University of California, Irvine (UCI) and, although updated for digital quality, it remained the same as the organization evolved (Fig. 6.1c). This logo was adopted as the LMSA National logo after the national unifica-

tion movement started in 2007–09. When the logo was updated in 2011 to reflect its new structure, the wings of an eagle were maintained as a homage to the West region's roots and to the UFW Movement (Fig. 6.1d).

Las Raíces: The Roots of a New Organization

In 1968, there were 20 Chicano and 3 Puerto Rican medical students matriculating into medical schools across the country [6]. As these numbers increased in the 1970s, the National Chicano Health Organization (NCHO) was established and began organizing Chicano medical students in California [5]. Robert "Bob" Montoya, a student at the University of Southern California, and David Hayes Bautista, a graduate student at the University of California, San Francisco, were among the early NCHO student leaders. The organization sought and received federal funding to staff an office in Los Angeles. Subsequently, under the leadership of NCHO Executive Director Fred Lopez, additional federal funding was sought and received, allowing the establishment of additional offices in San Jose, Albuquerque, Denver, San Antonio, and Chicago. Frank Meza, a pre-medical student at California State University Northridge and CCM leader, also became a leading member of the NCHO Board [5].

In the second half of the 1970s, the La Raza Medical Association (La RaMA) became the leading force in the recruitment and retention of Chicano health students. There were several student leaders who were critical to the success of La RaMA, including medical students Frank Meza, Jose Arevalo, Max Cuevas, Hector Flores, Laura Solorio, and pre-medical students Raquel Arias, Tina Nevarez, and Elena Rios [5]. Rios, a graduate of the University of California Los Angeles School of Medicine, would go on to establish National Hispanic Medical Association (NHMA) in 1994 and help facilitate the growth of the National Network of Latin American Medical Students (NNLAMS) shortly thereafter [7].

Students from NCHO and La RaMA began meeting as an informal group in the Fall of 1982. Recognizing the mutual goals of increasing the number of Chicano/Hispanic/Latino students in the health professions, the organizations decided to coalesce and the Chicano/Latino Medical Student Association (CMSA) was established. The new CMSA was introduced as a network of medical students throughout the entire state of California during the National Association of Minority Medical Educators Conference in September 1984. The original founding schools of CMSA were the California medical schools (as reflected in Table 6.1), which were then divided into the Northern and Southern Regions of California. The organization soon would welcome a chapter in Arizona and eventually in other Western states, such as Utah, Oregon, and Washington.

Table 6.1 List of States and School Chapters (stand alone or connected) in the LMSA West Region (as of December 2022)

Alaska: None
Arizona: A T Still University School of Osteopathic Medicine, Mayo Clinic Alix School of Medicine - AZ, Midwestern University - Arizona College of Osteopathic Medicine, University of Arizona - Phoenix
California: California Northstate University-COM (CNU), Charles Drew University of Medicine and Science (UCLA), David Geffen School of Medicine at UCLA, Kaiser Permanente Bernard J. Tyson School of Medicine (KPSOM), Keck School of Medicine of USC, Loma Linda University School of Medicine, Stanford School of Medicine, Touro University COM - CA, University of California - Davis School of Medicine, University of California - Irvine School of Medicine, University of California - San Diego School of Medicine, University of California - San Francisco School of Medicine, University of California, Riverside,
Hawaii: University of Hawaii John A. Burns School of Medicine
Idaho: None
Montana: None
Nevada: Touro University COM - NV, University of Nevada - Las Vegas, University of Nevada, Reno School of Medicine
Oregon: Oregon Health & Science University
Utah: Noorda-COM, Rocky Vista University College of Osteopathic Medicine- Southern Utah, University of Utah School of Medicine
Washington: Pacific Northwest University Health Sciences, Washington State University Elson S. Floyd College of Medicine
Wyoming: None

Affirmative Action

In 1977, Allan Bakke filed a lawsuit against the University of California with the argument that he was denied admission solely on the basis of race. Bakke, a Caucasian male, had twice applied for admission to the University of California, Davis (UC Davis) School of Medicine and was rejected both times. The school reserved sixteen places in each entering class of one hundred for "qualified" minorities, as part of the university's Affirmative Action program, in an effort to redress longstanding, unfair exclusion of minority students from the medical profession. Bakke's college grade point average and test scores exceeded those of any of the minority students admitted in the 2 years Bakke's applications were rejected. In 1978, the U.S. Supreme Court ruled that Mr. Bakke should be admitted to medical school, yet still allowed the use of a student's race as a factor in admissions criteria [8]. Minority students were thrust into the media spotlight, and several, including Frank Meza, testified in the hearings. The negative impact of this unwanted attention was felt by the students; however, it also made them a very tight-knit group and united in their mission.

Affirmative Action and a number of subsequent policies have continued to impact the communities and students for whom LMSA exists. A notable example includes California's Proposition 187 (1994), which aimed to make immigrants residing in the country without legal permission ineligible for public benefits. California's Proposition 209 (1996) eventually eliminated Affirmative Action, by prohibiting public institutions from discriminating on the basis of race, sex, or ethnicity. Arizona's Proposition 200 (2004) sought to suppress voters by imposing additional requirements on proof of identification. Although some elements of this latter proposition were overturned in 2013, anti-immigrant and anti-Mexican rhetoric began to expand. Margarita Loeza, MD, MPH, reported, "We were very concerned about Prop. 187, [Gov.] Pete Wilson, and the end of affirmative action." As a medical student and leader at the University of California, San Diego (UCSD), Dr. Loeza served

as Medical Student Representative (MSR) of her school's CMSA chapter, as well as Treasurer, Secretary, Southern CEO, and Conference Coordinator for the organization's 1997 regional event. Her views were shared by many of her counterparts. Awareness of the impact such policies have on the welfare of their communities, their peers, and their patients has influenced generation after generation of LMSA members, as well as the activism in which these student and physician leaders have engaged.

Student Activism and Las Clínicas

The Brown Berets, founded by David Sanchez in 1967, represented a pro-Chicano community-based youth organization that advocated for social justice and played a significant role in El Movimiento [9]. Its members were largely motivated to protest by the police brutality faced by Chicanos in East Los Angeles; however, the Brown Berets would tackle a range of social and political issues that plagued Chicano neighborhoods, including political invisibility, educational inequality, and limited healthcare access. One major accomplishment of the Brown Berets was the establishment of El Barrio Free Clinic [10]. The Clinic was located on Whittier Boulevard in East Los Angeles, and operated from 1968 to 1970. It was operated by an all-volunteer staff headed by Gloria Arellanes, a prominent female leader among the Brown Berets. While clinic operations were run by the Brown Berets, the medical staff consisted of volunteers from various schools and hospitals—including pre-medical and medical student volunteers. Conflict within Brown Beret leadership led to a split in the organization in February 1970. The female members resigned from the Brown Berets and formed their own organization, Las Adelitas de Aztlán. Ultimately, the clinic closed its doors in December 1970. Las Adelitas then opened a clinic a short distance away on Atlantic Boulevard in March 1971 with a similar name, La Clínica del Barrio. Many of the same volunteers remained involved, including then pre-medical student Frank Meza. The clinic prospered and eventually became a community health center under the leadership of Dr. Cástulo de la Rocha. Subsequently, it became AltaMed Health Services, which has grown to be the largest federally funded Community Health Center in the country [5].

Students at the University of California, Davis established La Clínica Tepati in 1974 to provide healthcare to the underserved Mexican-American community of Sacramento [4, 5]. Deriving its name from Tepatli, the Nahuatl word for "healer," the clinic was only the second student-run clinic in the nation. The clinic's medical student leaders included Randy Clarke, Antonio Velasco, and Frank Meza, who was active in the Brown Berets and establishment of the Los Angeles-area clínicas. Still in existence at the time of writing, this free clinic is staffed each Saturday with physician volunteers and has provided services continuously to underserved Latino patients in the Sacramento area for over 45 years [11]. It has also provided clinical experience and support to hundreds of pre-medical students who have gone on to become doctors or pursue other health professions.

> The clinic is one of the most important things I've done. I started as an undergrad as a "blueberry" or volunteer in blue scrubs. I was able to meet a lot of UC Davis medical students and get mentoring. I was able to learn about the medical journey and now I am a medical student. We have students who are in pre-law, interested in the arts, just people who want to help people. I'm able to practice with people who remind me of my family and a lot of the conditions I see are really similar to what I see in my own family.
> —Dagoberto Piña, Medical Student, UC Davis & volunteer for La Clinica Tepati

Following the inspiration of Clínica Tepati, medical students at UCI established Clínica Cariño. The students were led by then medical student Mario San Bartolome, who completed undergraduate studies at UC Davis. The UCI students ran Clínica Cariño in partnership with Loaves and Fishes Soup Kitchen in Santa Ana, California, a city whose population of 300,000 was approximately 80% Latino at the time. The clinic started with health screenings and referral services and was held once a month with plans to expand to a full-service free clinic. In 2001, UCI administra-

tors raised financial concerns about the sustainability of a free clinic, claiming that a full-service free clinic in Santa Ana was unnecessary, that there was adequate health care access in Santa Ana, and that undocumented immigrant patients would not come to seek healthcare services. Thus, student leaders under the direction of Dr. Emily Dow conducted a needs assessment report for the Santa Ana and greater Orange County communities, which concluded that "current evidence strongly suggests the 2001 administrative objections are either no longer valid or are surmountable." [12] After the report, the students secured a site in Santa Ana for a more permanent home but, due to landlord issues, ended up having to settle in the adjacent city of Tustin. After 10 years in operation, Clínica Cariño evolved and was renamed UCI Outreach Clinics in 2009.

As the number of minority students grew, so did the number of minority physicians. CMSA student leaders graduated from medical school, advanced through graduate medical education into physicianship, and began to establish and lead professional physician societies aimed at serving the underserved communities from which they hailed. Such physician organizations include the Pacific Medical Association, which later became the Chicano/Latino Medical Association of California; the California Latino Medical Association (CaLMA, est. 1998); and the Arizona Latin-American Medical Association (est. 1993).

> The issue is there are not enough culturally competent health-care professionals to meet the needs of the (Hispanic) community. Care is affected adversely because language and culture can create barriers for diagnosis and treatment,
> —Dr. Juan Villagomez, Chairman of the California Chicano/Latino Medical Association [13]

From Chicano to Latino Medical Student Association

In 2003, CMSA changed its name to the Latino Medical Student Association (LMSA) to better reflect the makeup of its members. The name change to the more inclusive Latino term reflected the growing diversity within Latino subgroups in medical schools, the developing Latino identity among U.S. Latinos, and the growing recognition of the Hispanic/Latino community as a political and economic force.

The rebranded organization maintained the majority of the governing structure from CMSA, composed of two medical student representatives from each medical school chapter. This body met quarterly to discuss business and to plan the future directions of the group. These quarterly meetings were to be attended by the Executive Council, made up of chapter MSRs along with the Regional Co-Chairs, Treasurer, and Secretary. There was also an annual conference hosted by chapters and traditionally open to medical and premedical students at any institution. The first conference was held in 1984 and hosted by the University of California, Los Angeles (UCLA). The conference included a celebration banquet to honor its graduating medical students. In 1993, donning of sarape stoles was introduced at the graduation banquet by student leaders at the time and was made by the mother of Javier Romero (UC Davis). Both of these traditions remain in practice through 2022.

Two key changes were made in the transition from CMSA to LMSA. First, realignment of the schools into Northern and Southern regions occurred alongside the introduction of a requirement for one leader to be elected from each and function as Co-Chairs. Previously, Co-Chairs could be from any school, leading to the potential for over-representation of southern California chapters, which often contained greater student numbers. Moreover, with the establishment of new chapters outside the state of California, this change was made to ensure chapter diversity in top leadership. Of note, the Northern and Southern Co-Chairs promote communication among the region's chapters and their MSRs, as well as with other health organizations as needed for project development. The second change was an accountability clause, which came about from the inconsistent involvement among the individual CMSA chapters. Prior to this clause, some of the chapters would have no regularly scheduled chapter meetings and intermittently participate in the CMSA board meetings. The change required each chapter's leaders to submit a signed contract to LMSA that stipulated the requirements and expectations in order to continue being recognized as an active chapter (Fig. 6.2).

LMSA Inc. was incorporated as an official organization under the nonprofit public benefit corporation law for charitable purposes on January 22, 2005. Those indispensable to achieving this task included Ms. Emma Ledesma, UCI LMSA advisor, and the initial directors of the corporation: Jose Mayorga (UCI), Moses Salgado (UC Davis), Lucio Loza (UCLA), and Fernando Antelo (UCLA) (Fig. 6.3). The organization soon began to have influence by dual-degree student leaders, such as Eunice Rivas (Stanford), Efrain Talamantes (UCLA), Eric Sandoval (UC Irvine), and Omar Guzman (UC Irvine), and advisers such as Dr. Mario San Bartolome, who helped reshape the organizational structure with corporate titles such as Chief Executive Officer and Vice President for various aspects of the organization's programming. The goal was to present LMSA Inc. as a forefront leader in professional development for Latino medical students and to facilitate communication with potential sponsors. These changes were reflected in the initial Bylaws when LMSA Inc. received its 501(c)(3) nonprofit organizational status on May 16, 2007 (Fig. 6.4). The new 501(c)(3) status launched an era of increased fundraising that included small grants from the California Wellness Foundation and California Endowment, as well as corporate sponsorships from Southern California Kaiser Permanente and Molina Health Group. This allowed the organization to afford travel reimbursements for regional leaders, chapter development mini-grants, scholarships for pre-medical and medical students, and the new annual LMSA leadership conference at the beginning of the academic year.

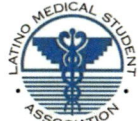

Latino Medical Student Association

LMSA Chapter Contract
2006-2007

In order to implement a consistent LMSA mission throughout our respective chapters, we have developed the following contract to help you understand what steps you need to take to be recognized as an active LMSA Chapter.

The following requirements will be implemented during the 2006 – 2007 academic year. An evaluation of your chapter will be conducted bi-yearly (January, May). Failure to meet these requirements will result in a thorough review of your chapter by the LMSA Regional Board. The LMSA Regional Board will then make several recommendations in order to get the chapter to abide by the requirements. If these recommendations are not followed up by the chapter, they will be subject to further penalty that will be decided by our Medical Student Representatives (MSRs) at the proximate LMSA Board Meeting.

Sign Contract → Abide by requirements → 1ˢᵗ Evaluation* (January) → 2ⁿᵈ Evaluation* (May)

*Failure to meet requirements → LMSA Board Review → LMSA Recommendations
*LMSA Recommendations not followed → Penalty will be determined at LMSA Board Meeting by our MSR's

1. **LMSA Leadership Conference:** (2) Medical Student Representatives and (2) Co-Chairs
   If MSR's or Co-chairs are not available to attend, they must send other chapter leader representatives.
   Total (4) chapter representatives.

2. **General Meetings:** 2 chapter meetings/quarter, or 3 chapter meetings/semester.

3. **LMSA Regional Dues:** Must be collected by deadline stated.

4. **LMSA Mentorship Program:** establish a mentorship program within the first 4 weeks that the undergraduate or high school students begin coursework.

5. **LMSA Newsletter:** Submit (3) articles/year by deadlines stated.

6. **LMSA Regional Conference:** Strive to get 100% of your chapter members to attend our yearly LMSA Regional Conference. All chapter leaders are expected to attend.

7. **Communication:** Medical Student Representatives (MSR's) are responsible for responding to any LMSA Regional correspondence. If MSR's do not respond on time- co-chairs will be notified and expected to reply immediately.

8. **LMSA Board Meetings:** Medical Student Representatives (MSR's) must attend all (4) Regional Board Meetings. If MSR's are unable to attend, another chapter representative must attend. (ex. Co-Chair, Secretary, Treasurer, etc).

LMSA Chapter School: _____

_____   _____
Medical Student Representative (1)   Medical Student Representative (2)

_____   _____
Co-Chair (1)   Co-Chair (2)

Drew ● UCLA ● UCSF ● UCD ● UCSD ● Stanford ● USC ● UCI ● Western ● U of A ● Utah
U of Washington

www.lmsa.net

Fig. 6.2 LMSA Chapter Contract (©LMSA)

Articles of Incorporation
Of
Latino Medical Student Association
A California Public Benefit Corporation

Article I
The name of this corporation is **Latino Medical Student Association**

Article II
This corporation is a nonprofit public benefit corporation and is not organized for the private gain of any person. It is organized under the Nonprofit Public Benefit Corporation Law for charitable purposes. The specific purposes for which this corporation is organized are to promote minorities entering the medical field thereby enhancing the quality of minority health care. To support undergraduate students and medical students who are interested or currently pursuing a career in medicine.

Article III
The name and address in the State of California for this corporation's initial agent for service of process is 2550 Corporate Place Suite C202 Monterey Park, California , 91754.

Article IV
(a) This corporation is organized and operated exclusively for charitable purposes within the meaning of Section 501 (c) (3) of the Internal Revenue Code.
(b) Not withstanding any other provision of these Articles, the corporation shall not carry on any other activities not permitted to be carried on (1) by a corporation exempt from federal income tax under Section 501 (c) (3) of the Internal Revenue Code or (2) by a corporation contributions to which are deductible under Section 170 (c) (2) of the Internal Revenue Code.
(c) No substantial part of the activities of this corporation shall consists of carrying on propaganda, or otherwise attempting to influence legislation, and the corporation shall not participate or intervene in any political campaign (including the publishing or distribution of statements) on behalf of, or in opposition to, any candidate for public office.

Fig. 6.3 First Page and Signatures of LMSA Articles of Incorporation (©LMSA)

Article V

The names and addresses of the persons appointed to act as the initial Directors of this corporation are:

Name

José Mayorga

Address

6324 Adobe Circle Road

Irvine, CA 92617

Moses Salgado

3317 Broken Branch Court #119

Sacramento, CA 95834

Lucio Loza

11634 Bos St.

Cerritos, CA 90703

Fernando Antelo

1122 East Acacia Ave

Glendale, CA 91205

Article VI

The property of this corporation is irrevocably dedicated to charitable purposes and no part of the net income or assets of the organization shall ever inure to the benefit of any director, officer or member thereof or to the benefit of any private person.

On the dissolution or winding up of the corporation, its assets remaining after payment of, or provision for payment of, all debts and liabilities of this corporation, shall be distributed to a nonprofit fund, foundation, or corporation which is organized and operated exclusive for charitable purposes and which has established its tax-exempt status under Section 501 (c)(3) of the Internal Revenue Code.

Date: January 22, 2005

José Mayorga, Director

Moses Salgado, Director

Lucio Loza, Director

Fernando Antelo, Director

Fig. 6.3 (continued)

Appointment of Initial Directors
and Adoption of Bylaws of
LATINO MEDICAL STUDENT CORPORATION
a California Nonprofit Public Benefit Corporation

The undersigned, being the Sole Incorporator of Latino Medical Student corporation, a California nonprofit public benefit corporation (the Corporation), adopts the following resolutions on behalf of the Corporation:

WHEREAS, no bylaws have been adopted for the regulation of the affairs of the Corporation;

WHEREAS, it is deemed to be in the best interest of the Corporation that the bylaws be adopted as the bylaws of the Corporation; and

WHEREAS, under California Corporations Code section 5134, the Sole Incorporator is authorized to adopt bylaws:

IT IS RESOLVED THAT the bylaws attached to these resolutions are adopted as the Corporation's bylaws; and

IT IS FURTHER RESOLVED THAT the Chief Information Officer (secretary) of the Corporation is authorized and directed to execute a certificate of the adoption of these bylaws, to insert the bylaws as so certified in the minute book of the Corporation, and to see that a copy of the bylaws, similarly certified, is kept at the principal office to transact the business of the Corporation.

WHEREAS, under California Corporations Code section 5134, the Sole Incorporator is authorized to elect the initial directors of the Corporation; and

WHEREAS, the bylaws specify the offices of each director,

IT IS RESOLVED THAT the persons listed below are hereby elected as the initial directors and to the offices indicated, to serve until they resign or are removed or until their successors are duly elected and qualified.

Tony Arredondo	Director and Chief Financial Officer
Jorge E. De Amorim Filho	Director and Medical Student Representative
Brandon Dow	Director and Medical Student Representative
Andrea Friaz-Gallardo	Director and Medical Student Representative
Zulma Galvan	Director and Medical Student Representative
Courtney Gonzales	Director and Medical Student Representative
Ignacio Guzman	Director and VP of Conference and Regional Programs
Omar Guzman	Director and VP of Community Affairs
Natalia Isaza	Director and Medical Student Representative
Cynthia La Morgese	Director and Medical Student Representative
Jeff Mora	Director and VP Conference & Regional Programs
Berenice Nava	Director and Medical Student Representative

Fig. 6.4 LMSA Inc. 501(c)(3) Not-for-profit Corporation Bylaws (©LMSA)

Johnny Orozco	Director and Medical Student Representative
Don Portocarrero	Director and VP of Scholarships
Joel Ramirez	Director and VP of Mentorship
Eunice V. Rivas	Director and Northern CEO
Rudy Rodriguez	Director and Medical Student Representative
Dennise Rosas	Director and Undergraduate Representative
Alberto Ruvalcaba	Director and VP of Communications
Eric Sandoval	Director and Southern CEO
Michelle Shuff	Director and Medical Student Representative
Efrain Talamantes	Director and VP of Website
Mario Diego Terán	Director and Medical Student Representative
Jesus Ulloa	Director and Medical Student Representative
Veronica Vasquez	Director and Medical Student Representative
René Venegas	Director and Medical Student Representative

Date: ___5/16/07___

Eric Sandoval, Sole Incorporator

Fig. 6.4 (continued)

Community, Continuity, Collaboration: The Formation of Regional Leadership Retreats

The first leadership retreat of the organization was created by leaders Omar Guzman (Southern CEO, UCI) and Natalia Isaza (Northern CEO, Stanford) and took place in 2007 at UCI. Ms. Emma Ledesma, the UCI Chapter advisor at the time, was instrumental in helping the LMSA leadership carry out the retreat. Medical student representatives and the various VPs of the organization were invited to attend this retreat and help plan out the organization's agenda and priorities for the upcoming year, in line with the organization's core values (Fig. 6.5). Recognizing the challenges faced by student leaders when they transitioned each year, the leadership was focused on maintaining the stability of the organization, preserving its nonprofit status, building its infrastructure further, and continuing to improve its ongoing programming. The theme selected that year was presented as the 3 C's: "Community, Continuity, Collaboration."

In line with this theme, leadership retreats have been repeated and expanded in subsequent years, with students gathering for one weekend in the summer. Traditionally, these meetings started with a welcome social event on Friday night. A full agenda of meetings would follow on Saturday. During this time, leadership provided historical context of the organization and other professional development activities to the medical student leaders who were part of the executive board. Mentorship and guidance were usually provided by physician members of the organization's Advisory Board, many of whom were alumni of LMSA or its antecedents. Once the theme was set for the year, it would be presented at the summer leadership conference. The co-chairs and MSRs of each chapter were invited to attend with reimbursement for their travel. The first leadership conference took place at

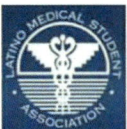

LATINO MEDICAL STUDENT ASSOCIATION, INC.

"Fostering Diverse Physicians for a Changing Society"

LMSA Core Values

The challenges that healthcare professionals face today require dynamic leadership capabilities and a strong commitment to key Core Values. LMSA is dedicated to preparing future health professionals for this rigorous journey. Our members practice these values in every aspect of their medical and personal lives. LMSA'ers share a common vision of serving those in need and dedicate their lives and careers to ensure everyone has access to healthcare. We provide our members with life-changing experiences that reaffirm and instill our Core Values:

1. **Community / Comunidad**

   Community or comunidad manifests itself when individuals from diverse backgrounds come together with a common dream or goal and build a safe environment based on mutual respect, trust and support. These elements create a passionate and perseverant family that can face and overcome adversity as individuals and in unison. LMSA's passion resonates throughout our lives and our commitment extends beyond healthcare to create a better world for all who live in it.

2. **Courage / Valor**

   Courage or valor is the quality or state of mind or spirit that allows one to act with confidence, resolve, and self-possession in the face of uncertainty and risk. LMSA is a community that seeks individuals who have the courage to make tough decisions and lead by example. Courage can be leaving ones friends and family to get an education, taking the most challenging courses at ones undergraduate or professional school, taking 8 hour exams on a Saturday morning, or making a commitment to help human kind by dedicating ones life to healthcare. LMSA continuously fosters courage by advocating for communities that have no voice or often ignored by society.

3. **Leadership / Liderazgo**

   Leadership or liderazgo is the capacity or ability to lead others under any condition, most importantly in-light of hardship. LMSA was founded by courageous leaders who compromised their medical educations to ensure that future underrepresented minorities receive fair educational opportunities, with the end-result of providing underserved communities with culturally competent healthcare. This leadership legacy has given our organization the drive to address educational and healthcare disparities at all levels. We know when to follow and get the job done, but we also know when to take the lead and make change happen!

4. **Consciousness / Conocimiento**

   Consciousness or conocimiento is a sense of one's personal or collective identity, including the attitudes, beliefs, and sensitivities held by or considered characteristic of an individual or group. LMSA is aware of the issues that affect underserved populations and the community at large. Our members continuously provide each other with opportunities to make a difference through community service. We reinforce our understanding of the Latino community by actively working in these communities. We serve our communities with pride and treat everyone with the up-most respect, constantly reminding ourselves of the communities we come from.

5. **Commitment / Compromiso**

   Commitment or compromiso is a state of being bound emotionally or intellectually to a course of action or to another person or persons. LMSA is committed to serving underserved communities and changing the face of healthcare to better meet the needs of a growing Latino population. Our LMSA'ers have committed themselves to challenging health professions and still maintain their commitment to serving others!

UCLA • UCSF • Drew • UCD • UCSD • Stanford • USC • UCI • Western • U of A • Utah

Fig. 6.5 Core Values of LMSA Inc. (2006) (©LMSA)

UCI in 2003, again with the help of UCI Chapter Advisor Ms. Ledesma. In 2007, then-VP of Mentorship Alvaro Galvis, MD, PhD, added a pre-medical component to the existing leadership conference structure; through this, pre-medical student leaders in their own organizations were invited to take part in professional development activities and networking events with medical students.

LEAP Year: The Enactment of Longitudinal Initiatives for LMSA Inc. Growth

Listen to the call of your brothers and sisters. The chains of oppression are strong- be it the MCAT, a guidance counselor, a professor or an economic situation. They have been left behind while we have become medical students. I joined LMSA to give that helping hand and create an attitude that

no man or woman will be left behind. This is the essence of LMSA's mission.
—Alvaro Galvis, MD, PhD, Southern CEO, in his election speech delivered during the 2008 LMSA Inc. Conference at UCD

By 2008, LMSA Inc. had achieved a transformation into a professional development organization. The infrastructure was in place to focus back on its roots of activism and mentorship for pre-medical students while becoming a leader in the struggle for national unification. In 2008, the medical student leaders of LMSA Inc. launched a new initiative to leverage this newly developed infrastructure and create meaningful and sustainable programs for the benefit of fellow trainees. Deriving its theme from 2008 being a leap year in the Gregorian calendar, the initiative was named LEAP Year, for Leadership, Evolution, Accountability, and Professionalism (Fig. 6.6). The LEAP year leadership was largely influenced by medical students Mario Teran (Northern CEO); Alvaro Galvis (Southern CEO); Jose Anaya (Chief Financial Officer); Minerva A. Romero Arenas (VP of Scholarships); Tatianne Velo (VP of Mentorship); and Karen Espino, who held a newly created position (VP of Policy).

Becas y Reconocimientos

Keeping in line with building the pipeline, LMSA Inc. continued to focus on providing scholarships to pre-medical students. The Sí Se Puede Scholarship was established in 2004 in partnership with Kaplan, Inc. to fund preparatory courses for the Medical College Admissions Test (MCAT). The agreement with Kaplan, Inc. was originally agreed upon in the 1980s with Stanley Kaplan himself, although later agreements would be handled between the students and Kaplan's executive leadership. The award was later renamed Janine Gonzalez, MD Scholarship, although the Kaplan courses remained as the award. The Amanda Perez, MD scholarship was established in 2008 and funded by Dr. Perez, an alumna of LMSA at the Charles Drew University Chapter. She served as MSR and later was in charge of the Scholarship Program when she served on the Executive Board for the Western Region. It would provide scholarships to high school seniors who were among the first generation in their families to attend college. Each year, at least 2 students were selected, though more could be awarded depending on annual fundrais-

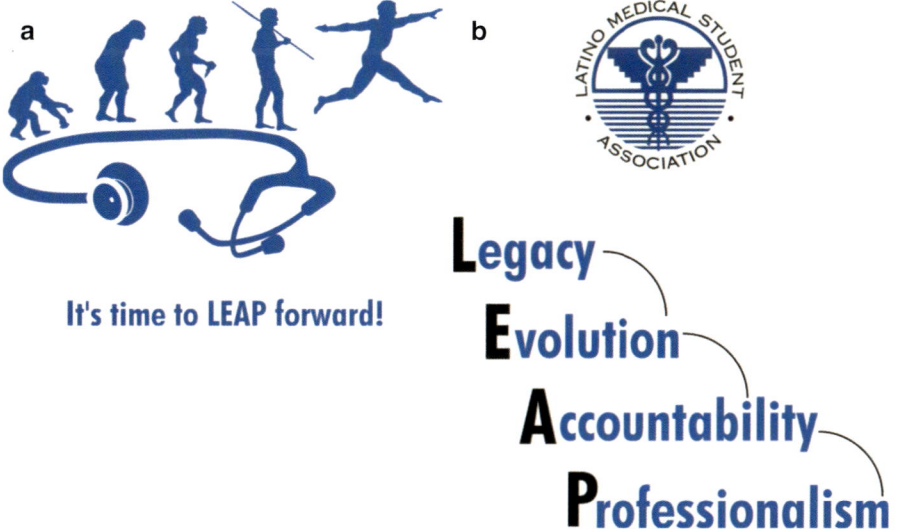

Fig. 6.6 LMSA Inc. LEAP Year, 2008–2009 (©LMSA), The logos shown were used as part of the LMSA Inc. Leadership Conference in 2008. (**a**) Front logo, as inspired by evolution theory. (**b**) Back logo defining the LEAP acronym

ing. A third scholarship, the Sí Se Puede AMCAS/AACOMAS® Scholarship, was established and funded through proceeds of the annual conference. This scholarship was designed to assist pre-medical students mitigate the financial burden of applying to accredited U.S. Medical Schools and to increase the pool of underrepresented students entering the medical profession.

In addition, LMSA also established awards to recognize and offer some support to the medical student members of the organization. These awards included the LMSA Community Service Award, the LMSA Medical Student Representative of the Year, and the Richard Juarez Commitment to the Community Award. Richard Juarez was a UCLA-Drew medical student who died unexpectedly during his fourth year of medical school. He was very involved in his school's chapter and a well-known student at other schools, as he held a medical student representative position on the regional board. Each chapter would submit its own nominees for the final vote by LMSA Inc. leaders, as organized by VP of Scholarships.

> The year I took over, we voted in having a scholarship for medical students. Before that we only had an MCAT scholarship for pre-medical students. The scholarship was based on merit, leadership, [and] commitment to the mission of LMSA. Everything was under supervision and evaluation was done by the advisors - like the LMSA Faculty/Community Advisors. Dr. Zapanta, Dr. Frank Meza, Emma Ledesma, Dr. Hector Flores.
> —Donald Portocarrero, DO, Western University; LMSA VP of Scholarship (2006–2007), MSR (2005–2006, 2007–2008)

Finally, the LMSA Faculty/Advisor Service Award was given to a faculty or administrator who was considered instrumental in supporting the goals and mission of LMSA throughout the year.

In 2006–2007, there were two new awards named after longtime LMSA mentor Bob Montoya, MD. He was an alumnus of the University of Southern California, where he was instrumental in establishing the Office of Minority Affairs (OMA) and the NCHO. He was known for his ability to work collaboratively with other groups, and this helped push for legislation at the federal, state, and local levels. He initiated and directed California's Health Profession's Career Opportunity Program and developed partnerships with the state's nine medical schools, four dental schools, and three public health schools in existence at the time, directly contributing to the establishment of the OMA's at the University of California medical school campuses. Dr. Montoya also initiated and directed the Minority Medical Education and Training Shortage Area Elective/Preceptorship and the California Shortage Area Medical Matching Programs, whose purpose was to prepare medical, physician assistant, and nursing students and residents for practice in medical shortage areas and then match them to jobs at clinics and practices in those areas. Dr. Montoya inspired and helped countless trainees with his efforts to strengthen the pipeline of medical education for minority students and bolster care provided to communities in need.

These awards were initiated by the 2006 leadership and the first awards were granted in 2007. The medical student award was to be granted to candidates who demonstrated a desire to advance the state of healthcare and education in Latino communities through leadership in extracurricular activities and/or membership in civic organizations and commitment to the mission of LMSA Inc. The Lifetime Achievement Award was awarded to senior physicians or other health professions faculty who demonstrated consistent dedication to the advancement of the Latino community and Latino medical students as voted by the LMSA Inc. chapters. The first award was presented to Dr. Montoya in 2007. The second was awarded to Dr. Frank Meza in 2008, who, in addition to being a tremendous mentor and earning many accolades as a physician, was a founder and served as National Chair of Chicanos for Creative Medicine (1972–1975), was on staff at the Brown Beret Barrio Free Clinic (1969–1970), and contributed to the organization tremendously. The third was to Dr. Hayes-Bautista in 2009.

Minerva Romero Arenas, VP of Scholarship (circa 2009), restructured the LMSA scholarship and award programs. These changes were meant to meet the changing needs of the students served and to increase the sustainability and quality of these programs. Such changes included revising application materials for pre-medical students to help use the LMSA scholarships as a test-run of their application to medical school, and providing detailed feedback to all undergraduate students who applied. The partnership with Kaplan, Inc. was also expanded to increase benefits to LMSA members and more undergraduate students.

Building the Pipeline: El Futuro

To create closer ties between LMSA Inc. and other pre-medical student societies, LMSA Inc. created new positions in its leadership team. These included the VPs of undergraduate relations (one each for the northern and southern regions of LMSA), who would work closely with the VP of Mentorship. These positions were filled by premedical students who served as liaisons between LMSA and the Latino premedical student groups, particularly the largest groups in California: CCM and CHE. These positions would help provide opportunities for leadership to pre-medical students and mentorship from current LMSA medical students. In addition, the VPs of undergraduate relations developed more mentoring opportunities locally and worked to increase participation in the pre-medical track at the LMSA conferences. Additional positions including the VP of Community Affairs, Newsletter, and Website were modified to allow leadership by premedical students. Moreover, any board position could have pre-medical interns that work closely with the board member in carrying out the duties of that office, again with the goal of providing opportunities for mentorship and leadership to the students who would eventually be applying to medical school themselves. The annual leadership conference created a completely funded and separate program for undergraduate/premedical student leadership development. In addition, selected premedical students from across the region were funded to attend the conference and registration was free for all premedical students.

La Política: LMSA Delves into Policy

In 2009, LMSA created the VP of Policy to oversee a full committee with 5 members and eventually initiate a policy summit in the fall. Karen Espino was the first person to hold that leadership position. The first step was to provide a Physician Advocacy Training and Action, which was done in collaboration with the American Medical Students Association. Student members of LMSA were invited to join the Policy Committee, which was charged with developing an agenda and set of stances for LMSA Inc. to support, with approval from MSRs across the region. In the following years, LMSA Inc. began to take formal policy stances ranging from endorsing universal health care as a right to affirming support for women's right to choose abortion.

Activism flourished in the organization. Efforts were made to collaborate with organizations such as Border Angels and Flying Samaritans to help provide medical treatment for undocumented immigrants on the California border with Mexico. LMSA Inc. became a co-sponsor with the California Health Professionals Student Alliance (CaHPSA) for lobby day, an event in which medical students from across the state lobby in Sacramento in support of legislation towards healthcare equality and the establishment of a fundamental right to healthcare. The organization joined the Unite Here Local 2 union boycott of all Starwood Hotels in San Francisco. At that time, hotel workers that had a Latino majority were being asked to work without a new contract that had expired in 2004 without any health insurance benefits or raise in wages. LMSA had previously made contractual agreements with a Starwood Hotel to host the regional conference but the event was moved in solidarity with the union at the cost of losing a deposit of $5000 paid to the hotel. This new activism became a launching pad for the organization. As LMSA West coalesced with LMSA

National, this would also influence the eventual creation of a National Policy Summit and the LMSA National Policy Chair.

National Unification: LMSA Inc. Becomes LMSA West

> See the moment, seize the moment.
> —Hector Flores, MD, at the 2008 NNLAMS GLAS and LMSA Inc. Leadership Conference

As LMSA Inc. in the West grew in their operations and programming, so did its counterparts in other regions of the U.S. Since the turn of the twenty-first century, regional entities had been collaborating with each other through a national consortium known as the National Network of Latin American Medical Students (NNLAMS). While an initial push for the creation of a unified voice for Latino medical students and physicians led to the establishment of NNLAMS, later pushes called for an even greater extent of national unification. As part of this later struggle, Dr. Phil DeChavez, NNLAMS executive director, and Ruben Font, Jr., then the National Coordinator of NNLAMS, attended the 2008 LMSA conference and met with the new regional CEOs to launch a concerted effort for national unification. At this meeting, leaders made arrangements to utilize LMSA as the national name and outlined the process of unification that was advocated for over the next few years. Additionally, the leaders arranged for the NNLAMS' Garcia Leadership and Advocacy Seminar (GLAS) to take place in conjunction with the 2008 LMSA Inc. summer Leadership Conference hosted by UCSD in San Diego, CA.

By the end of March 2009, all other NNLAMS regions had voted in favor of unification under one common name and selected Galvis, then the LMSA Southern CEO, to serve as the first LMSA National Coordinator. LMSA Inc. leadership then voted at their 25th Annual Conference hosted by UCLA to change their name to LMSA-West, give the LMSA name, website, and entity to NNLAMS, and make the official name change effective at the end of the 2010 fiscal year. The 2011 conference, titled "Uniting our Voices for Justice in Healthcare," represented a culmination of the unification efforts and celebration of all aspects of LMSA (Fig. 6.1). It was the first conference for which all regions and the national organization officially shared the LMSA name. This event also represented the 27th now LMSA West Regional Conference, as well as the 12th annual UCI LMSA-West chapter premedical conference—which, at the time, was the largest premedical student conference in California. The conference itself was the largest to date for LMSA, with 120 exhibitors; 250 high school students bused in from the Santa Ana Unified School District; 1100 premedical students overall; 500 medical students; 110 residents; and numerous physicians. There were conference tracks for high school, community college, college juniors and seniors, post-baccalaureate premedical students, medical students, and residents. By the end of the conference, everyone was part of the LMSA familia.

> I had the opportunity to be elected as a Northern CEO during my last year of medical school. I was the first openly gay person elected to this position. I am very proud of how accepting and inclusive LMSA is.
> —Manuel Mendoza, MD, LMSA Inc. Northern CEO (2009–2010)

Overview of LMSA West

The Latino Medical Student Association West (LMSA-West) was established in 2009, after a series of name changes and the formalization of a national unification movement amongst various medical student organizations catering to Hispanics/Latinos. The mission of LMSA West is to recruit and support individuals in the health-care professions who will strive to improve the access and delivery of healthcare to Latinos and medically underserved populations. The LMSA West Region encompasses medical schools from Alaska, Washington, Oregon, Idaho, Montana, Wyoming, California, Nevada, Utah, Arizona, and Hawaii. As of the academic year 2019–2020, there were 19 active chapters, as shown in Table 6.1.

The LMSA West continues to carry out its mission with the LHS+ community through leadership, mentorship, and professional development. In addition to the chapter leadership and MSRs, the LMSA West Regional Board includes 17 leadership positions for medical students and 2 for pre-medical students (see Table 6.2). The CEO positions were renamed Co-Directors, though the designations of one for each of the Northern and Southern regions of LMSA West remain and the Director-Elect was added to help provide an opportunity to learn more about the role. Several positions have been doubled to allow for co-leadership, such as the VP of Policy (North/South), VP of Mentorship (North/South), and VP of Scholarship (Co-VP). The VP of Undergraduate Relations positions was renamed Northern and Southern Undergrad Representative (Table 6.3).

The regional executive board continues to encourage individual chapter events and programming. Chapters may apply for the mini-grants program through LMSA West to fund innovative projects and programs that help LMSA meet its mission. Each year, active LMSA-West Chapters are eligible to receive up to $1000 in mini-grant funding.

The region continues to hold two major annual events for professional development and networking: the Summer Leadership Conference and the Annual Regional Conference. Both are attended by several hundred premedical, medical students, and alumni. Many LMSA alumni seek to give back to the organization and have come back to serve on its Advisory Board to help provide advice, guidance, and organizational memory to LMSA West. Current Advisory Board Members include Drs. Amanda Perez, Margarita Loeza, Daniel Cabrera, Donald Portocarrero, Amy Garcia, and Lisa Montes. Other alumni who previously served as members of the Advisory Board include Drs. Richard Zapanta, Fernando Antelo, Jose Avalos, Alberto Manetta, and Mario San Bartolome.

Table 6.2 Current LMSA West Regional Board Leadership Positions (as of December 2022)

1. Northern Co-Director
1. Southern Co-Director
2. Director-Elect
3. Chief Financial Officer
4. Chief Information Officer
5. VP of Internal Affairs
6. VP of Medical Education
7. VP of Research and Analytics
8. VP of Policy (North)
9. VP of Policy (South)
10. VP of Mentorship (North)
11. VP of Mentorship (South)
12. VP of Community Affairs
13. Co-VP of Scholarships [2]
14. VP of Conference
15. VP of Development
16. VP of Social Media & Outreach
17. Southern Undergrad Representative
18. Northern Undergrad Representative

Table 6.3 LMSA (West) Annual Conference with Titles, Host Institution, and Artwork. (All artwork property of LMSA) (©LMSA)

Year	Conference Title	Host School	
2022	Nuestra Gente Resiliente: Empowering Our Communities and Building Our Future	UCSD	
2021[a]	Potenciar El Cambio: Empowering Interconnection In Healthcare to Create Change	UCI, OHSU	
2020	Potenciar El Cambio: Empowering Interconnection In Healthcare to Create Change [Canceled due to COVID-19 Global Pandemic]	UCI	
2019	We Belong! Luchando por Nuestro Lugar. Stanford	Stanford	

Year	Conference Title	Host School	
2018	Breaking Borders, Building Bridges: Paving the Future of Medicine	UCLA	
2017	Unidos en Acción: Calling to action, Moving to action, and Sustaining action with our communities	UCSF	
2016[a]	Prevenir es Curar: Addressing New Obstacles and Improving Healthcare in our Communities	WUHS	

Year	Conference Title	Host School	
2015	Manteniendo Nuestras Raíces, Branching Towards Success.	USC	
2014	Transforming our script in medicine: advancing leadership, policy, research, and community	UCD	
2013	Waves of Change: Improving the Health of our Community	UCSD	

Year	Conference Title	Host School	
2012	At a Crossroads: Ensuring a Healthy Future	Stanford	
2011[a]	Uniting Our Voices for Justice in Healthcare	UCI	
2010	Welcoming Change: Bridging Gaps for Latinos by Changing Health Policy	UCSF	

Year	Conference Title	Host School	
2009	The Power of 25: The Healing Legacy Continue	UCLA	

[a] The 2011, 2016, and 2021 Conferences served as both the LMSA National and the LMSA West Regional Conference

Unidos Podemos Más: Collaborations

While the students who join LMSA West tend to be Hispanic/Latino in ethnic origin, the organization is open to all students who share the vision of the organization. Students of LMSA West often have formed alliances with other student organizations. These collaborations have been particularly lasting when made with student organizations from backgrounds considered Underrepresented in Medicine, such as the Student National Medical Association (SNMA) and the Association of Native American Medical Students (ANAMS). Seeing similar problems in their communities, the lack of representation in medicine, and interests in bringing about social justice and change, common programming was sought.

One example was the Pre-Health Conference co-hosted by LMSA and SNMA at UC Irvine. The conference offers undergraduate students a wide variety of workshops to expose them to various health career pathways. The 18th annual conference was held in November 2019. At chapters including Arizona, Utah, Oregon, and Washington, the students of the various racial and/or ethnic minoritized groups like ANAMS, SNMA, LMSA, and the Asian Pacific American Medical Student Association (APAMSA) have routinely held social events and supported each others' lectures, fundraisers, and conference events.

At Stanford, a coalition formed of medical student representatives from APAMSA, LMSA, SNMA, Stanford American Indigenous Medical Association (SAIMA), LGBTQ-Meds, and Stanford Muslim Medical Association (SMMA). Named the Stanford University Minority Medical Alliance (SUMMA), its annual pre-medical student conference aims to increase diversity in the health professions in order to better care for underserved communities. The annual SUMMA pre-medical conference is one of the oldest on the U.S. West Coast and draws hundreds of students from throughout the Bay Area. The SUMMA is supported by the Center of Excellence for Diversity in Medical Education (COEDME). Established in 1993 with the assistance of a grant sponsored by the U.S. federal Health Resources and Services Administration, the goal of the

COEDME is to prepare the next generation of medical leaders to address the health issues of a diverse society.

Recently, LMSA West has also worked closely with the Alliance in Mentorship (Mi Mentor). This 501(c)(3) non-profit network was formed in 2012 by LMSA alumni, who envisioned peer-to-peer mentoring in addition to medical students to pre-medical mentorship. The Mi Mentor partnership led to the "Get on the Bus" Campaign, whereby students are able to attend the annual LMSA Regional Conference with travel (chartered bus), lodging, and conference registration provided at a very low cost ($30 USD, in 2019).

> We also collaborate with MiMentor because we get to see these pre-med students and it's amazing to give back to people who have gone through the same things that you have and you are able to inspire them to become a physician.
> —Maria Zepeda, Medical Student, UC Davis LMSA Chapter Co-Chair

Additional LMSA West Programming

The LMSA West region continues to engage actively in health policy affecting the Latino and other vulnerable and/or underserved communities. The VP of Policy position was expanded to have one leader in each of the Northern and Southern regions of LMSA West. Some of the issues that the organization has delved into in the last decade include advocacy in support of people who are undocumented but brought to the U.S. as minors, commonly termed DREAMer or DACA-students after the acronyms for legislation (Development, Relief, and Education for Alien Minors Act or Deferred Action on Childhood Arrivals). More recently, students have also delved into advocacy regarding the treatment of asylum-seekers.

Lastly, the LMSA West Scholarship program continues to offer several of the original scholarships, including the Amanda Perez, MD scholarship; Janine Gonzalez, MD MCAT scholarship; and the Sí Se Puede Scholarship. More recently, the organization established the High School Pipeline Program Scholarship for pre-medical students, the Cinthya Felix Scholarship for pre-health students, and the DREAMers of Tomorrow Scholarships to support undocumented medical and pre-medical students attending school in the states served by LMSA West. Additionally, the Latino Health Research Scholarship was developed in 2017 to support, encourage, and facilitate scholarly research and academic engagement by LMSA-West medical students. In recent years, the scholarship program of LMSA West has received significant support from AltaMed Health Services Corporation.

El futuro: LMSA West 2022 and Beyond

LMSA West has demonstrated tremendous growth in its first decade of existence following unification. Its success is rooted in the long history of student activism present in the region since the 1960s. This activism has driven generation after generation of LMSA students to advocate for their communities. Moreover, activism represents such an important aspect of the organization's values that not one but two members of the regional board are to focus on policy. Individual LMSA chapters each continue to develop mentorship programs with local premedical organizations and individuals, many funded through the mini-grants that the regional organization provides. Regional conferences and the LMSA National Conference continue to provide opportunities for mentorship and networking along the pipeline of medical education.

Minerva Romero Arenas, MD, MPH, FACS (former VP of Scholarships) recounts:

> I was a member and student leader in LMSA (West) at the University of Arizona—Tucson. The connections I made and the valuable leadership skills I developed while in LMSA placed me in a position to confidently become one of the four founding members of the Latino Surgical Society (LSS) after residency. Two of the other three founding members of LSS, Joseph López, MD and Gezzer Ortega, MD, were student leaders of LMSA a their respective institutions, during their medical school tenure. The fourth founding mem-

ber, Joseph Fernández-Moure, MD, was an ally and supporter of LMSA. The benefits of LMSA are not for medical school days alone.

Through the innovative use of digital platforms such as Mighty Networks and Zoho, LMSA West strives to connect pre-medical and medical students to physician mentors for career advice, allows members to engage with each other virtually, and build community throughout the year. Collectively, these efforts will continue to improve the landscape of healthcare for LHS+ trainees, physicians, and patients in the West and beyond.

> LMSA gives a lot of motivation to the pre-medical students. My cousin and I were the first ones to pursue any education, much less higher education in my family. My mom was undocumented immigrant and had not even primary education and my dad did not go to elementary school. My tío, my cousin's dad, was a bracero. What my cousin and I did was a huge leap for my family. LMSA kept me motivated. It was really important for me to see someone who looked like me graduate.
> —Margarita Loeza, MD, UCSD alumna and LMSA Inc. leader [MSR, Treasurer, Conference Coordinator, Southern Co-Chair]

References

1. The Chicano Civil Rights Movement. The Library of Congress; 2011. https://www.loc.gov/item/ihas.200197398/

2. Michals D. Dolores Huerta; 2015. National Women's History Museum. https://www.womenshistory.org/education-resources/biographies/dolores-huerta

3. Rosales FA. Dictionary of Latino Civil Rights History. Houston, TX: Arte Publico Press; 2006.

4. Renteria TH. The Familia: cohesion and conflict. In: Chicano professionals: culture, conflict, and identity. London: Routledge; 2013.

5. Montes L. A Tribute to Dr. Frank Meza. Latinx Physicians of California; 2020, January 24. https://latinxphysiciansofca.org/drfrankmezatribute/

6. Castillo-Page L.. Diversity in Medical Education: Facts & Figures 2016. Association of American Medical Colleges; 2016.

7. National Institutes of Health. Changing the Face of Medicine | Elena V. Rios. U.S. National Library of Medicine. Retrieved January 30, 2023, from https://cfmedicine.nlm.nih.gov/physicians/biography_270.html; 2015, June 3.

8. Regents of the University of California v. Bakke, 438 U.S. 265, 98 S.Ct. 2733, 57 L.Ed.2d 750; 1978.

9. Brown Beret Headquarters | Los Angeles Conservancy; 2019. LAconservancy.org. https://www.laconservancy.org/locations/brown-beret-headquarters

10. El Barrio Free Clinic | Los Angeles Conservancy; n.d. LAconservancy.org. https://www.laconservancy.org/locations/el-barrio-free-clinic

11. History of Clínica Tepati; n.d.. Clinica-Tepati. Retrieved January 30, 2023, from http://clinicatepati.com/about-clinica/history-of-clinica/

12. Our History – UC Irvine Outreach Clinics; 2023. UCIoutreachclinics.org. https://www.ucioutreach-clinics.org/about/our-history/

13. Doctor Addresses Minorities' Health-Care Needs; n.d. Chicago Tribune. Retrieved January 30, 2023, from https://www.chicagotribune.com/news/ct-xpm-1999-06-07-9906070161-story.html

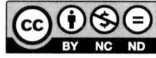

A Unified National Organization: The Budding of LMSA

Elizabeth Homan Sandoval, Edgar Figueroa,
Victor Cueto, Donald Rodriguez, Julia Su,
and Alvaro E. Galvis

"Wisdom lies neither in fixity nor in change, but in the dialectic between the two."

— *Octavio Paz*

On the Brink of a National Union

In order to set the stage for the creation of a national Latino medical student association, political advocacy and advancement for Latinos in the United States had to occur. The GI Bill, the 1958 National Defense Education Act (NDEA), and the 1964 Higher Education Act (Civil Rights Act) opened new opportunities for low income and minority students to attain higher education, especially Chicanos [1]. The "blowouts" and "walkouts" led by high school students of East Los Angeles during March 1968 helped spark the rise of the Chicano Rights Movement [2]. Student-led organizations flourished, with examples including La Raza Unida; Organization of Latin American Students; the Hijas de Cuauhtémoc; the Mexican American Youth Organization; and the United Mexican American Students (UMAS), which later became El Movimiento Estudiantil Chicano de Aztlán (MEChA) [2–4].

By the late 1960s, there were Latino students in medical schools across the U.S. who saw a need to organize, support each other, and mentor premedical students aspiring to pursue medicine. In 1972, Jaime Rivera, MD, and Emilio Carillo, MD—then Harvard medical students and members of the political and social action organization known as the Young Lords [5]—founded the Boricua Health Organization (BHO). BHO went on to form a network of student chapters at other medical schools in the Northeast, eventually becoming the National Boricua Latino Health Organization (NBLHO) and then the Latino Medical Student Association (LMSA) Northeast.

E. H. Sandoval (✉)
University of Iowa Hospitals and Clinics, Iowa City, IA, USA
e-mail: elizabeth-homan@uiowa.edu

E. Figueroa
Weill Cornell Medical College, New York, NY, USA

V. Cueto
Department of Pediatrics and Internal Medicine, University of Miami, Miller School of Medicine, Miami, FL, USA

D. Rodriguez
The University of Chicago Pritzker School of Medicine, Chicago, IL, USA

J. Su
Donald and Barbara Zucker School of Medicine at Hofstra/Northwell, Long Island, NY, USA

A. E. Galvis
Department of Pediatrics, Division of Pediatric Infectious Diseases, Loma Linda University Children's Health, Loma Linda, CA, USA

© The Author(s) 2024
J. P. Sánchez, D. Rodriguez (eds.), *Latino, Hispanic, or of Spanish Origin+ Identified Student Leaders in Medicine*, Sustainable Development Goals Series, https://doi.org/10.1007/978-3-031-35020-7_7

Around the same time, a group of medical and dental students from California, Arizona, Texas, Colorado, and New Mexico met at the University of California, San Francisco (UCSF); these pre-health, medical and dental school Chicano students came together to form the National Chicano Health Organization (NCHO) [6–8]. A similar organization called La Raza Medical Association (abbreviated La RaMA) emerged at a Fresno meeting of medical students from many California medical schools on December 18, 1976 [9]. In 1983, NHCO and La RaMA merged to create the Chicano/Latino Medical Student Association (CMSA), now known as LMSA West. While these organizations looked to other established national medical student organizations for inspiration, their beginnings differed greatly.

Early Steps Leading to the National Network of Latin American Medical Students

While LMSA had its beginnings from student efforts at individual medical schools, other national medical student organizations were off-shoots from larger parent organizations. For example, the American Medical Association (AMA) formed the Student American Medical Association, the precursor to today's American Medical Student Association (AMSA) in the 1950s as a way to get students involved in organized medicine [10]. The National Medical Association (NMA) was formed in 1895 as the major professional organization for African American doctors and health professionals who were excluded from white organizations like the AMA. The NMA played an important role in the passage of the Civil Rights Act of 1964 and the president of this organization helped establish the Student National Medical Association (SNMA) as a means of supporting students and encouraging them to pursue a career in medicine [11, 12].

AMSA and SNMA, though distinct, shared a parallel history, where the student sections "broke off" from the parent organization for various reasons; these included a mix of differences in political ideology, desire for programmatic autonomy,

administrative demands and funding. Today, both organizations are thriving, well-established, independent non-profit organizations with large student members in medical school chapters across the country. The two organizations also have numerous staff, property including stocks, and gross receipts of over $1 million (SNMA) and $3 million (AMSA) according to recent 2018 IRS tax records [13, 14].

Latino medical student groups had a different developmental experience. As outlined in other chapters of this book, Latino medical students formed their local and then regional organizations in response to personal and community needs using grassroots approaches. These organizations were rooted primarily in ethnic enclaves with strong cultural identities: Puerto Ricans in the Northeast, Cubans in the Southeast, Chicanos in the West, Mexican Americans in the Southwest, and Puerto Rican and Chicanos in the Midwest. Later waves of immigration would eventually introduce other Latino groups into the medical student pool. These regional Latino medical student groups each had their own rich history, had differing extents of reach and popularity within their respective geographical areas, and had variable financial stability. Some were plagued by the usual issues that student groups face (e.g. diminished student interest and lack of institutional support). They struggled with yearly turnover of leaders on the chapter, regional and national levels. Another challenge was the lack of infrastructure, such as permanent staff or offices. Moreover, there was also limited advising and mentorship on how to grow an organization due to lack of connection to a 'parent' organization.

In 1994, the National Hispanic Medical Association (NHMA) was founded to unify physician leaders around the country to address Hispanic health [15]. Co-founder, Elena Rios, MD, MSPH, had been instrumental in the founding of the West regional medical organization as a medical student in 1982. Dr. Rios also organized regional student leaders to form a national network of Latino medical students in 1987. This network, however, never took hold nationally among medical students, as reported by alumni from the mid-1990s—to the point that NBLHO and CMSA leadership in 1998 had no awareness of it. Years later, with the formation of NHMA, there was increased enthusiasm in revisiting the idea of a national organization for Latino medical students.

By the late 1990s, NHMA had reached out and encouraged student leaders from the various regional groups to attend the first NHMA conference held in Washington, DC in 1997. Due to rumors among the student leaders that NHMA was considering starting their own medical student group, the existing regional medical student organizations (e.g., CMSA, NBLHO, etc.) wanted to preserve the integrity of their regions. The conference created a natural opportunity for the student leaders from the various organizations to come together to discuss their regional organizations, successes and opportunities, and learn more about the NHMA. While there are no known records from those gatherings, meeting notes in an email to an NBLHO member indicated that, by 1998, the regional organizations agreed towards working together as a consortium with the aspiration to form a national organization (E. Figueroa, personal communication, 2020). The two largest groups, the CMSA, representing the West coast, and NBLHO, representing the Northeast, would participate under the conditions that neither organization would give up their history and autonomy and that there would **not** be a new organization dictating how their regions must operate. The other three regions agreed.

Rise of the National Network of Latin American Medical Students (NNLAMS)

> We cannot seek achievement for ourselves and forget about progress and prosperity for our community…Our ambitions must be broad enough to include the aspirations and needs of others, for their sakes and for our own.
> —César Chávez

In March of 1998, the leaders of the five regional groups agreed to form the National Network of Latin American Medical Students (NNLAMS).

The leaders of the following five regional organizations would serve as the ruling body of the organization called the NNLAMS Board of Directors: Latino Midwest Medical Student Association (LMMSA; Midwest), National Boricua Latino Health Organization (NBLHO; Northeast), Hispanic American Medical Student Association (HAMSA; Southeast), Texas Association of Latino American Medical Students (TALAMS; Southwest), and Chicano/Latino Medical Student Association (CMSA; West). As the inaugural National Coordinator, the board selected Fausto Meza, MD (Table 7.1), from the University of Texas Medical Branch at Galveston. Though there was agreement to align, the discussion was heated and lengthy to find a consensus on the national name. Fidencio Saldaña, MD, served as Fundraising Chair for

Table 7.1 History of NNLAMS and LMSA National Coordinators & Presidents

Regional Designation Key: MW, Midwest; NE, Northeast; SE, Southeast; SW, Southwest; W, West
1999–2000 Fausto Meza, MD- SW (First NNLAMS National Coordinator)
2000–2001 Nicholas Arredondo, MD-SW
2001–2002 Luis Humberto Macías, MD-W
2002–2003 Daniel Macías, MD-W
2003–2004 Omar Rashid, MD, JD-SE
2004–2005 Eddie Machado, MD, MBA-NE
2005–2006 Tony Olivera, MD, PhD-SW
2006–2007 Gerardo Solario, MD- NE
2007–2008 Daniel Correa, MD-NE
2008–2009 Ruben Font Jr., MD-MW
2009–2010 Julia Bregand-White, MD-MW (First Latina National Coordinator)
2010–2011 Alvaro Galvis, MD, PhD-W (First use of the term "National President")
2011–2012 Raymond Morales, MD, PhD-MW
2012–2013 Emma Olivera, MD- MW
2013–2014 Alvaro Galvis, MD, PhD-W
2014–2015 Amanda Hernández, MD, PhD-NE
2015–2016 Abner A. Murray, MD, PhD-MW
2016–2017 Eric R. Molina, MD, PhD-SW
2017–2018 Eric R. Molina MD, PhD-SW
2018–2019 Lucas Warton, DO-NE (First DO medical student National President)
2019–2020 Julia Su, PhD (MD Candidate)-NE (First self-identified ally elected as National President)
2020–2021 Donald Rodríguez, PhD (MD Candidate)-MW
2021–2022 Karina Diaz, PhD (MD Candidate)-W
2022–2023 Gualberto Muñoz (MD Candidate)-SE; Roxie Lazo Gonzalez (MD Candidate)-SE

NNLAMS from 1999 to 2001. As an attendee of NNLAMS's first Garcia Leadership & Advocacy Seminar (GLAS) in Galveston, TX (Table 7.2), Dr. Saldaña recalls the debate surrounding which organizational name to use:

> In our sense, it was the first time recognizing the importance of national connections and blending a Latino diaspora across the United States. It was a recognition of the importance of coming together, how big our Latino community was, and that GLAS was recognizing how to foster these leaders, the first steps.

However, there was deep concern about loss of regional autonomy, finances, history and identity in the movement to unify nationally.

The politics of identity is a particularly repetitive theme when organizing Latinos/Hispanics, as linguistic, socioeconomic, and numerous other differences exist within this single demographic. Although many Latino students are Spanish speaking, not all are; even within the Spanish language, different accents, phrases, and word definitions are used depending on country of origin. In terms of immigration status, some students were born in the United States to families who have resided for

Table 7.2 History of NNLAMS/LMSA National GLAS and LMSA Policy Summit Conferences

2000, 2001 University of Texas Galveston 1st and 2nd GLAS
2002 University of California Los Angeles 3rd GLAS
2003 University of Texas Galveston 4th GLAS
2004, 2005 Duke Durham, NC 5th and 6th GLAS
2006 Mt. Sinai School of Medicine NY 7th GLAS
2007 GLAS canceled due to lack of financial support
2008 University of California San Diego 9th GLAS
2009 University of Illinois at Chicago 10th GLAS
2010 Boston, Massachusetts 11th GLAS
2011 Duke Durham, NC 12th GLAS
2012, 2013, 2014, 2015 Doctors Hospital Renaissance Edinburg, TX 13th to 16th GLAS
2014. 2015 1st and 2nd National LMSA Policy Summit at NHMA National Conference in DC
2016 3rd National LMSA Policy Summit at George Washington University DC
2017, 2018, 2019 4th to 6th National LMSA Policy Summit at Association of American Medical Colleges DC
2020 LMSA National Virtual Policy Summit
2021 LMSA National Virtual Policy Summit
2022 (moved to Spring 2023)

generations on land that formerly existed under Mexican or Spanish rule. Other students whose families more recently immigrated from Cuba, Mexico, Venezuela, El Salvador, or other Latin American countries have had vastly different lived experiences, especially with the U.S. immigration system. Some students have had one parent who identifies as Latino and another parent who has not, representing broad diversity in cultures and ethnicities. Some of the students were the first in their family to attend college, while others came from generations of physicians. It is with this background of differences that the members came to the table to negotiate an organizational name. The words in the name NNLAMS were carefully considered, as each conveyed identity and/or hierarchy; both of these needed to be balanced. Thus, it was agreed that the national structure would be a "network" and that the national leader would be a "coordinator"—not a president. In addition, the identity term chosen was not Hispanic, Chicano, Boricua, or Latino, but rather Latin American.

The 1999–2000 academic year saw significant progress towards building a unified, national Latino medical student organization. During this time, there was ongoing two-way communication between NNLAMS and the regional organizations, consisting of regular conference calls and emails. For the first time, all regions were coordinating small scale projects to deploy simultaneously, such as student surveys, bone marrow donor registration drives, and leadership development conferences. One of the NNLAMS national officer positions was the American Medical Association/Council of Medical Student Organizations Liaison (AMA/CMSO). From its inception in 1999, NNLAMS had a vote in the AMA Medical Student Section. In February 2000, NNLAMS leaders were invited to attend the 4th annual NHMA conference in Washington, DC, and were provided conference space and a time for meeting to discuss organizational matters and network. Over 150 pre-medical and medical students were registered to participate in NNLAMS at the NHMA conference. By March 2000, the

NNLAMS board had drafted their own constitution, and regional organizations began the process to update their own organizational documents to reflect their membership in the consortium. Importantly, NNLAMS clarified that they were not, nor never had been, the official student arm of the NHMA.

Per its constitution's mission statement, NNLAMS was "founded to represent, support, educate, and unify U.S. Latino/a medical students." The organization's objectives were as follows:

- "To unify the body of Latino medical students in the U.S.;
- To actively promote recruitment and retention programs at all levels for Latinos;
- To educate Latino medical students on health issues; to protect and advocate for the rights and interests of Latinos in health care, both as providers and consumers;
- To promote leadership opportunities for Latinos in medicine; and
- To promote volunteerism in the Latino community." (See Fig. 7.1.)

N.N.L.A.M.S.

National Network of Latin American Medical Students

NNLAMS Newsletter   **Vol I Issue 1 - Fall 2005**

NNLAMS History	**GLAS 2005**	**Dr. Hector Garcia**	**Duke University**	**NNLAMS 1st National Conference 2006**	**Next Newsletter**
Learn about NNLAMS, an important national organization for Latino medical students. **Page 1**	Latino medical student leaders nationwide are invited to further their careers with leadership and advocacy skills. **Page 1**	Bio of the physician that is honored by our leadership seminar, GLAS. **Page 2**	Learn about Duke University's Support of GLAS & NNLAMS! **Page 2**	Read about the historic NHMA and NNLAMS partnership to develop the conference for us! **Page 2**	We're making plans for the next edition. See how you can get involved! **Page 3**

NNLAMS

For over thirty years, Latin American medical students have been organized in regional organizations, pursuing their goals to eliminate disparities in health care.

In 1987, regional Latin American medical student entities formed a National Network of Latin American Medical Students (NNLAMS) in order to:

- Unify all Latino medical students in one organization.
- Actively promote recruitment and retention of Latino Students at all levels.
- Educate medical students on Latino health issues.
- Act as advocates for the rights of Latinos in health care.
- Provide leadership opportunities for Latinos.
- Promote volunteerism in the Latino community.

In 2003 all five regional organizations incorporated under one national name and filed as one unified national non-profit, tax-exempt organization.

In 2004, NNLAMS, Inc. established an NNLAMS Alumni Board of Trustees, with long-term tenure, that is composed of

physician alumni involved with NNLAMS for over ten years.

With this infrastructure, we can ensure the stability, continuity, permanence and long-term vision of NNLAMS.

6th Annual G.L.A.S

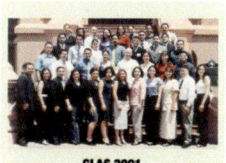

GLAS 2001

You've heard about it. We're excited about it. Now time to find out more!

Committee Chair Ali Rashid MS, USF-SOM MSI, NNLAMS alumnus Philip DeChavez MD MPH, and Omar Rashid, Duke-SOM/SOL MDc/JDc organized the NNLAMS' 6th Annual Dr. Hector P. Garcia Leadership and Advocacy Seminar (GLAS) at Duke University's Fuqua School of Business R.D. Thomas Executive Conference Center on September 9th - 11th, 2005. The focus of the event was to further develop the national Latino physician leadership of our country to improve the quality of and access to health care and medical education for all.

Participants included Latino medical student leaders and alumni physicians from across the country, including Dr. Elena Rios, President of the National Hispanic Medical Association, Dr. Rene Rodriguez, President of the Inter-American College of Physicians and Surgeons, Dr. Jaime "Gus" Rivera, Director of the Division of Public Health of the Department of Health and Human Services of the State of Delaware, and Dr. Kevin Schulman, Director of Fuqua's Health Managment Sector Program. The Keynote Speaker was Dr. Joxel Garcia, the Deputy-Director of the Pan-American Health Organization, the oldest international health organization on the planet. Sponsors of this event included Duke University School of Medicine, the National Institutes of Health and the California Endowment.

Thank you for taking the time to read this first issue of our newsletter.

Will there be more? Actually, Yes! We want to keep our members and sponsors informed about NNLAMS events.

Stay tuned for details on the 1st NNLAMS National conference, local events in your regions, and much more in our next newsletter!

Best Wishes,
Vanessa Villacorta MSIII
NNLAMS Publication Chair

Fig. 7.1   Cover Page of First NNLAMS Newsletter, 2005 (©LMSA)

The NNLAMS constitution also established roles for its national officers and enabled its national board members—that is, the leaders of the five regional organizations—to make organizational decisions. This allowed regions to set the vision of NNLAMS and direct unified efforts among Latino medical students nationwide.

Moreover, in 2000, NNLAMS leaders created an additional forum to meet, the Garcia Leadership and Advocacy Seminar (GLAS), which continued annually until 2015. The creation of GLAS was led by Fausto Meza, MD, with the aim to train regional student leaders and national student officers in effective leadership and advocacy skills. He noted "these students were leaders, and would go on to be leaders as physicians," and so he wished to help better arm them for that role. He also had the goal in mind of bringing student leaders together in person to build bonds and trust, in order to foster national collaboration. From 2000 to 2003, NNLAMS leaders convened in person annually at GLAS and at NHMA's annual meeting. While the regional organizations continued to focus on activities within their respective regional territories, NNLAMS began to function as an umbrella under which regions could more closely network. Moreover, as the annual turnover of leaders often jeopardized the survival of a national union, each meeting also served to reemphasize reasons to unify nationally and build trust between regions. NNLAMS leadership during these years kept the organization in existence, and created the opportunity for leadership and advocacy training at the GLAS conferences.

In 2003, these efforts culminated in the formal incorporation of NNLAMS as a consortium of five regional organizations under one national name. At that time, NBLHO and CMSA kept their regional names, while the other regions changed to NNLAMS Midwest, NNLAMS Southeast, and NNLAMS Southwest. Philip DeChávez, MD, MPH, then a 2003–2004 Morgan Commonwealth Fund Fellow in Minority Health Policy at Harvard University, led the efforts to acquire non-profit status, with advice from Dr. Rios of NHMA. While in medical school, Dr. DeChávez was a national leader of Latino medi-

cal students, serving as NBLHO President from 1998 to 1999. Dr. DeChávez was ultimately appointed by NNLAMS student leaders as the organization's National Executive Director, though he had been serving as a physician advisor for several years. NNLAMS obtained federal recognition as a 501(c)(3) nonprofit organization in 2004, which facilitated more concerted fundraising and unification efforts.

NNLAMS held its first national conference in 2006, in conjunction with the NHMA annual meeting that year (Table 7.3). Thanks to the efforts and support of multiple individuals, including National Coordinator Anthony Oliva, MD, PhD, and Dr. Rios of NHMA, NNLAMS developed a 2-day conference attracting over 200 medical and health professional students from all over the country. The conference provided an opportunity for NNLAMS student leaders to reflect upon the previous year's work, network with other students and health professionals, and organize the organization's operations, vision, and strategic plan. NNLAMS was also able to fundraise $1000 from that first conference, facilitating the enactment of future programming. Moreover, the first conference furthered the organization's goal of inspiring the next generation of Latino physicians. Lorena Del Pilar Bonilla, MD, 2005–2006 NNLAMS Secretary, recalls "being so impressed with the keynote speaker, Joxel García, MD, Deputy Director of Pan-American Health Organization (PAHO)." She remembers 14 years later how his words inspired her to "be a physician that can be a catalyst for positive change and go above and beyond to address Latino health disparities even as a medical student." NNLAMS continued to receive physical space for its programming at the NHMA National Conference through 2009. Each year, conference attendees increased in number, and NNLAMS was growing in strength, participation, and aspirations.

Alongside its growing events, NNLAMS added a slew of other national initiatives from 2006 to 2009. These initiatives included a national community service day, titled NNLAMS César Chávez National Latino Health Day, and several publications geared at growing organiza-

Table 7.3 Themes and Locations for LMSA National Conferences, 2006–2022

Year	Location	Theme
2006	Washington, DC NHMA	Somos Unidos: United to Eliminate Health Disparities for Hispanics
2007	San Antonio, TX NHMA	Celebrando La Diversidad: Bicultural Health Care is a National Priority.
2008	Washington, DC NHMA	La Leyenda Continua
2009	Brooklyn, NY NHMA	Tomorrow's Doctors: Leading Advocacy and Activism in Medicine
2010	Chicago, IL University of Illinois at Chicago	Latino Medical Student Association: A United Voice (first independent national conference)
2011	Irvine, CA University of California, Irvine (UCI)	Uniting Our Voices for Justice in Healthcare
2012	Boston, MA Harvard Medical School	Nuestro Futuro en Nuestras Manos: Empowering the Next Generation
2013	Miami, FL Miami-Dade College	Tomando Acción: Ensuring Health Equity for All
2014	Houston TX Baylor and UT Houston	Creciendo Juntos: Improving Health for and by Latinos
2015	Cleveland, OH Case Western Reserve Univ.	Llegamos, Seguimos: Celebrating a Decade of Progress
2016	Pomona, CA Western University of Health Sciences	Prevenir es Curar: Addressing New Obstacles and Improving Healthcare in Our Communities
2017	Hempstead, NY Hofstra	¡Aquí Estamos! Our Journey and the Climb to Greater Heights
2018	Miami, FL Miami-Dade College	Siempre Unidos: Celebrating Diversity and Bridging the Gap
2019	Lubbock, TX Texas Tech University Health Sciences Center	Todos Tenemos Valor: Building Solidarity Through Healthcare
2020	St. Louis, MO Washington University School of Medicine	Unidos por Medicina y Más: A Multidisciplinary Approach to Latinx Health
2021	Virtual UCI & Oregon Health & Sciences University	Potenciar El Cambio: Creating Interconnection in Healthcare to Create Change
2022	Philadelphia, PA The Logan Hotel	Cincuenta Años de Comunidad: Fostering Service, Health Equity, and Leadership

tional funds and providing additional resources to medical students across the country. Daniel Turner Lloveras, MD, then a medical student at the University of Chicago, championed the idea of a service day alongside César Chávez's niece and NNLAMS member Christina Chávez, MD; both proposed the initiative at the 2007 NNLAMS conference and the event was launched that year. One day a year, all NNLAMS chapters across the U.S. would volunteer, work towards, and advocate for the improved health of Latino communities. Then a medical student at the University of Illinois at Chicago (UIC), Elizabeth Homan Sandoval, MD, MPH created the NNLAMS Residency Guide as a mechanism to raise funds

for the organization. Launched with the help of then-students Anika Backster, MD; Michael López, MD, PhD; and Gerardo Solorio, MD; the annual guide garnered sponsorships from medical schools wanting to advertise to Latino medical students. This generated a major source of revenue for NNLAMS until 2010. Additional publications included the NNLAMS National Newsletter started in 2005 by then-UIC student Vanessa Villacorta, MD (Fig. 7.1). Lastly, with the help of Dr. DeChávez, NNLAMS sought out grants and increased fundraising efforts to maintain its operations in the absence of national dues or regional contributions. While dues would later be instituted as the organization continued to grow, this rising NNLAMS—led primarily by students, for students—sowed the seeds for programs that would last for decades.

Unification: The Struggle and Compromise for a Shared National Identity

NNLAMS represented the first steps toward creating a national identity for Latino medical students. It had achieved this goal by setting the foundation of a national board and a means to communicate among the various regions. However, a major limitation was that the organization served merely as a "network" among various regional organizations, leaving NNLAMS with limited potential to grow. The identity and loyalty of most individual members rested firmly with their respective regional organizations, not with NNLAMS. Throughout the early 2000s, the engagement of various regions with NNLAMS waxed and waned depending on the priorities of the individual regions. For example, CMSA in the West was undergoing major internal restructuring from 2003 to 2007 that led to the name change into LMSA Inc.; its leadership had minimal to no desire of participating in the further development of NNLAMS. The West region created the junior executive position of NNLAMS Representative to attend national events and vote on behalf of the West rather than have their CEOs directly involved. Moreover, there was difficulty in recruiting members from all the regions to be part of the national leadership board, as medical student leaders felt that their time was best spent working to develop their regional organization. An exception to this was the NNLAMS Midwest region, which had student leadership involved in growth of both the Midwest and the national entity. A pivotal moment in greater unification occurred with the development of the first NNLAMS national conference, occurring in conjunction with NHMA in 2006 (Table 7.3). Many NNLAMS leaders saw the conference as a unique opportunity to develop its own workshops, programming materials and fundraising avenues independent of regional support. Moreover,

Latino medical student leaders had a new avenue to come together in a setting outside their regional events where they could get excited about a national identity. With each new NNLAMS national conference, the number of participants increased, to the point where, eventually, an independent conference was needed.

Moreover, around the mid-2000s, conflicts began to emerge between NHMA and NNLAMS. First, while NNLAMS faced reduced room rental and food expenses by sharing a venue with NHMA for the organizations' annual meetings, profit sharing was minimal. The joint event arrangement left NNLAMS with no revenue from conference attendee or exhibitor registration and only funds raised through advertising in the Residency Guide. This threatened long-term organizational growth. Secondly, NNLAMS faced competition from NHMA in the quest to represent Latino medical students nationwide. At the time, NHMA was working to form its own national medical student arm, in order to represent Hispanic physicians at every level of training—from premedical students to retired physicians. To achieve this goal, NHMA launched its own local medical student organization in the Washington, DC, metropolitan area. This organization primarily worked on mentorship for premedical students, helping to create the premedical student exhibitor fair and medical student panel held as part of the NHMA conference. The students involved with NHMA's medical student section were invited to be part of the NNLAMS national conference in 2007. That year, NHMA medical student section representatives communicated that the eventual goal for NHMA was to have NNLAMS merge with the medical student section of NHMA, with NHMA maintaining control of the student section's finances and leadership structure. For several reasons, many NNLAMS leaders worried such an arrangement would lead to a loss of historical identity, autonomy, flexibility, and ability to effectively serve students. Third, as the NNLAMS conference expanded, there was an increased need for larger rooms, additional time slots for educational and leadership sessions, and better coordination of conference planning than had been afforded by

NHMA leadership. In interviews, several former NNLAMS leaders remarked that unnecessary logistical difficulties arose due to hosting the annual conference jointly with NHMA, kickstarting conversations regarding a standalone NNLAMS event.

A critical turning point between NHMA and NNLAMS took place at the 2008 national conference. Students complained that the NNLAMS workshops at the conference were overcrowded and hot, jeopardizing involvement in future events. Moreover, students involved with NHMA's local medical student arm were introduced at the NHMA conference gala as national medical student leaders, with concomitant disregard of NNLAMS and NNLAMS' established, autonomous leadership. Despite these two organizations existing separately from one another, leaders involved with the NHMA medical student section attempted to take part in the closed-door meeting of the NNLAMS board; this move was largely perceived by NNLAMS as encroachment. Based on the previously existing agreement between NNLAMS and NHMA, the final joint conference was set to take place in 2009. As NNLAMS Executive Director, National Coordinator, National Coordinator-Elect, and LMSA-NNLAMS Liaison, respectively, Dr. DeChavez, Ruben Font, MD, Julia Bregand-White, MD, and Mario Teran, MD, proposed the launch of a fully independent NNLAMS national conference in 2010. The proposal rapidly garnered broad approval.

Soon thereafter, the NNLAMS Board held further discussions about pursuing unification rather than remaining a network of regional organizations. Talks resumed at the LMSA Inc. conference in the West, hosted by the University of California, Davis. Mario Teran, MD, and Alvaro Galvis, MD, PhD, had just been elected as northern and southern CEOs for LMSA Inc. in the West. Working with Dr. DeChávez and student doctor Font, they devised a strategy to launch final unification of all the regions under the LMSA name. Several NNLAMS leaders felt the organization could no longer remain static, given the climate in which the organization found itself: one of rapid growth necessitating a robust long-

term strategy and being recognized as an independent 501(c)(3) organization representing the national voice of thousands of Latino medical students. Regarding the name to use for the national organization, significant debate emerged regarding the differences between the terms "Hispanic" and "Latino." The former was considered an English-language term that generally referred to the way that Latin Americans are united through their connection to Spain and their links to Spanish culture and tradition [16]. While Spaniards would be included under this term, Brazilians would not. The term had been used politically by White House administrations to distinguish Hispanics as a different type of "white" from Anglo descent, and was preferred by most Baby Boomers and older Generation X members. On the other hand, the term Latino was viewed as a Spanish-derived word that referred to the way that Latin Americans are connected to one another via their common history of colonization. Spaniards, then, would not be part of this formulation, while Brazilians would be. This term had been popularized in the late 1900s and early 2000s, appealing to younger members of Generation X and early Millennials. While these terms are often perceived as interchangeable in broader society, many students preferred using Latino based on their association with the common history of colonization rather than with a European power. Moreover, Latino as a Spanish/Latin word created an additional distinction from NHMA. Throughout the entire history of organizing by Latino medical students, all of the formal student groups that emerged at the regional and national levels chose words other than Hispanic in their titles (e.g., NBLHO, CMSA, La Raza Medical Student Association, LMMSA, LMSA). Thus, it came with little surprise that LMSA emerged as the name behind which all regions could rally.

The process by which unification would occur was developed by the "unification team," consisting of student doctors Galvis, Teran, Font and Bregand-White, alongside Executive Director Dr. DeChávez. These individuals created a full presentation delineating the model for unification, which would serve as part of the strategic planning for the organization for the following year. The model was first presented at the combined NNLAMS GLAS & LMSA Inc. Leadership Conference, held in the summer of 2008 at University of California, San Diego. The model divided unification into four phases: acceptance, name change, integration, and completion. Phase 1—acceptance—had already been fulfilled, with the promotion of a national identity, the increased collaboration between regional organizations, the creation of NNLAMS, and the accomplishments of this national entity. Phase 2, scheduled to be finished in 2010, involved the adoption of the LMSA name by all regions, with the West region transitioning its name fromLMSA Inc. to LMSA West. Phase 3—integration—was originally presented to take place between 2011 and 2013, and entailed pursuing several opportunities for greater interconnectedness between LMSA National and its regions. Internally, this phase would involve the creation of a constitution and bylaws document for the new LMSA National, allowing the organization to define and synchronize the roles of its executive officers and governing Board of Directors. Externally, all regional websites would show a unified front by becoming subdomains of lmsa.net, using the same template and design, and hosting all content on a national server. Finally, national profits and fundraising would become more centralized, with some distribution of funds going to the regions. To be completed after 2013, Phase 4 was pitched as the culmination of unification efforts, with LMSA National in a position to seek funding to have permanent paid staff, seek other avenues of political involvement as a nonprofit with 501(c)(4) or 501(c)(6) status, and be on par with peer organizations such as SNMA and AMSA.

The process of the name change transition from start to finish took almost 2 years (2008–2010). From Fall 2008 to Spring 2009, the unification team traveled to all regional board meetings, presented the unification model, and addressed questions and concerns from regional leadership. Intense debate took place at the

regional levels, particularly in the Northeast and West, as student leaders discussed concerns about loss of local and regional identity and history. As National Coordinator in 2009, Julia Bregand-White, MD, released a letter titled "State of the Network'' along with a video address; in both, she grounded the evolution of NNLAMS to LMSA in the need to further unite those dedicated to changing the "Face of Medicine and the way health care is delivered in our country." According to Dr. Bregand-White, the transition from NNLAMS to LMSA was rooted in the desire to give Latino medical students a national presence, voice, power, and recognition. To do so, NNLAMS needed to trade siloed regional efforts to one national identity. Framing the transition in this light helped convert staunch opponents of the change into some of the transition's most favorable proponents. Ultimately, the greater gain of a unified identity for a stronger national voice superseded the apprehensions that were passionately considered and debated. Over the 2009–2010 academic year, each region formally approved the name change to LMSA and executed said change in its legal and financial documents. The spring of 2010 marked two key milestones: the launch of the first independent national conference in Chicago, IL; and the rebranding of all regions to LMSA Midwest, LMSA Northeast, LMSA Southeast, LMSA Southwest, and LMSA West.

However, the work was not yet over. National student leaders at the time of the NNLAMS-LMSA transition focused heavily on further unifying regions and generating greater visibility for the organization on a national stage. At GLAS 2010, led by National Coordinator Galvis, the LMSA National leadership team moved to create new initiatives focused on a renaissance of the organization's brand and reach. In line with the previously defined Phase 3 component of the unification plan, the organization pursued four major undertakings: (1) clarifying and redefining its relationship with NHMA; (2) fundraising as a unified entity; (3) restructuring national leadership and programming; and (4) rebranding the new LMSA National organization.

Upon completion of its name change, the new LMSA became the premier organization for Latino medical students. To mitigate ensuing tension with NHMA, National Coordinator Galvis and Dr. DeChávez traveled to Washington, DC, after GLAS to meet with Dr. Rios. In that meeting, NHMA agreed to halt its own independent medical student organization and LMSA agreed not to pursue its own physician organization. A new Memorandum of Understanding was created in which the National Coordinator of LMSA became an *ex officio* member of the NHMA Board. NHMA would recruit graduating medical students to become members of their organization through the NHMA Council of Residents (COR) and the latter entity's involvement in LMSA meetings. LMSA agreed to send its National Board and National Coordinator to participate in the NHMA annual meeting with travel support by NHMA. LMSA and NHMA also agreed to coordinate so that their conferences and major events did not overlap, and to promote each other's activities to their respective members.

In order to fundraise for the rebranded organization, LMSA National created a dedicated fundraising committee in 2010. This committee transformed the existing LMSA newsletter to the more formal Journal of the LMSA (JLMSA), with Orlando Sola MD, MPH, as editor. With its first edition launched at the 2011 LMSA National Conference at the University of California, Irvine (UCI), the JLMSA provided additional opportunities for fundraising, through advertisements from medical schools and residency programs, and for showcasing LMSA members' scholarly work. The fundraising committee also created the first LMSA National prospectus and began fundraising efforts for both the National Conference and the organization as a whole. Notable new sponsors during this period included the California Endowment and the Doctors Hospital at Renaissance (DHR), which subsequently

became the major sponsor for both GLAS and National Conference from 2011 to 2015.

Furthermore, the LMSA National leadership structure underwent its first major restructuring during this period. This included the formation of a new LMSA National Policy Chair and Committee. Led by student doctor Sola and then-LMSA West Southern CEO Tatianne Velo, MD, the Policy Committee sought to create policy stances for the organization, explore new avenues of activism for LMSA, and file for designation as a U.S. 501(c)(4) or 501(c)(6) nonprofit organization. With this updated designation, LMSA could engage in lobbying and political activities to champion important causes for medical trainees. Keeping this in mind, LMSA was invited to join the National Association of Hispanic Healthcare Executives (AHHE) by their president and founder, George Zeppenfeldt, MD. National Coordinator Galvis spoke at the AHHE National Legislative Summit in New York and the AHHE/Hispanic Congressional Causes Healthcare Summit about Hispanic health care disparities and the lack of support for Latinos to enter medical schools.

For rebranding, LMSA created a Branding Committee in 2010. Led by Victor Cueto, MD, MS, then a medical student at Drexel University College of Medicine, this working group spearheaded a number of new initiatives based on perspectives from all the regions. The committee invited each region to provide representatives, independent of the national leadership, and tasked committee members to help take stock of their region's viewpoints. The most lasting and impactful work of the committee was the design and adoption of a new logo, which LMSA has continued to use through 2022 (Fig. 7.2). The decision to adopt a new logo was a practical, yet extremely symbolic and momentous change. At the time, the logo used at the national level was the original logo used by LMSA Inc. in the West. However, the digitized original work of this logo had been lost over time; hence, there was no available high-resolu-

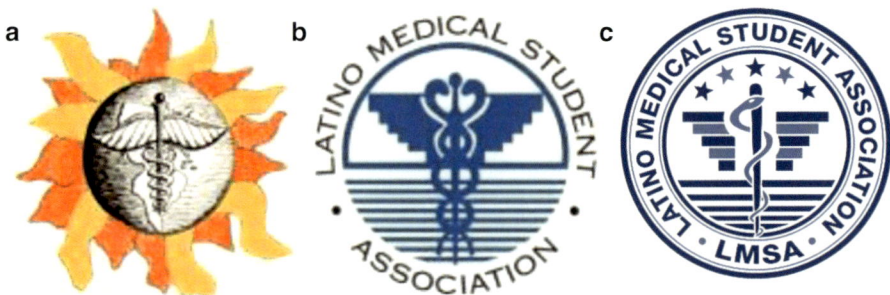

Fig. 7.2 NNLAMS & LMSA National Logos (©LMSA). (**a**) NNLAMS Logo prior to national unification and renaming in 2010. (**b**) Logo used by LMSA National between 2010 and 2011. (**c**) Updated LMSA logo, approved in 2011 and in use through 2022

tion copy that could be utilized for merchandising and printing purposes. In crafting the new logo, the branding committee and national leadership aimed to not break with tradition, but rather build on its strong foundation. After 1 year of discussion and debate at the local, regional and national levels, the executive board voted on a new logo with updated features that represented all regions, while honoring the tradition of the former logo, such as the UFW águila (eagle) and its important place in the cultural roots of the West region. The new logo had a familiar circular shape and blue color, yet the caduceus at its center was replaced by the rod of Asclepius, a more appropriate symbol of medicine. The rod of Asclepius was flanked by eagle's wings on a background of a rising sun, and newly crowned with five stars representing the new unified organization of five sister regions. The logo was approved at the 2011 LMSA National Conference held at UCI, the largest LMSA conference to date with over 1000 attendees. By the fall of 2011, a year after the effort began, the new symbol of a unified LMSA began to be widely used in official publications. In the spring of 2012, it was officially introduced to members in the form of a commemorative pin. After a long and arduous transition process to assume a common name, website, logo, and identity, LMSA headed into a new decade with five regions and thousands of members – stronger and more united than ever before (Fig. 7.3).

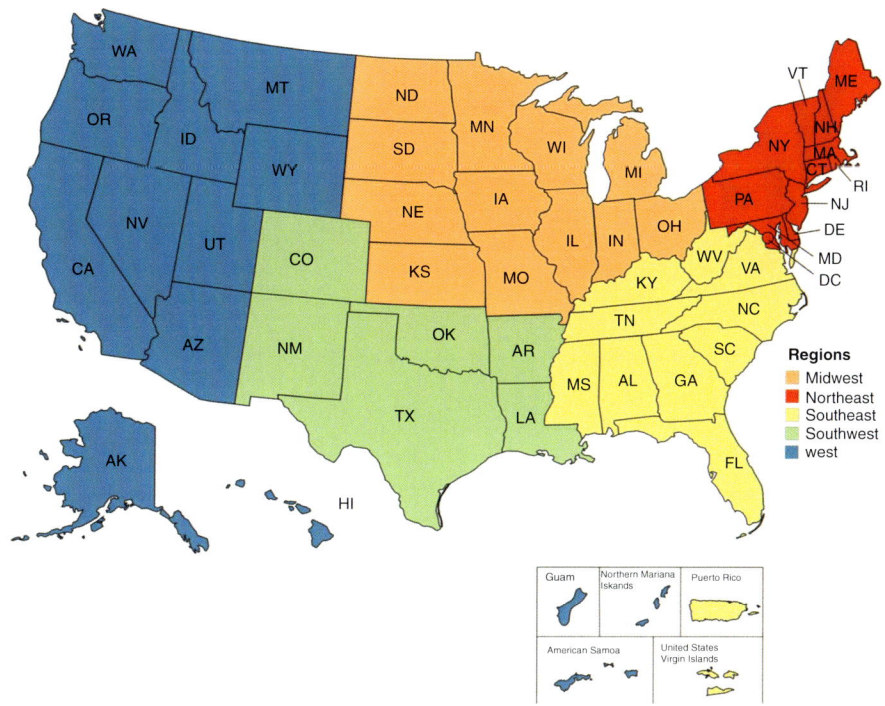

Fig. 7.3 LMSA National Regions (©LMSA)

Over a Decade of Evolution: LMSA National, 2009–2022

The following section will discuss the development and growth of the national organization's identity specifically as LMSA. It should be noted that LMSA's development process has, by no means, remained static since the organization's renaming in 2009–2010. As alluded to above, LMSA continues to evolve each year with changing leaders and members, and its flexibility and dynamism imbue the organization with unique strengths, as well as distinct challenges.

Julia Bregand-White, MD, and subsequent National Coordinators/Presidents continued to prioritize unity over the years that followed, through deliberate attempts to have the national organization deliver clear benefits to LMSA members and regions. Such benefits included the creation of infrastructure and documentation so that students at individual medical schools could start their own chapters, thereby growing the LMSA network. Moreover, LMSA National

sought to collaborate with AMSA, SNMA, and other peer organizations to establish joint programming that members of all organizations could attend. NHMA was tapped in order to create a list of physicians willing to advise LMSA students, regardless of geographical distance. LMSA continued to utilize its vote and voice at the AMA MSS; notably, through the efforts of AMA and LMSA leaders such as Dr. Homan Sandoval, voting participation of all Underrepresented Minority National Medical Student Organizations was codified by the AMA House of Delegates in 2008. National leaders over the years have sought to leverage these and other partnerships and collaborations to provide members and regions with the resources needed to thrive.

Simultaneously, LMSA began crafting new national priorities, in addition to those set in place by NNLAMS predecessors. Among the first of these was medical Spanish. In 2011, Ray Morales, MD, PhD, became National Coordinator after serving as NNLAMS Midwest Co-Director, and was elected on a platform of bringing medical Spanish curricula to the forefront of undergraduate medical education. From there, a national medical Spanish committee quickly came to be, and was led by student doctor Morales and Lauren N. Rodríguez, MD, with mentorship from longtime LMSA advisor Monica Vela, MD. Not only did LMSA develop and disseminate a medical Spanish curriculum that its chapters could implement, but the organization also conducted a national survey on the "state of medical Spanish curricula at U.S. medical schools," obtaining responses from 83% of U.S. medical schools [17]. Though 66% of schools had some form of medical Spanish instruction incorporated into their curricula, very few of them had validated instruments to measure proficiency after course completion. This study was the first to discuss the expanding medical Spanish curricula in the U.S. and is thus cited repeatedly as a landmark article on the topic.

As another national priority, LMSA aimed to make the organization—and medical school in general—more accessible to students. At the 2012 LMSA National conference at Harvard, then-VP of Scholarship Jimena B. Alvarez, MD, presented the first LMSA National Scholarship, after fundraising for it and organizing for a year. This was also the first LMSA conference that had its own commercial, which was filmed and streamed thanks to National Coordinator Morales. That same year, the LMSA Regional Development Committee—led by then-Yale School of Medicine student Amanda Hernández, MD, PhD—sought to develop a structure for the formation of premedical student chapters. Through the proposed Pre-Medical Association of Latino Students (PALS), LMSA sought to develop pre-medical student groups that would branch off of LMSA medical school chapters, enabling the strengthening of relationships to pre-medical students for the provision of support, mentorship, and opportunities for involvement in LMSA events. The LMSA Regional Development Committee envisioned implementing PALS through a series of phases. Phase 1 was to gather information on existing Latino pre-medical programs and how LMSA could be supportive,

creating momentum for the project. Phase 2 was to centralize and strengthen already existent premedical organizations and their relationships with medical students. Then a student at the University of Miami, Daniella Delgado, MD, did much in the role of Pre-Med Liaison to advance the initiative from the undergraduate side. Dr. Delgado shared, "Throughout my undergraduate years, LMSA involvement was one of my most formative experiences and helped me develop many of the skills I needed as a physician. For these reasons I love LMSA!" By 2012, with Emma Olivera, MD, as National Coordinator and Miguel Gosalbez, MD, as Membership Co-Chair, the pre-medical chapter program was launched as the LMSA Premedical Latino Undergraduate Society (LMSA PLUS).

Collaborations were continually emphasized during this period. In 2012, multiple memoranda of understanding (MOUs) were signed, updating and establishing relationships with partners such as the National Hispanic Medical Association, National Hispanic Serving Health Professions Schools (HSHPS), Student National Medical Association (SNMA), and Dr. First. SNMA invited National Coordinator Olivera to speak at their 2012 national Annual Medical Education Conference on the topic of Eliminating Health Disparities: Partnerships with a Purpose. Likewise, then-SNMA President Michael Knight, MD, MSHP, was invited to the LMSA National Conference that year. A much needed database software program was developed through collaboration with UIC to better track LMSA members and alumni. In 2012, Doctors Hospital at Renaissance (DHR) commenced their generous support of GLAS events for 4 years. Notably, this relationship with DHR was critical for the advancement of LMSA National. During GLAS, the mission and vision of LMSA were repeatedly reviewed, debated, and updated, as the leadership felt it was necessary to continue to clarify and agree on the future path of LMSA and its five regions. This discussion continued for another few years, culminating in significant updates to the constitution and officer positions.

When student doctor Galvis returned for a second term as National President in 2013, the task of evolving infrastructure to meet organizational demands was of the utmost priority. At that time, the Southeast and Southwest regions were having difficulties with recruitment and fundraising. To support them, a new profit sharing proposal was created that would not only give every region a certain portion of funds from National Conference profits but would also dedicate additional funds for regions that needed further development. Moreover, as NHMA had started to develop regional infrastructure modeled on LMSA's regions, LMSA asked NHMA regional liaisons from the latter's COR, Council of Young Physicians (CYP), and senior physicians to serve as advisors to LMSA regional leaders. To bolster scholarship fundraising efforts and amounts, a guaranteed portion of conference profits was set aside to fund scholarship recipients. Lastly, LMSA National expanded both its Policy Committee and its relationship with NHMA to facilitate the launch of the LMSA Policy Summit. Set to take place during the NHMA National Conference, the LMSA Policy Summit attracted students who would participate in the advocacy training sessions offered by the summit, as well as legislative visits with their respective elected representatives on Capitol Hill. NHMA facilitated the scheduling of these Hill visits, filling a key operational need at that time.

Enacting Structural Changes to Set a New Path Forward

The process of unifying regions into one national entity and identifying a new path forward for the organization highlighted the need for significant structural changes to leadership positions at both the regional and national level. In seeking to establish a more unified national organization, leaders after 2011 needed to develop an initial mission, vision, and structure of LMSA National, such that the organization's core components embodied the shared goals and values of its diverse membership. Under the leadership of the National Coordinator Olivera and National Coordinator-Elect Galvis, LMSA voted at GLAS 2012 to simplify the mission statement, turn most

of the NNLAMS old mission statement into objectives, and establish a vision of the organization. The approved proposal read as follows:

The **Latino Medical Student Association** unites and empowers medical students through service, mentorship and education to advocate for the health of the Latino community.

Our vision is: Unifying Medical Students to promote Latino health.

Part of our objectives include:

- To unify all Latino medical students into one organization;
- To provide a voice for underrepresented medical students;
- To actively promote recruitment and retention of Latino students at all levels;
- To educate medical students on Latino health issues;
- To advocate for the rights of Latinos in health care;
- To provide leadership opportunities for Latinos; [and]
- To promote volunteerism in the Latino community [18].

Leadership positions at the national level reflected the aforementioned priorities: of 15 officers in 2011–2014, 3 focused on membership and regional development; 2 on health policy, one of which served as LMSA representative to the American Medical Association Medical Student Section (AMA MSS); 2 on publications, the positions of which oversaw the creation and maintenance of the Journal of the Latino Medical Student Association; and 1 on coordinating a nationwide community service day, termed Latino Health Day and timed to coincide with César Chávez Day.

As LMSA National's programming, fundraising, and outreach expanded, so did the responsibilities of the National Coordinator. This, combined with growing trust between the regions and the national organization, led to the renaming of the top leadership position to National President for the 2013–2014 term and beyond. The increased frequency of in-person national meetings, between GLAS, leadership retreat, and a national conference assisted in the upswing of trust. In reflecting on the differences between his two terms at the helm of LMSA National, Dr. Galvis states:

> My first term [as Coordinator] was about creating the new normal LMSA National with our motto of 'strength in numbers.' In my second term, [as President,] it became about infrastructure building: how to make an organizational impact for the next ten years. The energies between the groups were completely different. But that is the beauty of a constantly evolving organization.

The National President title more appropriately reflected the significant responsibilities of the position on the student's curriculum vitae and residency applications. There was also a contraction of elected national officer positions to simplify elections at the LMSA National Conference. Many positions were shifted to appointed positions to save time for other business at the meetings. The National Coordinator-elect position was eliminated and the Vice President position was split into two: Internal Affairs and External Affairs.

Ultimately, LMSA sought to create a new organizational model and constitution which would better align regional leadership positions and improve efficiencies across the organization. This effort also aimed to harmonize regional and national leadership structures, as well as enhance collaboration between these bodies. In 2015, under the leadership of National President Amanda Lynn Hernández, MD, PhD, LMSA unveiled an updated constitution that ushered in a number of key changes. Notably, the updates formalized the LMSA National Executive Committee, creating a structure for the group of officers tasked with overseeing the national organization's operations and programming. The Executive Committee was distinct from LMSA National's Board of Directors (BOD), which consisted of two directors from each of the five regions. As was the case in NNLAMS, the BOD represents LMSA National's voting body, such that initiatives LMSA seeks to implement at the national level must obtain approval by regional directors. This two-tiered governance structure has existed through 2022.

Within the Executive Committee, new positions were created to reflect both the growing ventures at the national level and the successful models at the regional level. Some of these positions fell under the newly formed External Affairs branch, which focused on outward-facing aspects of LMSA, such as public relations, digital media, and partnerships with other organizations. Other positions were added to the Internal Affairs branch, charged with managing all membership matters and business operations, such as finances and record-keeping. This expanded structure of the LMSA National Executive Committee remained as described in place until 2022, when it was further elaborated into Operations, Programming, and Communications branches (Fig. 7.4). Moreover, since 2015, regional leadership structures have also changed in order to mirror positions at the national level and promote collaborations between national and regional organizations. National committees have aligned with regional positions to ensure that all regional officers for a given position would sit on the corresponding national committee, mentor and be mentored by their peers and counterparts, and synergize national and regional efforts. Such changes, while seemingly minimal, have had significant implications for organizational unity and for increasing leadership opportunities for trainees from underrepresented backgrounds in medicine.

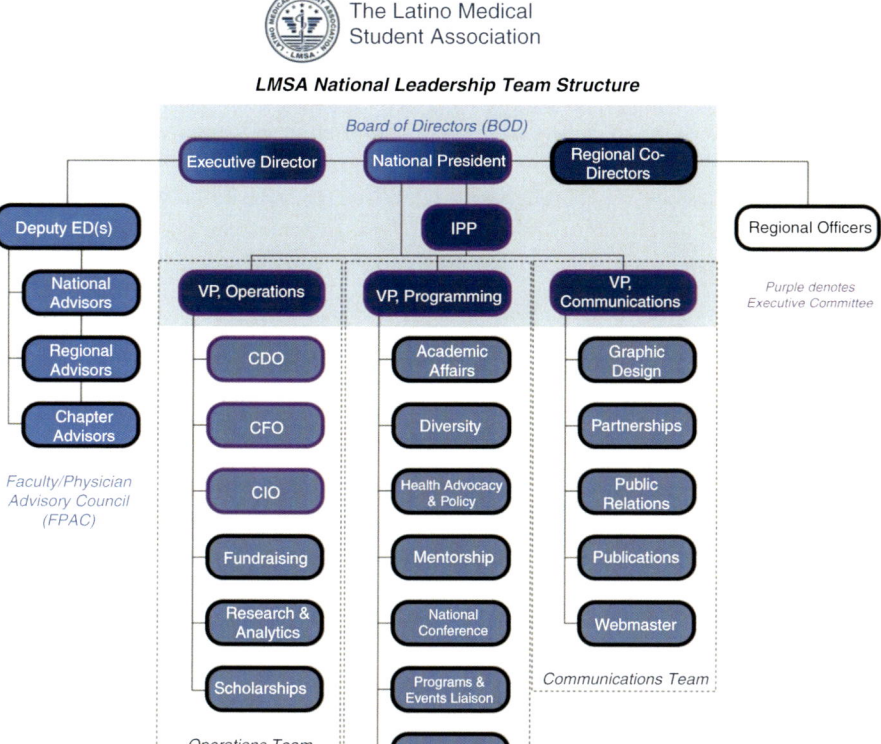

Fig. 7.4   LMSA National Leadership Structure as of December 2022 (©LMSA)

Expanding Advisory Support: The Role of Professional Advisors & Faculty

Historically, although each chapter had to have at least one faculty advisor, LMSA and its national precursors operated with few official faculty or physician advisors. In the decades since the formation of NNLAMS, the roles and structures of advisors have been revised multiple times. When Dr. DeChávez led the initiative to establish NNLAMS as a 501(c)(3) organization, he became the organization's first National Executive Director (ED) in 2003. That position has remained the main advisory role to the organization even through 2023, and has always been filled by a volunteer physician. In 2004, NNLAMS established an Alumni Board of Trustees composed of

physician alumni who had been involved with the organization for over 10 years. The objective of this alumni board was to ensure the stability, continuity, permanence and long-term vision of the organization. As listed in the NNLAMS 2007 and 2008 National Conference programs, advisors included Fausto Meza, MD, Phillip DeChávez, MD, MPH, and Louis DiBernardo, MD. Unfortunately, the Alumni Board of Trustees petered out over time.

Thus, in 2010–2011, National Coordinator Galvis created an Advisory Council which included Dr. DeChavez as National ED; Monica Vela, MD, as Physician Advisor; Richard Zapanta, MD, as NHMA Advisor; Ruben Font, MD, as Alumni Advisor; and Julia Bregard-White, MD, as Alumni Advisor. However, this council experienced frequent turnover and dissolved. Following the passing of Dr. DeChavez,

Dr. Font was selected to serve as National ED in 2013. Following Dr. Font's departure from the role, Elizabeth Homan Sandoval, MD, MPH, was selected by the LMSA National Board in 2015 to become the third LMSA National ED. As former LMSA Midwest Co-President, National leader, and Southeast Advisor during residency, Dr. Homan Sandoval had been highly involved with the organization for almost a decade. In 2017, John Paul Sánchez, MD, MPH, was selected as National Co-ED. While the plan at the time was for the position to become a two-person role, Dr. Homan Sandoval stepped down in Spring 2018.

Chosen for his instrumental role in the creation of NHMA COR and CYP, along with his extensive national and regional involvement in LMSA as NMHA COR Chair, Dr. Sánchez as National ED set out to develop a strong national advisor reservoir for LMSA leadership. During the LMSA National Conference at Hofstra in the spring of 2017, he created the first LMSA Advisor Orientation and Training programming to entice more chapter advisors to attend. In November 2017, alongside then-LMSA National President Eric Molina, Dr. Sánchez successfully established a formal LMSA Faculty/Physician Advisory Council (FPAC), with clearly defined and documented structure and objectives. Overseen by the National ED, LMSA FPAC was formed with physician and faculty advisors from each of the five regions. National advisors bear considerable knowledge and expertise in LMSA structure and history, and serve as content experts for varying responsibilities of the organization and topics of particular importance to the LHS+ medical student community.

LMSA National Faculty/Physician Advisory Council (LMSA FPAC)

As of this chapter's development in 2022, FPAC consists of nine distinguished academicians, possessing dean, chancellor, and/or full professor with tenure designations, from across the coun-try. Led by the LMSA National Executive Director, FPAC works to:

- Support and refine the strategic plan of LMSA National each year;
- Increase discussion of ongoing and emerging Hispanic-related health issues;
- Promote more engagement by LMSA local medical school chapters in regional and national programming;
- Empower local chapters and their advisors to develop the personal and professional interests of LMSA members and cultivate the next generation of Latino leaders; and
- Identify strategies to bolster the promotion and tenure efforts of LMSA chapter advisors.

While NNLAMS and LMSA student leaders routinely consulted physicians and professionals for advice on various organizational matters, many of these same leaders emphasized the central role for students in dictating the organization's direction. LMSA ultimately arose as a product of arduous grassroots organizing by medical students, fighting for collective recognition at the level of medical schools, states, and regions prior to national unification. As such, inherent in LMSA is an acute awareness of the balance between student leadership and advisor oversight. Moreover, student leaders have frequently debated the roles and responsibility of LMSA advisors, creating carefully crafted language and parameters for delineating the scope of advisor oversight and privileges.

However, LMSA's growth, combined with the inevitable turnover of student leaders, necessitates the long-term involvement of physician and faculty advisors, the majority of which are LMSA alumni. Advisors provide institutional memory that extends beyond the 4 years of typical medical school training and are able to develop expertise around national organization professional responsibilities in order to mentor and foster successive generations of student leaders. Ultimately, the long-term involvement of physician, faculty, and alumni advisors in LMSA National has helped student leaders, across the years, maintain their focus and alignment on LMSA's core values: unity, service, mentorship, education, and advocacy for patients and communities in need.

Embracing Allies

In recognizing the contributions of numerous student and faculty leaders, each with differing backgrounds and perspectives, it is important to acknowledge that LMSA would not be where it is today without the help of allies and allyship. In this section, allies will be defined as people who do not belong to a marginalized group but recognize the struggle of the marginalized group and are willing to:

> …stand up and take on the problems borne of oppression as their own, without remove or distance…even if allies cannot fully understand what it's like to be oppressed for their race or ethnicity, gender, sexuality, ability, class, religion, or other marker of identity.
> —Roxane Gay, On Making Black Lives Matter [19]

Allyship is "a lifelong process of building relationship based on trust, consistency, and accountability with marginalized individuals and/or groups of people." [20]

The growth of LMSA has benefited from mentors, members, and student leaders who do not identify as Latino. In 2019–2020, for the first time in the organization's history, the LMSA National President position was filled by a self-identified ally: Julia Su, then an MD/PhD candidate at the Donald and Barbara Zucker School of Medicine at Hofstra/Northwell. During her term, National President Su expanded the organization's dialogue around allyship, and promoted similar discussions at other national organizations. Such discourse emphasized the importance of collaboration across racial, ethnic, and other identities in promoting the development of a diverse physician workforce and the improved health of all medically underserved communities.

Every year, many LMSA chapter leaders struggle with a common issue: they may be one of a few Latinos in their medical school and feel they do not have enough members to plan all the events they want while maintaining academic success. In working to plan initiatives ranging from Medical Spanish events to health fairs for immigrant communities, LMSA leaders may occasionally feel disempowered by the thought that their few numbers preclude them from accomplishing all the initiatives they set out to do. In such instances, allies and allyship have greatly benefitted LMSA. LMSA chapters often collaborate with their local SNMA counterparts to host events and programs that help reduce overall administrative burden. At some institutions, LMSA and SNMA chapters exist as combined entities. Additionally, allies join to learn about the health care disparities affecting Latinos and the ways they can better serve this population; sessions on cultural humility and Medical Spanish represent just a few examples of workshops that should extend beyond the walls of LMSA. Involving allies in such conversations is critical because, as future physicians, we all must learn to take care of patients from many diverse backgrounds.

LMSA activities play a critical role in developing this symbiotic relationship. With the help of allies, including, but not limited to, the SNMA, Asian Pacific American Medical Student Association (APAMSA), the Association of Native American Medical Students (ANAMS), and the AMA Medical Student Section, LMSA can better carry out its mission and goals to create a more diverse physician workforce that includes Latino individuals and allies and that—as a whole—better serves the Latino population. LMSA faces a serious task in 2023 and beyond of creating a clearer vision for its role in the world, particularly as the LHS+ (Latina/o/x/e, Hispanic, or of Spanish Origin+) community confronts exacerbated disparities in healthcare, immigration, education, and finances in the post-COVID-19 era. Allies will continue to be vital partners in LMSA's fight to eliminate injustice.

National Initiatives & Programming for LHS+ Medical Students: Past, Present and Future

Since its inception as NNLAMS, LMSA National and its medical student leaders have sought to bolster the success of LHS+ individuals in medicine through the development and implementation of specific initiatives and programs, described further in this section.

Promoting Professional and Leadership Development of LHS+ Medical Students: The Garcia Leadership & Advocacy Seminar (GLAS)

In 2000, the Garcia Leadership and Advocacy Seminar (GLAS) was designed to cultivate and develop the leadership, organizational, and advocacy skills of recognized LHS+ medical student leaders from across the United States. As the architect of GLAS, NNLAMS National Coordinator Meza named the program in honor of Hector Pérez García, MD. Dr. García was a Presidential Medal of Freedom awardee in 1984, the first Mexican-American recipient of said award, and the subject of the Public Television documentary titled "Justice for My People: The Dr. Hector P. Garcia Story." An important underlying objective of the conference was to formally develop national leaders and help unify leaders from across the U.S. in their work to build a national organization.

GLAS was hosted by the University of Texas at Galveston, Duke University in Raleigh, NC, and by Doctors Hospital at Renaissance (DHR) in Edinburg, Texas. In 2010–2011, Alvaro Galvis, MD, PhD, Ray Morales, MD, PhD, and Dr. DeChávez collaborated with Dr. Meza, who had gone on to become Chief Medical Officer at DHR. From 2012 to 2015, DHR was a generous supporter of LMSA National, hosting dozens of students for a 3-day conference each year and sourcing hotel rooms, conference space, support staff, and outstanding speakers. Speakers over the years that GLAS was held at DHR included former NASA astronaut Jose Moreno Hernández; Congressman José Ruiz, MD; Texas State Representative Veronica González; and several DHR hospital administrators, such as Carlos Cardenas, MD.

Annual National LMSA Conference

Over the years, there have been many outstanding accomplishments produced by dedicated medical student members volunteering their time to create a National Conference. The first great feat was in 2006 with the inaugural conference. In 2010, the next giant leap occurred with an independent conference. A year later, the largest National Conference in the organization's history thus far took place at UCI. In 2014, the first round of 5 regions hosting the event was completed. By 2022, National Conferences have been held in each region twice, at allopathic and osteopathic medical schools, with average attendance of 200–500 medical and premedical students (Table 7.3).

Consistently, National Conferences have been packed with programming to build attendees' knowledge base for advocacy and leadership, as well as clinical skills. The scientific poster sessions at every National Conference have provided a place for LMSA students to showcase their work and receive professional feedback on their posters and presentations. Awards presented at each poster session have helped students build their Curriculum Vitaes and their self-confidence. In 2018, a TED Talk-like session was started called "8 for 8" to highlight incredible scholarly works and service endeavors of LMSA members. One of the topics covered in the 2018 LMSA National Conference—hosted in conjunction with LMSA Southeast—was the Puerto Rico Task Force, which provided grants, textbooks, and other support to medical students in Puerto Rico severely impacted by Hurricane Maria. The 8 for 8 session was a chance for students to share the details of their extraordinary work, be recognized for their efforts, and inspire others.

Fostering Growth of Physician-Advocates: LMSA Policy Summit

> Young people have a duty to defend their country with weapons of knowledge
> —Pedro Albizu Campos

Since its inception in 2014 (Table 7.2), the LMSA National Health Policy Summit brought together LMSA members from around the country. Attendees have learned about timely health policy issues facing U.S. LHS+ communities, have gained exposure to leadership development strategies and opportunities, and have evaluated organizational resolutions and stances for LMSA National to adopt. The Summit was originally held in conjunction with NHMA's annual meetings in 2014 and 2015. In 2016, the Summit became a stand-alone LMSA event and was held in-person at Association of American Medical Colleges (AAMC, Washington D.C. As the Summit grew, the event incorporated funding and objectives from GLAS, with the latter's phasing out in 2016. The Summit has occurred in partnership with AAMC through 2022.

In its most recent format, the Summit takes place over 3 days, which include legislative visits with Democratic and Republican congressional offices; plenary sessions and workshops focusing on advocacy, leadership, and health policy; and review of potential LMSA resolutions. This review occurs during a formal business meeting in which LMSA leadership uses parliamentary procedure to vote on resolutions covering a wide range of health policy-related matters submitted by LMSA members across the country. This exercise provides member-originated feedback on LMSA National priorities and familiarizes members with meeting structures commonly used in other outlets of organized medicine, such as the AMA. Once passed, resolutions are often published in peer-reviewed medical and medical education journals recognized by the U.S. National Library of Medicine. The first resolution to be published in a medical education journal focused on a joint decision by LMSA, NHMA, and HSHPS to acknowledge the unique health issues and disparities of Latinos who identify as a part of the LGBT+ community [21]. Subsequent resolutions have encouraged even greater emphasis on supporting and mentoring subgroups within the Latino community, such as undocumented immigrant students and those from low-income or first-generation backgrounds.

Efforts to Strengthening the Pipeline of Underrepresented Racial and Ethnic Minoritized Trainees

LMSA members share a passion for ensuring that LHS+ patients and their families receive culturally and linguistically concordant and humble care by healthcare providers. To bring this vision forward and deliver the best care to an increasingly diverse patient population, the medical profession must invest in trainees from diverse backgrounds. Organizations like LMSA exist to support those who embrace the challenge of reducing health disparities across multiple medical specialties. In this vein, LMSA has continued to encourage its members to identify mentors for themselves, while serving as mentors for others; to seize opportunities for presenting, publishing, and disseminating original work; and to partner with allies in the pursuit of health equity.

Mentorship has been a core pillar of what LMSA does and why it exists. There are two parts to mentorship in LMSA: (1) LMSA members serving as mentors to premedical students (via LMSA PLUS or through partner organizations) and (2) LMSA members receive mentorship through mentors who guide them on their journey to residency and beyond. As mentorship is a critical part in what LMSA does, the National leadership team has often had two Mentorship Co-Chairs. These officers collaborate with their regional counterparts to provide programming for premedical and medical students at the chapter, regional and national levels. Moreover, all LMSA National Conferences have a premedical school track, which often include mock interviews, medical student panels, and personal statement workshops. Lastly, LMSA works closely with NHMA, HSHPS, and physician organizations centered around medical specialties (e.g. AAFP, AAOS, APA) to create additional opportunities for LMSA members to meet potential mentors.

One of the great success stories of LMSA in mentoring a student through the pipeline involves Emma Olivera, MD, who started as a premedical student attending a NNLAMS Midwest regional conference. Dr. Olivera went on to matriculate to UICOM at Rockford, and held many positions on the national level, including LMSA Midwest Co-President, LMSA National Coordinator, and NHMA COR Chair. She now serves a primarily Latino patient population in the Chicagoland area, and is a mentor to medical students. In addition to Dr. Olivera, many former LMSA leaders and award recipients go on to "pay it forward," providing mentorship to trainees across the continuum of medical education and supporting the next generation of diverse U.S. physicians.

Recognizing the Exceptional: LMSA National Awards

As of 2022, LMSA bestows at least three National Awards upon outstanding individuals who have made great strides in supporting the mission and objectives of LMSA.

The first of these is the Phil DeChávez LMSA National Mentor of the Year Award. In the summer of 2012, the LMSA National Board and Officers were devastated to learn that National ED Dr. DeChávez had died unexpectedly. Dr. DeChávez was a devoted mentor to student leaders. He uplifted their spirits when doubt crept in, and when failures and setbacks occurred. He was a constant kind soul that had deep belief in the students and their ideas. His humble upbringing on the West side of San Antonio influenced him to always support those that had the world against them, and to speak for the voiceless until he had helped them find their voice. He is deeply missed by all who were mentored by him, and his mission and memory live on in the spirit of mentorship in LMSA. In recognition of his steadfast service and myriad accomplishments on behalf of Latino students, LMSA grants the Phil DeChávez LMSA National Mentor of the Year award annually to the organization's most highly

regarded mentor. Award recipients since 2013 are as follows:

Year	Recipient
2013	Philip DeChavez, MD, MPH
2014	Ruben Font Jr., MD
2015	Fernando Mendoza, MD, MPH
2016	(*no award information available*)
2017	Rebeccah R. Rodriguez Regner, D.O.
2018	Maria L. Soto-Greene, MD, MS-HPEd, FACP
2019	Monica B. Vela, MD
2020	Sunny Nakae, PhD, MSW
2021	Juan Robles, MD
2022	Denise A. Martinez, MD

At the 2014 LMSA National Policy Summit, the LMSA J.P. Sánchez LGBTQ Award was announced in honor of another beloved and outstanding mentor and advisor. The students honored National ED Dr. Sánchez's LGBTQ educational, research, clinical, and service advocacy work by naming the scholarship after him. This award is presented annually for outstanding work in the field of LGBTQ Health serving Latino LGBTQ communities in the United States. Recipients have included David Alejandro Sanchez (2017), Alec Gibson (2018), Aileen Portugal (2019), Antonio Flores (2020), Mauricio Franco Jr. (2021), Joshua Soler (2022), and Delia Sosa (2023 SALUD Summit).

The LMSA National Scholarship was created by Jimena Alvarez, MD, after several years of fundraising and hard work. Financial prizes are given to outstanding LMSA students annually at the National Conference to help offset recipients' costs of medical education. As of December 2022, over 50 students have received this award.

In March 2022, at the 50th Anniversary of LMSA's first chapter, LMSA honored distinguished LHS+ leaders who have made considerable contributions for the LHS+ community during each decade between 1970 and 2019. Recipients of the LHS+ Leader of the Decade Award included David Hayes-Bautista, PhD (1970–1979 Award); Helen Rodriguez-Trias, MD, MPH (1980–1989 Award); Elena Rios MD, MSPH (1990–1999 Award); Jose Manuel de la Rosa, MD (2000–2009 Award), and J.P. Sánchez, MD, MPH (2010–2019 Award).

Conclusion: The Spark Became a Flame of Hope to Carry into the Next Decade

The scope of LMSA's accomplishments and evolution is best understood through the challenges LMSA has faced over its lifespan. As noted throughout this chapter, the lack of full-time staff, coupled with the turnover of student leaders and advisors, has increased the difficulty of maintaining long-term initiatives and documenting impact. In the absence of financial support from U.S. government agencies or parent organizations, funding has varied significantly based on the national organization's success in recruiting sponsors and exhibitors to LMSA events. Moreover, addressing the tug-of-war between regional and national identities remains a unique task for LMSA in comparison to its peer organizations and partners.

Yet, in spite of these hurdles, LMSA continues to provide conferences, webinars, publications, scholarships, mentorship, leadership opportunities, and other programming to empower the next generation of diverse physicians in the U.S. LMSA possesses immense untapped potential, waiting to be realized through the support of partner organizations that fund, collaborate, and enhance the visibility of LMSA; medical schools and faculty that invest in LMSA to the same extent as other medical student organizations; and students dedicated to growing a strong and more unified organization and maintaining institutional memory.

Over decades, LHS+ medical students have been able to bridge vast differences in geographic location, country of origin and heritage, socioeconomic status, immigration status, and even language, keeping their eye on the bigger picture of what they have in common, and the values they hold in union. The many years of empowering and inspiring conference themes demonstrate that shared hope and motivation. Examples include: "Todos Tenemos Valor: Building Solidarity through Health Care;" "Unidos por Medicina y Más;" "Tomando Acción: Ensuring Health Equity for All;" and "Nuestro Futuro en Nuestras Manos."

The power to overcome all obstacles has always emerged from the shared vision of medical student leaders, joining together to decrease health disparities, increase representation of Latinos in medicine, support each other through the rigor of medical training, and form even stronger future leaders. Their hope will be a flame to carry into the next decade as *la lucha continúa*.

Personal Narratives:

Gerardo Solorio, MD

National Coordinator (NC) 2006–2007, NC Elect 2005–2006

The NNLAMS National Coordinator of 2006–2007, Gerardo Solorio, MD, shared that he became involved in NNLAMS because he had been part of LMSA at UCLA as a premedical student. Yet, when he left California for Washington, DC, to attend George Washington University (GWU), he had no family or friends in the area. He was craving support and connection to a community. He attended the NBLHO conference at Temple University in Philadelphia, PA, in 2003; there, he met NNLAMS National Coordinator Eddie Machado, MD, who then became a mentor to him. "Now when I deal with issues and how to solve them, I have my leadership skills to fall back on from NNLAMS." He notes he owes his leadership development to his experiences with GLAS and NNLAMS conferences and to the mentoring he received, including advice from Philip DeChávez, MD, MPH. Dr. Solorio helped build the NBLHO and NNLAMS chapter at GWU, went on to become NNLAMS National Coordinator-Elect, and then served as National Coordinator. He stated that, at the time, "NNLAMS was in state of infancy." As leaders of NNLAMS, "we wanted to do these things for our people, our members, our community." The biggest accomplishments during his years of involvement were:

> Organizing for the first NNLAMS conferences, the launch of the Residency Guide… [the] approval of initiation of César Chávez National Latino Health Day, [the] start of the NNLAMS newsletter, the rebuilding of the Southeast region, and the Name Change Committee to attempt to unify regions under one name.

On the topic of campaigning for a single name across regions, he states:

> [NNLAMS] is a complex organization, there are different views, different regional cultures and issues, there was a lot of passion behind the past names from historical standpoint and what they wanted to identify with. There were different names and each [region] wanted to identify to their names, but some of us understood that, in order for us to become mature and known as an organization, we probably needed to have a unifying name, unifying logo and websites. In the past each region had a different name, a different logo, a different website look; that did not work well when speaking with sponsors. There was a lot of blood, sweat and tears during these discussions. We had to go through that, we all had to go through that, it was part of the organic process of becoming a mature strong organization.

He adds:

> What makes me proud when I go to the website is seeing that LMSA has not only continued what we built but it has expanded—it has exploded! It's good to see new medical schools involved, new residency program sponsors, and new projects. Who would have thought we would have a stand alone national conference, we would have a unified name? Now 20 years later, we are leaders; we are the ones speaking up for our patients and our communities.

Dr. Solorio ends with stating he is proud to say LMSA leaders have remained steadfast to that ideal.

Julia Bregand-White, MD
National Coordinator (NC) 2009–2010, NC Elect 2008–2009

Early in my life I saw the struggles of a family living without higher education or advanced training. The financial struggles and barriers to change grew as my parents had more children at such a young age. Early on I knew that I wanted something different for my own life. I wanted to make a meaningful impact on people's lives in a career that had personal and financial rewards. My parents hadn't gone to college and I often felt isolated as a student without a clear path. With the constant love and encouragement from my family I paved my own way. I had a natural tendency towards science and found medicine fasci-

nating. We didn't know how to navigate the typical road to medicine so I started at a junior college and tried to use every opportunity I could, throwing on the track team while working full time hours and volunteering to build my CV. When I was accepted into medical school, I knew my hard work had only just begun but that, if I was able to keep up my momentum, I would be able to fulfill my dream of becoming a physician.

Many people are surprised that I am Latina when they meet me, and I often found myself explaining how or why I considered myself as such. I am of mixed heritage with a Puerto Rican paternal grandfather and otherwise European grandparents. My Stepmother is Puerto Rican and Stepfather is Ecuadorian so I have a diverse family in many ways. I know the community I was raised in, the struggles we faced, and the shared goal of making our lives better in each generation. I find great satisfaction in caring for the Latino community, the peace they feel when their doctor can speak to them in their own language, and the efforts I make to relate to their circumstances and create options for their care.

My time in LMSA allowed me to investigate my own ethnicity and culture. We had so many deep conversations about how race and ethnicity impacts medical care and outcomes and how we can work together to improve the health of the Latino community. We also had colorful conversations about the name of the organization. During my year as National Coordinator, I led a national movement to organize and unify all our regions under one name to optimize the impact we could make at local, regional and national levels. We had to take into consideration the history of the organizations before that time, [along with] the meaning of the words Latino, Hispanic, Latin American, and Boricua. During my role as National Coordinator, I learned even more about the passion our members had for their identity and—while we were hoping to work together as a unified organization—we could not and should not discount the diversity of the community we represented.

References

1. Gandara P. Over the Ivy Walls. New York: State University of New York Press; 2012.
2. Muñoz C. Youth, identity, power: the Chicano movement. London. Verso, 2007.
3. Blackwell M. ¡Chicana Power! Austin: University of Texas Press; 2016.
4. Ramirez LG, Flores Y, Gamboa M, González I, Pérez V, Ramirez-Castañeda M, Vital C. Chicanas of 18th Street. Chicago: University of Illinois Press; 2011.
5. Partida MG.. Research Guides: A Latinx Resource Guide: Civil Rights Cases and Events in the United States: 1968: The Young Lord's Organization/Party; n.d.. Guides.loc.gov. https://guides.loc.gov/latinx-civil-rights/young-lords-organization
6. Lopez RW, Madrid-Barela A, Flores Macías R. Chicanos in higher education: status and issues. Chicano Studies Center Publication, Monograph No. 7. In: ERIC. Chicano Studies Center-Publications. Los Angeles: Univ of California; 1976.
7. Hayes-Bautista D. La Nueva California. Los Angeles: Univ of California Press; 2004.
8. Montes L. A Tribute to Dr. Frank Meza. Latinx Physicians of California; 2020, January 24. https://latinxphysiciansofca.org/drfrankmezatribute/
9. Bernadett T. First in State History Raza Students Organize Statewide. In Synapse – The UCSF student newspaper 5 May 1977—UCSF Synapse Archive; 1977. Retrieved January 30, 2023, from https://synapse.library.ucsf.edu/cgi-bin/ucsf?a=d&d=ucsf19770505-01.2.17&e=%2D%2D%2D%2D%2D%2D-en%2D%2D20%2D%2D1%2D%2Dtxt-txIN--------.
10. History. AMSA; n.d. Retrieved January 30, 2023, from https://www.amsa.org/about/history-of-amsa/
11. History - National Medical Association. The National Medical Association; 2019. https://www.nmanet.org/page/History
12. History. The Student National Medical Association; n.d.. https://snma.org/page/history
13. Suozzo A, Schwencke K, Tigas M, Wei S, Glassford A, Roberts B. Student National Medical Association Inc., Full Filing – Nonprofit Explorer; 2018. ProPublica. https://projects.propublica.org/nonprofits/organizations/520965479/201931349349308583/full
14. 2018 Form 990 for American Medical Student Association (AMSA) | Cause IQ; n.d. Retrieved January 30, 2023, from https://www.causeiq.com/organizations/view_990/362222695/ed6d5e02c97b9d94a1d28bb0225fa425
15. History. National Hispanic Medical Association; n.d. Retrieved January 30, 2023, from https://www.nhmamd.org/history
16. Lopez MH, Krogstad JM, Passel JS. Who is Hispanic? Pew Research Center; 2022, September 15. https://www.pewresearch.org/fact-tank/2022/09/15/who-is-hispanic/
17. Morales R, Rodriguez L, Singh A, Stratta E, Mendoza L, Valerio MA, Vela M. National Survey of Medical Spanish Curriculum in U.S. Medical Schools. J Gen Int Med. 2015;30(10):1434–9. https://doi.org/10.1007/s11606-015-3309-3.
18. LMSA National Mission; 2016, February 18. Web.archive.org. https://web.archive.org/web/20160218222943/http://lmsa.net/org/mission
19. Gay R. On making black lives matter. Marie Claire; Marie Claire; 2016, July 11. https://www.marieclaire.com/culture/a21423/roxane-gay-philando-castile-alton-sterling/
20. Atcheson S. Allyship – the key to unlocking the power of diversity. Forbes; 2018, November 30. Retrieved January 30, 2023, from https://www.forbes.com/sites/shereeatcheson/2018/11/30/allyship-the-key-to-unlocking-the-power-of-diversity/?sh=76a29d2049c6
21. Sánchez JP, Sola O, Ramallo J, Sánchez NF, Dominguez K, Romero-Leggott V. Hispanic medical organizations' support for LGBT health issues. LGBT Health. 2014;1(3):161–4.

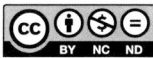

Tu Lucha es Mi Lucha: The Evolution of a Student-Driven LHS+ Health Policy Initiative

8

Orlando Sola, Franklyn Rocha Cabrero,
Ankeeta Mehta, Maria Paola Santos,
and John Paul Sánchez

History of Latino and Student Advocacy

> The revolution is not a quenepa that falls when it is ripe. You have to make it fall.
> —Modified from Che Guevara, MD

Introduction

Latino history in the Americas is a pastiche of indigenous and African identities seen through the aperture of European cultural assimilation.

O. Sola (✉)
Department of Family Medicine, Chase Brexton
Health Services, Baltimore, MD, USA

F. R. Cabrero
Adult General Neurologist & Clinical
Neurophysiologist (Epilepsy/NIOM), Diplomate of
the American Board of Psychiatry and Neurology,
Long Beach, CA, USA

A. Mehta
UT Southwestern Medical Center in Dallas,
Dallas, TX, USA

M. P. Santos
Family Medicine, Duke Family Medicine and
Community Health, Durham, NC, USA

J. P. Sánchez
Diversity, Equity, and Inclusion, University of New
Mexico Health Sciences, Albuquerque, NM, USA
e-mail: exec.director@lmsa.net

The nascent story of advocacy within the Latino Medical Student Association (LMSA) builds on this identity, evolving from a long history of Latino health advocates.

Current trends in Latino advocacy within the United States have evolved as a response to U.S. militarization of its foreign policy within North America. These forces coalesced in the mid-twentieth century around a core of disenfranchised Mexican-American and Puerto Rican citizens who organized into advocacy groups such as the United Farm Workers (UFW) and the Young Lords Organization (YLO) to pursue health equity and social justice. Political movements led by cultural pioneers such as Cesar Chavez and Jose Jimenez created a precedent for prioritizing health care needs within Latino organized advocacy movements, but these efforts did not lead to meaningful Latino representation in political or academic institutions. Moreover, the heterogeneous characteristics of Latino communities in the U.S. promulgated ethnic and regional divides in advocacy initiatives. Political and healthcare trends since the 1960s highlight a need for physician leadership with training tailored to the Latino communities' needs across the U.S.

Communities that have succeeded in creating political agency often have social structures that support continued generations of leaders and community enrichment. Failures to create similar Latino resources were not due to deficiencies of individual leaders, but reflect the lack of resilient

© The Author(s) 2024
J. P. Sánchez, D. Rodriguez (eds.), *Latino, Hispanic, or of Spanish Origin+
Identified Student Leaders in Medicine*, Sustainable Development Goals
Series, https://doi.org/10.1007/978-3-031-35020-7_8

academic structures that can galvanize organized policy development and community advocacy. Expanding on historical traditions of community advocacy LMSA developed policy programming that would allow physician trainees to advocate for Latino patients not only as clinicians, but also as community advocates, policy experts and leaders of academic health centers.

Recent health care reform in the United States has focused on policy solutions to rising epidemics of chronic disease, including several sections of the Patient Protection and Affordable Care Act (PPACA) that target disparities in underserved and marginalized communities [1]. Successful implementation of these and future systemic reforms will require a highly dedicated physician workforce with literacy in health policy. Latino health advocacy presents specific challenges, as Latinos are likely to have lower levels of health care access than comparable minority groups [2–4]. As the Latino community continues to grow to represent approximately 1 in 3 individuals in the U.S. by 2050 [5], so do the challenges of recruiting and training physician advocates.

Students and educators have shown interest in increasing their exposure to health policy training, [6, 7] and the Liaison Committee on Medical Education mentions health policy and advocacy within its current curricular standards [8]. However, few institutions have integrated the academic skills necessary for successful physician advocacy within their medical curricula. Physician advocacy organizations such as the American Medical Association (AMA) do provide practical health policy training opportunities for medical students, yet no educational setting focuses specifically on the healthcare needs of Latino communities, or attempts to foster an environment of creative policy innovation based on the Latino identity. Into this void stepped LMSA, creating a platform for Latino leadership development and community advocacy.

History of Medical Student Political Advocacy in the United States

In the 1950s the AMA developed a forum for students to participate in medical advocacy. The Civil Rights Movement, peace activism during the Vietnam War, and a push for systemic reform in health care led a group of progressive students to break from the AMA, forming the American Medical Student Association (AMSA). As a student-run organization without a physician counterpart, AMSA created a blueprint for the infrastructure needed for students seeking social change through student-driven discourse, legislative debate, and community advocacy.

Student advocacy did not end with the growth of AMSA, but rebounded across the country as various constituencies organized and advocated for the growth and improvement of the U.S. healthcare system. In 2014 students in the University of California San Francisco, Mount Sinai and Harvard collaborated over virtual platforms to protest worsening trends of police violence. Connected by shared ideals and a growing social media network, students coordinated seminars, protests and academic publications to advance the national discourse on race and ethnicity in both healthcare and medical education. Their work, and the contribution WC4BL made to the #BlackLivesMatters movement was reflected not only in reputable academic publications, but in the political debates that began to recognize the role race plays in U.S. society. If AMSA awakened the political consciousness of medical students in the United States, WC4BL showed how, armed with versatile social media platforms and reinvigorated beliefs in justice and humility in medicine, students could effectively change their surroundings. The rise of WC4BL lit a fire in the hearts and minds of medical students across the United States. The question now was whether the Latino community could harness the flames of creative destruction for the benefits of their education, patient care and public health.

Latino advocacy in health care during the Civil Rights Movement suffered from a lack of Latino leaders in leadership positions within the medical industry. The cohort of Latino medical students who were tasked with creating the LMSA policy process thus faced the challenge of building organizational infrastructure without institutional precedents or cultures of policy development. Educational theories of Frierer and Dewey further exemplified how policy programming can synergize with effective experiential educational content. The LMSA policy process strove to center scholastic programming on these ideals, integrating advocacy, structured mentoring, and competency development into a conference geared towards community advocacy and leadership development.

Maturation of Student Advocacy: Exploring the Basis for Latino Medical Student Advocacy

Medical students and residents have increasingly represented a progressive political reform agenda through their organizational advocacy work. The disruptive nature of rising generations of physicians in training, individuals who have yet to forget the ideals of humility, empathy and collaborative health that marked their initiation into medicine, drives the innovations and political reforms in medicine that has helped focus our health care systems on patients and the communities in which they live. However, prior to the development of policy programming, LMSA students existed without a clear educational forum for their growth and development as physician advocates. Organizations such as the Student National Medical Association (SNMA), with a historical grounding in the Civil Rights Movement and strong links to its physician counterpart, benefitted from an established professional network that provided mentoring and financial support. Without these resources Latino students could not easily avail themselves of educational curriculum based on their unified ethnic experience, participate in processes to share ideas and innovations tailored to Latino patient communities, or access national networks of Latino physicians who could role-model leadership in community advocacy and health politics.

In 2009 the national LMSA policy agenda was limited to its role within the AMA-Medical Student Section (AMA-MSS), where LMSA was awarded a position as an affiliated organization within its student House of Delegates. LMSA students were allowed to present resolutions and participate within the AMA-MSS's general legislative process and didactic sessions, but this pro-

gramming did not necessarily support the growth of Latino students as advocates for their communities. Scattered regional efforts to provide policy training within LMSA did take place, but were often sporadic and focused on regional priorities.

The years leading to the founding of the first LMSA sponsored advocacy programming in 2014 saw a political cataclysm that continues to define our society today. Students in LMSA saw the Latino voice ignored as neo-conservative constituencies attacked immigrant and minority communities, followed by legislative failures and continued militarization of U.S. immigration policy. Though progressive politicians gave voice to the travails of Latino communities, no successful legislative victories were obtained, and adoption of regulatory reforms such as Deferred Action Childhood Arrivals (DACA) received increasingly aggressive threats from conservative leadership.

Through these political trends grew the LMSA policy infrastructure, first implemented in the 2014 NHMA National Conference. Initially christened, the LMSA Student Policy Section (LMSA-SPS) conference programming allowed students to share their innovations in healthcare with their peers, and flourish in an environment that reaffirmed their cultural heritage. Unburdened by the social expectations as the only Latino representatives in a group of hundreds, as occurred in organizations such as AMA-MSS, LMSA students were free to grow and mature, to unlimber policy and academic skills that previously went unused or ignored. The LMSA policy process would grow into an annual policy conference that would cement the culture of policy education and community advocacy that continues today.

Developing LMSA Policy Programming

With just about every script (Orange is the New Black), in almost every corner of the set, I was faced with the truth: This was my parents' life. My mother had sat in handcuffs; my father had once worn an orange jumpsuit…for Mami and Papi, it could not have been any more real or painful…

they'd spent years handling the nastiest jobs, the ones often avoided by others. Manual labor. Low pay. No respect. They must've felt so trapped. It must've been so hard for them to maintain their dignity when others looked down on them or, worse, didn't see them at all [9].

—Diane Guerrero, In the Country We Love: My Family Divided

The Academic Basis of the LMSA Policy Programming

LMSA policy infrastructure has thrived due to the academic foundations that support the educational content training students in health policy. The Kern model was used to develop a common narrative running through conference didactic sessions as well as interactive health policy learning activities [10]. Student organizers found synergy between the Kern model's cognitive model for curriculum development and those used for policy development such as the CDC Policy Development Framework [11]. Combining these two frameworks allowed student facilitators to integrate educational and policy models into a single edifying experience where student growth coincided with community advocacy and systems reform. Through the non-traditional service-learning this engendered students participating in the LMSA-PS gained not only an understanding of the policy process and related topical content, but also practiced the skills of interpersonal communication, public speaking and leadership commonly used by successful physician advocates. The methodological approach of the Kern model also ensured novel curriculum met the needs of novice policy advocates, and evolved with the growth of an institutional culture grounded in health policy. These efforts created and maintained an active pool of students in LMSA who had the interest, understanding and ability to implement advocacy interventions in a professional, well organized manner.

Reflected in both policy and academic models, documentation and investigation of programming outcomes is a critical component of the Kern and CDC models. In addition to annual needs assessments, surveys embedded within LMSA educational and advocacy programming described participants general satisfaction as well as their perceptions of personal improvement in knowledge and competency-based learning objectives. Changes in behavior and tangible advocacy results was also monitored as participants experience in rally's, legislative visits and the COD drove both advocacy initiatives in LMSA and leadership within students institutions and regionals.

Administrative Logistics Behind LMSA Policy Programming

Though LMSA has a history of community advocacy, student engagement in the novel policy process was not guaranteed as many students were inexperienced in policy development. Existing leadership understood the theoretical role of health policy in addressing Latino health disparities, but without leadership development purposefully targeting student advocacy and policy training the political agency of LMSA constituents was rudimentary. To assist in the evolution of LMSA policy resources, a National Policy committee was created to supervise programming in health policy. An equally important goal of the national policy committee was to identify individuals in regional and chapter leadership with interest in health policy. As policy-related educational programming grew within LMSA, prospective student leaders were recruited from active participants to help build on institutional knowledge and competencies. This process engendered peer-to-peer and faculty mentorship and stimulated candid group discussions on ongoing political trends. Student leaders were then dispatched to their individual regions and chapters to develop policy projects guided by the national policy platform.

Implementing policy initiatives through regional infrastructure provided additional opportunities for student leaders to receive targeted organizational support, empowering each to become conduits of ideas, innovations and educational materials between regional and national governing bodies The academic context in which LMSA policy programming was created also ensured student leaders were taught how to evaluate and publish their advocacy work. With the organization primed for a pivot towards a proactive advocacy stance, the national policy committee began to develop and implement programming that would establish a longitudinal policy training and development process. These efforts lead to the founding of the LMSA-Student Policy Section (LMSA-SPS), a predecessor to the LMSA Policy Summit template used today.

The LMSA-SPS

The first LMSA-SPS took place on March 27th–30th, 2014 at the National Hispanic Medical Associations annual conference. To begin the process of developing student participants' foundational knowledge in health policy, the SPS hosted a brief series of conference lectures geared towards the novice student-advocate. Content was chosen based on an informal needs assessment which identified a deficiency of general health policy knowledge on historical political trends and advocacy-related competencies. The didactic series thus included sessions on basic policy nomenclature and definitions, the resolution writing process, and careers in health policy.

Following the scholastic series students were encouraged to participate in the first COD. Resolution submissions were limited to regional policy chairs to ensure a smooth inaugural event, and to help groom students for national policy leadership positions. Though resolutions were submitted by invitation only, the Congress was opened to all students. During the COD participants were encouraged to implement knowledge developed in previous lectures. In total 6 resolutions were proposed, debated and voted upon. The six resolutions submitted addressed the right to health care, health literacy, and diversity in medicine.

The SPS's agenda combined traditional didactic programming with the active learning activities hosted by NHMA, allowing students to develop a fund of knowledge that could be rein-

forced by participation in advocacy events. Efforts were made to involve high profile Latino role-models such as Julian Castro, the 16th United States Secretary of Housing and Urban Development, who gave a virtual key-note address. Collaboration with the NHMA also created opportunities for students to network with policy leaders in medicine, public health, and non-governmental organizations.

To help defray the costs of student attendance several strategies were implemented to raise funds. Scripts were created for students to solicit donations from their institutional deans or office of diversity. Students were also encouraged to approach faculty mentors to help fund individual travel scholarships for mentees. In the first year approximately $700 was raised, helping to cover attendance for over 30 students. The 2014 conference set the precedent for content development, organizational discourse and fundraising in subsequent years, culminating in 2016 when LMSA transitioned to hosting a stand-alone policy conference, the LMSA-Policy Summit (LMSA-PS).

The use of the Kern model allowed LMSA student leadership to identify the lack of health policy training for medical students on Latino health and provided a framework to develop an educational intervention that addressed existing inadequacies [12]. Student advocacy groups that serve underrepresented ethnic minority groups may also benefit from a venue that focuses on providing scholastic and practical training in health policy centered on their identity. The process of developing and implementing the LMSA-PS, and its positive outcomes, elucidates the benefits similar policy and academic resources can provide to students of all ethnic and cultural backgrounds.

Ankeeta Mehta, DO, University of North Texas Health Science Center of Osteopathic Medicine Co-Founder of the LMSA Policy Committee and Student Summit 2014.

The creation of the first policy summit provided many challenges and learning experiences. I understood that implementing a large change in an established organization would be challenging; however, the challenges faced were different than the ones I initially anticipated. Throughout the development of the summit, I was met with hesitation from LMSA board members as well as supporters of the organization. No one wanted LMSA to become an advocacy only organization with a largely political mission; however, the policy committee and I strongly believed that it was important to equip members with the skills in resolution writing and advocacy in order to advocate for Latino patients throughout their careers as physicians. As a non-Latina, my passion for LMSA stemmed from wanting to improve health outcomes in one of the most medically underserved populations in the U.S. In my opinion, advocating for patients in a structured way and empowering others to continue to do so was imperative. Though other organizations' infrastructures were used as guides to creating LMSA's own, creating the infrastructure that met the needs of LMSA to allow for equal representation of all members was important. Many regions had experience with policy, therefore uniting the regions who did, and engaging the regions who did not was crucial to the success of the summit. All documents used to train members in the process had to be created as no curriculum for policy and advocacy existed within LMSA at the time. Balancing medical school responsibilities as well as creating this infrastructure was difficult, but the support of the policy committee, and the conviction of each member that this was a crucial initiative, made it possible. Although the first policy summit was a minor footnote of the NHMA annual conference, it led to a much larger summit in subsequent years with the addition of legislative visits shortly after. Many students who participated in the first summit sought opportunities to be more involved with LMSA policy. The interest generated from the first policy summit grew quickly.

Dr. Franklyn Rocha Cabrero, MD, University of Illinois College of Medicine-Rockford, Past National VP of Policy 2015

I met Dr. Pamela Del Valle in 2014 at the national conference at the Baylor College of Medicine in Texas. She played a pivotal role in generating my policy interest. Dr. Del Valle, then a medical student, was part of the student policy leadership. The policy committee developed the national LMSA Policy Committee infrastructure, strategic vision and agenda, with support of the LMSA Board of Directors (Regional presidents). As a junior medical student finishing my term as an LMSA chapter president, I was ready to embark on a national leadership role in the organization. Although I had no experience, health policy captured my interest. The first LMSA-PS impacted my professional development forever, and was an impetus for personal and professional development. For me, this was an opportunity to develop the leadership structure of the Policy Committee. Dr. Mehta, Dr. Sola, and Dr. Del Valle participated in panel discussions promoting the accomplishments of the policy committee, including the successful development of policy committee workshops that sought to teach members how to be engaged in advocacy. This was developed in a time where policy curriculum in medical education focused in Latino health was non-existent.

Outcomes of the Inaugural LMSA Policy Conference

The success of the LMSA-SPS was measured by the level of student participation in the legislative process, as well as collaborative initiatives pursued by LMSA members after the policy section. The six resolutions submitted addressed the right to health care, health literacy, and diversity in medicine. Resolution authors were from an array of political, geographic and cultural backgrounds. Eight students and physicians acted as primary authors on resolutions, with an additional seventeen students providing testimony and expert witness during the COD. Only two contributors had past training in health policy, supporting the positive effect LMSA-SPS didactic programming had on participants' knowledge and confidence in participating in policy exercises. Students who gave testimony before the COD included premedical students, medical students, and physician faculty members.

The overall mission of the LMSA-SPS was to help train future leaders in Latino health policy, and set a foundation for further maturation of LMSA as an organization focused on community advocacy. Participants' increased involvement in policy activities represented an improvement in knowledge and competencies, and changes in behaviors and activities. Seven of the eight primary resolution writers gained further organizational policy leadership positions in addition to continued participation within the LMSA policy process. External collaborations blossomed, reaching into student and professional networks that provided important peer support, mentoring and role-modeling. In addition to a growing conference participation and policy leadership, the first LMSA policy conference helped engender collaborative advocacy initiatives that augmented future conference activities. External collaborations are discussed further in Sect. 5.

Post-Conference Activities

After the first conference, deliberate efforts were made to evaluate the policy experience of students participants at the SPS. Formal needs assessments were used to guide future educational and advocacy programming. Survey data showed an overwhelming interest in augmenting existing policy training curriculum and endorsed a belief that health policy is important to serve future patients. The inaugural SPS participants also showed increased confidence in their policy knowledge and competencies. Though these findings did not achieve statistical significance, they were useful in galvanizing support for further policy programming within LMSA.

Core objectives of the national policy committee evolved towards creating a streamlined, longitudinal, student driven policy development process that extended beyond a single annual conference. Regional leaders helped extend the effect of the SPS by inserting educational programming on health policy into subsequent regional conferences and local advocacy events. Students were encouraged to share their policy successes in peer-reviewed publications, develop collaborative projects with external student advocacy organizations, and expand innovative policy projects within home institutions. However, further growth would require dedicated administrative support from regional and national leadership. The national policy committee (2015) transitioned towards promoting policy committees within regional executive boards and creating sub-committees to work on specific policy projects. Educational materials were also distributed to LMSA chapters on the fundamental legislative policy skills, including resolution writing, testimony development and obtaining mastery of the parliamentary rules.

2015 LMSA-SPS

In March 2015, the second LMSA-SPS was held at the NHMA annual conference with similar educational and advocacy programming. With an opening of the legislative process to any student who wished to draft a resolution proposal, the number of submitted resolutions doubled. Topics addressed included the effects of social determinants of health, immigration reform, health in detention facilities, the founding of a scholarship supporting LGBTQ+ researchers, and school meals.

After a second year of organizational development, policy infrastructure in LMSA flourished into strong collaborations with external student organizations. Exciting alliances materialized with the BlackLivesMatter movement and by Students for a National Health Program (SNaHP), along with diversity initiatives sponsored by external advocacy organizations with interest in Latino leadership development. The policy committee structure continued to evolve in response to issues in Latino health relevant to participating medical students, including LGBTQ+ health and immigration reform. Health policy programming was codified through LMSA constitutional amendments, reinforcing not only policy-related didactics and the COD, but also collaborations with external advocacy organizations. These successes helped affirm the policy activities of LMSA and helped recruit ongoing support from institutions, faculty, and the growing LMSA student body.

Transition to the LMSA-Policy Summit (LMSA-PS)

Many factors contributed to the transition from the LMSA-SPS to the LMSA-PS. The transition started with the application of policies incorporated into the LMSA platform through the COD. In addition, a decision was made to search for alternative venues to the NHMA national conference. LMSA student leaders often felt that the sponsors of the NMHA National Conference at times perpetuated rather than remedied health inequities for Latino communities. For example, the decision by NMHA to have The Coca-Cola Company (TCCC) as a major sponsor, despite Latino children having higher childhood obesity rates than their peers at nearly all age groups [13], philosophically differed from how student leaders expected to champion Latino health equity. Student organizers of the 2014 and 2015 LMSA-SPS were also disappointed by the lack of partnership and collaboration afforded by NHMA. The student organizers were often given time slots that limited student engagement, inadequate meeting rooms (e.g. no AV equipment, limited spaces, lack of water), and last minute communication about changes in conference scheduling.

In response to these concerns, in 2016, LMSA student and faculty leaders, including Dr. Sola and Dr. Sánchez, met with Dr. Norma Poll-Hunter of the Association of American Medical Colleges (AAMC), leading to robust discussions on supporting health policy training amongst Latino communities. Sponsorship of the first annual, stand-alone LMSA health policy conference by AAMC in 2016, now titled the LMSA-Policy Summit (LMSA-PS), represented a major breakthrough. The AAMC was supportive of LMSA's vision of curriculum focused on experiential training in health policy, combining leadership development in policy and academia, community outreach, and advocacy activities in Latino health.

The LMSA-Policy Summit: Kern Model as a Theoretical Framework

Introduction

Based on the successes of the SPS, the LMSA-PS evolved in several significant ways. The conference included an exhibitor fair, expanded didactic sessions, a student-led rally, and legislative visits with congressional officials. This required new efforts in fundraising and development of interactive programming. Students worked to raise funds through a mix of outreach to local businesses, networking with national Latino advocacy organizations, and sponsorship by both academic institutions and individual faculty mentors. Organizational collaboration extended beyond the AAMC to include exhibitors from the Congressional Hispanic Caucus Institute (CHCI), medical schools and professional advocacy organizations such as the Hispanic Serving Health Professional Schools (HSHPS).

Inspired by the educational pedagogy of Dewey and Friere, LMSA used student advocacy activities to drive the broader scope of didactic content centered on community advocacy. Three educational tracks were created, divided into the core elements of Latino Health, Academia in Health Policy, and Health Policy Skills. Facilitators ensured educational content complemented experiential activities within the conference programming, such as legislative visits, rallies and the COD. In this manner, LMSA linked knowledge development with policy competencies that could lead to effective community action. Below is a discussion of novel programming developed for the inaugural LMSA-PS, a model followed with fidelity by future policy leadership.

Health Care Rally

To kick-off conference activities and to energize student participants, the LMSA-PS began with a public rally titled "Social Justice in Latino Health Care'', where students marched to bring exposure to the unjust trends in Latino communities. Rally themes were informed by student discourse and advocacy activities focusing on immigration reform. Organizers created posters with messages such as 'I'm a Bad Hombre", "Trump is an Immigrant", "Latinos Unidos for Health", and ensured permits were granted to march in public spaces on Capitol Hill. Additional messages trumpeted at the rally emphasized the importance of healthcare access, immigration status, cultural humility, and the institutional and structural contributors to the healthcare burdens affecting Latino communities. Prior to their planned march to the Spirit of Justice Park, students gave speeches to rally-goers highlighting student advocacy efforts and the growing challenges facing immigrant communities. Though the students marched in the present, they followed the path laid by generations of Latinos in the United States from whom a culture of action, advocacy and reform was inherited. Lasting a quarter-mile, the rally linked historical militarization of U.S. foreign policy and military conquests of Mexico and Puerto Rico to ongoing attacks on Latino culture perpetrated by the conservative republican leaders of the time. The social justice rally had a high level of student participation, creating a sense of righteous action that permeated the remainder of the conference. Building off the work of students who participated in the WhiteCoats4BlackLives movement, social media became an important conduit to promote rally speeches with medical students. LMSA rally's also became an important tool to advertise organizational priorities and stimulate civil action that was informed by ongoing student discourse.

Legislative Visits

Following the rally, students met to prepare for legislative visits with their elective officials. Senior student leaders on the policy committee identified elected officials who either came from a Latino background, represented large Latino constituencies or whose agenda included issues relevant to the LMSA policy platform. Scheduling meetings with elected officials presented a unique challenge for conference planners due to their busy agendas. Congressional offices were called and emailed regularly to stimulate engagement with congressional staffers and publicize the existence of LMSA and its activities in the Latino community. These efforts produced successful meetings with prominent Democrat and Republican leaders from multiple states including New York, California, Texas and Massachusetts. Congressional representatives included representatives Serrano, Napolitano, Warren, Cruz, and Cornyn, among others.

Prior to each legislative visit students discussed organizational priorities and best prac-tices in how to interact with congressional staff. Students then divided into smaller workgroups each assigned a set of elected officials. Within each workgroup, student participants were assigned specific roles that included discussion of the mission and history of LMSA, the reach of LMSA constituents, review of LMSA's advocacy priorities, and ensuring continued communication with elected officials over the coming year. More than 25 students representing political constituencies from 10 different states were trained rigorously on strategies to ensure a successful legislative visit, including the art of persuasion, political etiquette, and 2-minute "elevator speech" interpersonal communication skills. The policy committee provided biographies, legislative histories, talking points, and summary of issues for each work-group. These supporting documents were critical in ensuring student attendees were able to present professional expertise on the topics discussed, the organization's goal as policy advocates, and actionable items elected officials could take to address concerning trends in Latino health. Topics of discussion included healthcare access, DACA, immigration health, the Latino physician workforce, and mental health.

Networking and Mentorship

The first evening of the Policy Summit was an opportunity for LMSA members to meet, converse with peers, and share experiences from the day of marching on Capitol Hill and interacting with their Congressional representatives. At a networking activity sponsored by the AMA-Minority Affairs Committee, students had the opportunity to interact with physician and student leaders, sharing best practices on academic growth and professional development. The sponsored networking event represented an important organizational milestone where a professional advocacy organization legitimized the outstanding success of LMSA and reinforced the need for venues dedicated to policy-related leadership development within the Latino community.

Keynote Speakers and Panel

The second day of the LMSA-PS offered the first opportunities for students to meet policy leaders working in academic institutions, government agencies, and advocacy organizations through a series of addresses and didactic sessions. Karen Fisher J.D., Chief Public Policy Officer for the AAMC, welcomed students to the LMSA-PS, focusing on federal advocacy efforts to promote academic medicine. Captain Kenneth Dominguez M.D. M.P.H., a prominent public health leader involved in the HIV/AIDS epidemic, discussed trends in infectious diseases in marginalized communities and his professional arc as a CDC employee. Dr. Kathy Sykes Ph.D. gave the keynote address as the Senior Advisor for Aging and Public Health of the Environmental Protection Agency (EPA), discussing efforts to develop health policy regulations addressing Latino health disparities.

The morning session concluded with a panel discussion populated by veteran health policy advocates and the previous speakers, allowing interactive discussions with students on contemporary healthcare issues faced by Latino patients. Panelists accentuated their professional and academic experiences in health policy, including the pursuit of professional networks, influential mentors, and strategies to promulgate policy platforms into real impact in the Latino communities. This interactive panel prepared students for the subsequent small group breakout sessions offered within 3 tracks addressing Latino Health, Leadership and Academica, and Health Policy Skills (see figure for detailed list). Throughout the day participants were also invited to an exhibitor fair with over 20 booths representing academic and advocacy institutions. A poster fair held during breaks between sessions allowed students to share success in advocacy research and stimulated further evidence-based discourse on health care reform.

LMSA Congress of Delegates

Informed by health policy programming in external organizations, the LMSA policy development process centered on the legislative activities in the Congress of Delegates (COD), held on the third day of the LMSA-PS. The COD helped guide future LMSA advocacy programming, shaped policy-related educational offerings and set the boundaries for political activities within the organization. Within each congressional session students presented their resolutions for debate, which were then voted upon by nominated regional delegates. Potential actions taken on resolutions included adoption, non-adoption, tabling for further research, or referral to the National Board for discussion. A simple majority was necessary for adoption of most resolutions, though those involving reforms to the organizational constitution required support from two-thirds of voting delegates.

Though voting was limited to regional delegations, all students were invited to provide testimony for or against proposed resolutions. Representatives with relevant professional expertise from external organizations, as well as individuals with relevant professional expertise, were invited to provide testimony before the Congress. Like the U.S. political system, resolution language was actively amended while on the congressional floor using parliamentarian rules of order. Approved resolutions became part of the LMSA policy platform.

To ensure policy resolutions submitted to the COD met the organization's professional and academic standards, student participants were encouraged to work through a methodical preparatory process. After identifying a problem amenable to policy solutions, students were encouraged to share their research and policy proposals with regional leadership. Drafted resolutions were then presented to the virtual reference committee, an online forum allowing regional boards, national leadership, and topical experts to review and comment on proposed resolutions. Feedback provided to student participants can include general advice, suggested word-smithing and strategic planning that foreshadows likely points of debate on the floor of the COD. The national policy committee also reviewed each submitted resolution, providing commentary that contextualizes proposed policy actions within the historical precedent and ongoing policy activities of LMSA. Through this process students received expert opinion both on their resolutions topical content and the internal political and administrative levers that could be utilized to implement each proposal. The period between the virtual reference committee and the COD allowed regions to discuss submitted resolutions with voting delegates while students perfected their legislative proposals.

Procedural aspects modeled from the AMA-MSS included a modified parliamentary version of Robert's Rules of Order, and the infrastructure used to provide educational and mentoring programming necessary to support a student-run legislative process. AMSA structure was utilized less regarding procedural infrastructure but provided a template for a student-driven policy and educational process. Most importantly, adaptations ensured that the systems built around the LMSA policy programming centered on the experiences of Latino students and patient communities.

Resolutions submitted to the 2016 Congress addressed corporate influence on medical organizations, voting rights for Latinos, diversification of the workforce, and immigration health. After the energetic, organized chaos of legislative testimony and debate, LMSA delegates moved to approve 18 of the proposed resolutions. With these inputs the LMSA policy platform grew to reflect the needs and concerns of Latino medical students across the U.S.

Evolution of LMSA Infrastructure

If you're not careful, the newspapers will have you hating the people who are being oppressed, and loving the people who are doing the oppressing. El-Hajj Malik El-Shabazz Malcolm X

Evolution of Advocacy Strategies in the LMSA Policy Committee

The 2016–2017 years were notable for a divergence in the policy strategies and vision of LMSA leadership. The student founders of LMSA pol-

icy infrastructure had a goal of not only educating LMSA students in health policy, but also building specific competencies that could be actively applied. To date these goals coincided with the vision of academic development embodied within the mission and goals of LMSA. The nascent years of the LMSA policy infrastructure flourished within national political discourse guided by political leaders whose interest paralleled LMSA goals of health equity, immigration reform and public safety.

The rise, and electoral success, of conservative populism that culminated in the election.

of Donald Trump changed these factors. A group of student advocates within LMSA pushed for further political action, using LMSA resources and brand to counter the escalating vilification of Latino communities. Specifically, efforts were made to have LMSA actively advocate for students who had accepted DACA status by raising funds, actively contributing to the political discourse and creating a presence within rally's taking place across the country. However, as this evolution was seen as a transition to partisan politics that could place the organizations academic mission at risk, a chiasm grew in the organizational leadership that saw a small cohort of students leave LMSA to apply their efforts in external organizations with a higher focus on committing resources towards tangible outcomes within the Latino community. Academic development, peer-support and policy training became a larger focus within the organization, limiting resources dedicated to direct political action.

During this re-alignment towards an academic context, other caucuses hosted by LMSA also suffered. The 4 caucuses recognized by the LMSA policy committee in 2016, including those focused on LGBTQ+, immigrant and Latina communities, and health care equity, became inactive in 2017. Though these continue to be themes highlighted within the organizational policy platform, lack of structured support led many active students to migrate to external organizations. In lieu of these advocacy activities, further resources were dedicated to the development of academic resources addressing policy training.

Yaritzy M Astudillo, MD, New York Medical College'20, LMSA Chair of Policy 2018–2020, incoming fellow Ann & Robert H. Lurie Children's Hospital of Chicago

I was first invited to learn more about the policy resolution process by the 2016–2017 Chair of Policy, Tania Marin- Saquicela. My interest in the LMSA had been present as chapter president at NYMC and policy piqued my interest. I had not had any experience with health policy although I knew I wanted to learn more about the underpinnings of achieving healthcare goals within our system and I specifically wanted to understand this within and for the Latino community. Dr. Marin-Saquicela took me under her wing and exposed me to the community that is the LMSA and specifically the health policy committee. Through time I learned the resolution process, led the following year's effort, and was Chair from 2018–2020 leading two Health Policy Summits in Washington DC. I grew tremendously working on developing a space in which physicians-in-training could better inform their work and efforts in policy, advocacy, and community.

LMSA-PS Programming - 2017–2019

The purpose of LMSA-PS has remained to provide a venue for medical student leaders across the U.S. to share in the practical and scholastic lessons of health policy. Over the following years the LMSA Policy Summit became one of the most popular events of the LMSA calendar, attracting from 100 to 150 students for training, networking, and advocacy opportunities. It has led to widened interactions between the LMSA and medical students with government and local agencies. The second and third LMSA-PS continued along the in-person format, composed of a rally, legislative visits, didactic sessions and a legislative session over a 3 day period. Policy debates in the 2017 COD ranged from supporting internal resource development such as additional Medical Spanish curricula and anti-racism/anti-ethnoracism in medical education, to addressing specific legislation before the House and Senate such as the Resident Physician Shortage Reduction Act of 2017. Resolutions in 2018 were equally diverse, there was a continued focus on medical education as well as research with the

vision of advancing health equity. Academic medicine saw resolutions providing additional resources for the recruitment and development of faculty from under-represented minority backgrounds. Advocacy efforts had a strong focus on mental health and gun violence both on legislation and community work. There was also support for post-Hurricane Maria resources in Puerto Rico. The two conferences together accepted 28 resolutions that had the dual functions of introducing LMSA to new policy topics while building on common themes of Latino academic development, support for specific sub-groups within the Latino community, and general health care reform. The LMSA programming in this period saw growth and continued support from the academic community as students made it clear health policy was an area of importance to medical trainees.

LMSA Policy Process 2019–2021

2019–2020 saw the beginning of a changing tide with upheaval within the global community, as marginalized communities bore the brunt of the COVID-19 pandemic and mis-steps in the governmental response. Within this environment LMSA faced methodologic challenges, as requirements for virtual programming raised problems for a conference that was based on in-person, active participation. In response to the transition to virtual life, LMSA worked to develop virtual advocacy programming that could continue to honor learners' needs and address political trends affecting LHS+ communities. One example was a national virtual advocacy event held in response to family separations at ICE detention centers. Regional and national policy chairs organized a large advocacy effort titled: Cage-in: White Coats for Human Rights Nationwide Rally, a virtual rally where students provided testimonies to advocate for humane treatment of people in immigration detention centers. The 2020 and 2021 policy summits were also held virtually. Through the efforts of student leaders, fidelity was maintained to the original LMSA-PS conference template. Policy discussions continued to evolve with the ongoing political trends in the United States, focusing on immigrant health, resource allocation during the COVID-19 epidemic, and LHS+ leadership development. The creation of the LMSA Policy Curriculum in 2019 as a virtual educational experience complemented these moves towards the non-traditional approach to policy and leadership development taken by LMSA students.

Creation of the LMSA Policy Curriculum

To further enhance policy training, a longitudinal policy curriculum was developed and implemented in 2019. Curriculum development followed the Kern Model and was divided into two sections. Modules that addressed funds of knowledge, each composed of pre-lecture reading materials, recorded lecture and an in-person virtual review session. Content was driven by learners' needs assessments and included topics ranging from introductory health policy information to policy trends within the LGBTQ+ and immigrant communities, COVID policy responses and the pharmaceutical industrial complex. Student-run informal review sessions allowed learners to contextualize each module's learning objectives within the current political environment through candid, peer-driven discourse.

Workshops requiring active student participation were developed in concert with didactic programming, creating a space where students could apply foundational knowledge gained in previous didactics. Competency based workshops address health policy communications, developing advocacy programming, resolution writing and legislative debate. These workshops actively involved students using small-group breakout sessions where work-groups discussed specific policy topics and worked on drafting resolutions, communication, advocacy and legislative plans in more intimate settings. Each workshop ended with assignments that allowed students to work directly with faculty mentors on policy topics of personal interest. Efforts were made to ensure the

workshop schedule fit into organizational programming, improving the quality of legislative debates, communications with external organizations and constituents, and advocacy programming implemented at chapter and regional levels.

Curriculum facilitators strove to ensure educational content reflected the needs of learners as student interest frequently evolved. Ongoing surveys assessed students' interest in specific topics and the quality of scholastic programming using qualitative and quantitative methods within the Kern model of curriculum development. Adjustments continued to be made as students' interest followed policy trends of the day. Facilitators also made efforts to highlight the open nature of the curriculum, inviting students to create new content, lead review or workshop sessions, and modify curricular schedules to meet the specific needs of student learners. When paired with LMSA policy programming, the curriculum provided a powerful tool for leadership development and training.

LMSA Policy Outcomes

> Injustice anywhere is a threat to justice everywhere. We are caught in an inescapable network of mutuality, tied in a single garment of destiny. Whatever affects one directly, affects all indirectly.
> — Martin Luther King "Letter from Birmingham Jail," April 16, 1963

LGBTQ+ Caucus

The LGBTQ+ caucus exemplified how LMSA policy programming catalyzed both discourse and political action on health care issues important to Latino communities. In 2014, a group of students self-organized into the LMSA LGBTQ+ caucus after identifying an absence of policy language addressing Latino LGBTQ+ disparities in LMSA and other advocacy organizations. The caucus was able to gain an evidence-based understanding of Latino LGBTQ+ health trends and submit a policy resolution for the 2015 COD. They then educated their peers on Latino LGBTQ+ issues by contributing to conference programming development and encouraging organizational discourse on the role of LGBTQ+ communities within the Latino experience. The caucus grew, achieving recognition of the dual marginalization of Latino LGBTQ+ individuals and creating a funded scholarship to support LGBTQ+ research after the 2015 COD. Additional caucus activities included holding regular meetings to develop content and collaborate with external organizations such as GLMA, an advocacy organization representing sexual minorities in medicine. The LGBTQ+ caucus leveraged its organizational connections to successfully pursue adoption of policy language within advocacy organizations such as the NHMA and Hispanic Serving Health Professional Schools recognizing the role of LGBTQ+ individuals in ethnic-minority communities Participants in the caucus published their work in a pub-med listed journal LGBT Health [14], and created a template for additional caucuses to be developed including an Immigration caucus, Women in Medicine caucus, and a Puerto Rican caucus.

Immigration Caucus

In 2014, a group of Deferred Action Childhood Arrivals (DACA) -eligible students joined the LMSA policy committee, looking for peer support and a venue to advocate for their rights within the United States. This group of leaders became the seed of the LMSA Immigration Caucus, a collection of students, residents, and physicians focused on advocating for the rights of immigrant medical students and the patients they served. The immigration caucus was formally created in summer 2015 and was a driving force behind increasing LMSA activity in the immigrant-advocacy community. The immigration caucus worked to ensure LMSA continued to advance academic discourse on immigration, establishing immigration themes in newsletter and conference programming. Student leadership collaborated with advocacy organizations such as the PHD Dreamers, Loyola University medical school and Chicago Medical Association, among

others. They hosted community rallies, institutional teach-ins and published in local media.

The 2016 elections also energized student policy leaders to develop structured advocacy initiatives, leading to the creation of a GoFundMe campaign to support DACA students along with continued contributions to policy discourse and movements towards civil disobedience. These initiatives were eventually shelved in early 2017 to protect the academic agenda of LMSA and its institutional relationships, leading to an exodus of student leaders in the Immigration Caucus to alternative advocacy organizations more active in the ongoing political discourse on immigration policy in the United States.

Corporate Sponsorship

Students active in early LMSA policy programming honed many of their skills collaborating with student groups on the role of corporate sponsorship within medical advocacy organizations. Advocacy initiatives included the creation and distribution of marketing materials such as fliers and pins, soliciting signatories on petitions, and publications in regional medical newsletters. All these activities were aimed at increasing awareness of the business practices that feed into growing pandemics of metabolic disease in Latino communities. These initiatives created friction with NHMA, whose mission of reversing trends in Latino health care were seen to be at odds with direct and visible organizational sponsorship by companies such as The Coca-Cola Company (TCCC). Recognition given by NHMA to TCCC marketing highlighting lack of exercise as drivers of metabolic disease over consumption of sugar-sweetened beverages was also incompatible with the growing LMSA policy platform. Though both NHMA and LMSA were natural partners in policy development and implementation, these differences led to the organizational divergence after confrontations between students and TCCC marketing staff at the second LMSA-SPS, held in conjunction with the annual NHMA conference. In response to failed attempts to end the corporate relationship between NHMA and TCCC, LMSA students adopted policies in the 2016 COD that not only advocated against supporting the business model of the sugar-sweetened beverage industry, but also pushed Latino leadership to limit the industry's targeted advertising towards children in communities of color. Whereas TCCC and NHMA's relationship was evident at the NHMA Annual Conference, the group of student advocates were able to dissolve sponsorship relationships between medical organizations such as the American Academy of Family Physicians, a primary-care advocacy group, and TCCC.

LMSA External Policy Work: Coalitions with External Advocacy Organizations

While LMSA continued to develop internal policy structures and programming, the organization also enjoyed robust external collaborations on specific advocacy initiatives. An early collaborator was WhiteCoats4BlackLives, which had a presence in the 2014 LMSA-SPS. With the adoption of policy language in 2015 condemning the excessive use of police force in Afro-Latino and African American communities, LMSA had a platform from which organizational participation in the 2015 #ActionsSpeakLouder advocacy event could occur. #ActionSpeaksLouder called on academic medical centers to take action on social injustices perpetrated in their local communities. Medical students across the country were provided an advocacy toolkit to help develop and submit videos asking their institutions to promote equity in health care and education. Additional collaborators included Students for a National Health Program (SNaHP), AMSA, SNMA, and the NHMA-Committee of Interns and Residents (CIR). By leveraging the policy development process, LMSA students were able to guide internal policies that facilitated collaborations with national student movements that responded to unfolding cultural events.

SNaHP, a student organization focused on supporting universal health care in the United States, became an ongoing collaborator with LMSA. Student leaders from SNaHP partici-

pated in legislative sessions, leading to the adoption of resolution language pledging organizational support for a single payer system. The adopted policy allowed LMSA to be an active member in a SNaHP led national initiative titled "Ten One Medicare for All". Activities included a vigil and action day, along with programming promoting health equity, access to health care, and racial justice. LMSA joined numerous local, state, and national organizations in the push for health care reform.

The AMA had a historical reputation for failing to include the voice of historically marginalized communities in their political advocacy. Leveraging skills gained in LMSA policy programming, Latino students were able to challenge this organizational status-quo through the AMA-MSS resolution process. Writing resolutions, debating policies on the legislative floor, and establishing coalitions that would advance LMSA's organizational priorities allowed for recruitment of additional financial resources used in PS development, most tangible with sponsorship of policy networking events. Additional policies pursued within AMA student policy infrastructure included advocacy for DACA students, improving health care standards provided in immigrant facilities, limiting access to sugar-sweetened beverages, police brutality, and LGBTQ+ rights, among others.

An active advocacy presence within the AMA allowed LMSA contributions to the Young Health Pipeline Program Initiative, a mentoring program which supported collaboration between a wide range of advocacy organizations. Composed of representatives from AMA, SNMA, LMSA, the Asian Pacific American Medical Student Association and AMSA, the National Outreach Diversity Coalition worked on a common goal of supporting marginalized student communities pursuit of healthcare careers through structured mentorship and role-modeling. This initiative included strategic planning, awareness, and mentoring toolkits distributed to LMSA chapters across the country. Although the coalition was temporary, it showcased how students activated by the LMSA policy process were able to work across organizations to pursue equity and representation within medical organizations.

Publications

Academic and scholarly activity within the LMSA policy infrastructure became an important tool to validate, quantify and communicate the impact of the experiential policy curriculum. Ranging from peer-reviewed, data-driven publications to editorials and public communiques, students were encouraged to transform their policy work into publishable content. Publication of the successes of the LGBTQ+ caucus was discussed previously, but additional peer reviewed publications emphasized student interest and activity within LMSA. Adopted resolutions in the 2015 COD led to an editorial written by students interested in reform of firearm and policing policies. "Medicine, not Bullets for our Patients'', published in a blog hosted by the Huffington Post [15], described the case of Alan Pean, a patient receiving acute psychiatric care in a hospital in Texas who suffered from the effects of implicit bias, systemic racism, and aggressive escalation techniques inappropriate in a healthcare setting. Students advocating against corporate sponsorship published editorials in several state medical journals. Student facilitators also shared their educational innovations in peer-reviewed venues such as MedEdPORTAL and in evidence-based blogs such as PolicyRx.

In addition to external publications, LMSA sponsored several internal publications to ensure students could contribute to ongoing discourse on policy topics of interest. At different times these have included policy newsletters, journals, and regional communications. For example, in the LMSA Policy Committee 2016 newsletter, several members submitted policy papers on healthcare issues regarding the candidates Hilary Clinton and Donald Trump, police brutality as a social determinant of health, Texas's bill HB2 impact on Latina health access and rights related to conception, immigration law reform, and how to build coalitions within organized medicine.

Conclusion

Un pueblo ignorante es un instrumento ciego de su propia destrucción; la ambición, la intriga, abusan de la credulidad y de la inexperiencia de ciudadanos ajenos de todo conocimiento político (Ignorant people are the instrument of their own blind destruction…)
—Simón Bolívar, "El Libertador: Writings of Simón Bolívar"

The Latino medical student advocate in 2023 and beyond has a range of advocacy options to work on, from continued attacks from conservative leadership to increased levels of morbidity and mortality due to COVID-19 and other health stressors. It may be easy to loose hope in the morass of inequity and discrimination present in the U.S. Yet the need exists for continued advocacy efforts as political entities in the U.S. implement agendas contradictory to the general moral beliefs held by a majority of Americans.

The development of student driven policy infrastructure, including a longitudinal policy curriculum and the annual Policy Summit, has sparked enormous health policy interest in LMSA leaders and members, with an exciting trail of local, regional, and national advocacy events. To create a LHS+ physician workforce that has the tools to advocate for their community, it is important to provide early educational experiences in health policy and advocacy. The absence of policy curriculum in traditional medical education highlights the need for academic organizations such as LMSA to supplement existing scholastic resources. Challenges remain for medical students pursuing systemic reform. Limited protected time for advocacy within a rigorous clinical curriculum, lack of focus or funding for policy research and action in medical schools, the disparities in LHS+ matriculation, scarcity of LHS+ senior faculty mentors, and lack of structured programs that can help LHS+ students focus on their community advocacy projects all work towards the degradation of an empowered LHS+ physician workforce. This further emphasizes the importance of developing and training LHS+ student leaders that can obtain leadership positions in private and public institutions to influence policy trends in the United States. As we now stand on the shoulders of community LHS+ who fought for recognition during the Civil Rights Movement, future students will use the infrastructure developed by the early LMSA policy committee's to further improve the LHS+ experience in the United States.

The future for LMSA student leadership is bright. As we move towards a country that values diversity, equity, and inclusion of marginalized communities, it is imperative that we understand where we came from. A study of the past shows that history will repeat itself, and it is the duty of future LHS+ advocates to ensure our community prepares itself to face the bigotry, xenophobism, ethnoracism, and racism that will undoubtedly manifest in future political and social trends. With these tools the LHS+ community can only succeed, and ensure our children, and our children's children, are able to pursue the pan-American dream of freedom in actions and beliefs.

References

1. United States of America. Office of the legislative counsel. Compilation of patient protection and affordable care act. By Edward Grossman. N.p.: n.p., n.d. Print.
2. Tolbert J, Drake P. Key Facts about the Uninsured Population. https://www.kff.org/uninsured/issue-brief/key-facts-about-the-uninsured-population/. Accessed 5 Jan 2023.
3. Centers for Disease Control and Prevention. Health of Hispanic or Latino Population. https://www.cdc.gov/nchs/fastats/hispanic-health.htm. Accessed 5 Jan 2023.
4. Dominguez K. Vital signs: leading causes of death, prevalence of diseases and risk factors, and use of health services among Hispanics in the United States – 2009–2013. MMWR Morb Mortal Wkly Rep. 2015;64(17):469–78.
5. Passel JS and Cohn D. U.S. Population Projecttions: 2005–2050. Pew Research Center. https://www.pewresearch.org/hispanic/2008/02/11/us-population-projections-2005-2050/. Accessed 5 Jan 2023.
6. Riegelman R. Commentary: health systems and health policy: a curriculum for all medical students. Acad Med. 2006;81(4):391–2.
7. Agrawal J, et al. Medical students' knowledge of the U.S. health care system and their preferences for curricular change: a national survey. Acad Med. 2005;80(5):484–8.
8. Kassebaum DG. LCME accreditation standards for management of the medical school curriculum: a clarification. Liaison Committee on Medical Education. Acad Med. 1994;69(1):37–8.
9. Guerrero D. In the country we love: my family divided. Publisher Henry Holt & Co; 2016.
10. Kern DE. Curriculum development for medical education: a six-step approach. Baltimore: Johns Hopkins U; 2009. Print
11. Centers for Disease Control and Prevention. CDC's Policy Analytical Framework. https://www.cdc.gov/policy/opaph/process/analysis.html. Accessed 5 Jan 2023.
12. Sola O, Kothari P, Mason HRC, Onumah CM, Sánchez JP. The crossroads of health policy and academic medicine: an early introduction to health policy skills to facilitate change. MedEd Portal. 2019;15:10827.
13. The Dangerous State of Latino Childhood Obesity Salud America! https://salud-america.org/the-dangerous-state-of-latino-childhoodobesity/#:~:text=Latino%20kids%20have%20higher%20childhood,and%20Asian%20(7.3%25)%20peers. Accessed 7 Jan 2023.
14. Sánchez JP, Sola O, Ramallo J, Sánchez NF, Dominguez K, Romero-Leggott V. Hispanic medical organizations support for LGBT health issues. LGBT Health. 2014;1(3):161–4.
15. Palacios Y, Rocha-Cabrero F, Alvarez L, Penn A, Sola O. Latino Medical student association call to action: medicine, not bullets for our patients. HuffPost February 12th, 2016. Last Updated February 11, 2017.

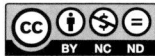

LMSA Faculty/Physician Advisors: A Critical Partner in Supporting LHS+ Medical Students

John Paul Sánchez, Elizabeth Homan Sandoval, Francisco Lucio, Pedro Mancias, Denise Martinez, Sunny Nakae, Hector Rasgado-Flores, Orlando Sola, Monica Vela, Deion Ellis, and Donald Rodriguez

J. P. Sánchez (✉)
Diversity, Equity, and Inclusion, University of New Mexico Health Sciences, Albuquerque, NM, USA
e-mail: exec.director@lmsa.net

E. H. Sandoval
University of Iowa Hospitals and Clinics, Iowa City, IA, USA

F. Lucio
University of Arizona College of Medicine, Phoenix, AZ, USA

P. Mancias
McGovern Medical School, Houston, TX, USA

D. Martinez
University of Iowa Carver College of Medicine, Iowa City, IA, USA

S. Nakae
California University of Science and Medicine School of Medicine, Colton, CA, USA

H. Rasgado-Flores
Chicago Medical School, Rosalind Franklyn University, Chicago, IL, USA

O. Sola
Department of Family Medicine, Chase Brexton Health Services, Baltimore, MD, USA

M. Vela
Hispanic Center of Excellence at the University of Illinois College of Medicine, Chicago, IL, USA

D. Ellis
Diversity, Equity, and Inclusion, Health Sciences, University of New Mexico, Albuquerque, NM, USA

D. Rodriguez
The University of Chicago Pritzker School of Medicine, Chicago, IL, USA

Introduction

All medical schools have physician and faculty advisors that supplement administrative staff (e.g. Dean of Student Affairs or Dean for Diversity, Equity, and Inclusion) to successfully guide trainees through medical school. Medical student advisors have the complex task of understanding their students holistically and managing their academic, personal and professional needs. Advisors to LMSA chapters have the added responsibility to handle the cultural aspects that influence their members' self-efficacy and success. As LHS+ medical students manage the interplay of their LHS+ culture and the culture of medicine, advisors must be ready to help trainees reflect on new experiences, adapt to a new culture, and achieve a new identity as self-assured and competent LHS+ physicians.

With the support of advisors, LMSA chapters and their preceding groups (e.g. BHO, CMSA, etc.) arose on medical school campuses to address the unmet developmental needs of LHS+ trainees and non-LHS+ trainees interested in serving LHS+ communities. There is a common expecta-

© The Author(s) 2024
J. P. Sánchez, D. Rodriguez (eds.), *Latino, Hispanic, or of Spanish Origin+ Identified Student Leaders in Medicine*, Sustainable Development Goals Series, https://doi.org/10.1007/978-3-031-35020-7_9

tion, and often a mandate at many medical schools, that medical student chapters have a faculty/physician advisor. Physicians and faculty typically assist students in understanding the policies and procedures to navigate the process of initiating, instituting, and funding chapters. Emilio Carrillo, MD, MPH, co-founder of the Boricua Health Organization (BHO), credited faculty advisors Dr. Poussaint, Dr. Einsenburg, Dr. Furshpan, and Dr. Kravitz for providing guidance and support in instituting BHO at Harvard Medical School and Dr. Rodriguez-Trias in building a regional presence.

The relationship between chapter leaders and advisors is mutually beneficial and necessary. An effective relationship can simultaneously meet the mission and goals of LMSA and fulfill the mission areas of the medical school. Trainees can achieve various scholarly outcomes such as receiving individual financial scholarships, applying for project grants, and presenting oral or poster presentations. They can also achieve leadership outcomes by serving in chapter, regional and national roles. Similar opportunities exist for faculty/physicians. When students and faculty collaborate, the aforementioned scholarly outcomes are more feasible and can allow for greater recognition of 'two-fers/three-fers' - the opportunity to achieve multiple outcomes from one primary activity. For example, successful chapters can apply for LMSA Chapter of the Year and faculty/physician advisors can apply for LMSA Regional or National Mentor of the Year. Students and advisors can write letters of recommendation for each other for promotion purposes. For medical students, this can increase their competitiveness for residency and for faculty to increase their promotion potential along a faculty (e.g. Assistant to Associate Professor) or administrative track (e.g. Director to Dean).

There are several factors that influence the success of the chapter and student-advisor relationship. **Prior and new chapter leaders must spend time discussing transition**. Chapter leaders usually serve one term in a position (e.g. chapter president) and have a short period to adapt. Advisors must ensure that there are transition meetings so new leaders understand facilitators of chapter success, mistakes to avoid, and

build on lessons learned. **Less is more.** It is critical for student leaders and faculty to consider what is realistic over an academic year regarding a feasible number of quality projects and events. These events must be properly advertised and documented, in order to showcase the chapter's successes to LMSA at large and to the medical school itself. Activities should align with the mission/strategic plan of the medical school and the LMSA organization. **Focus on members' needs.** Taking inventory of members' interests helps to ensure a greater level of engagement by members. **Aim for value-based alignment.** Advisors should help students appreciate how their efforts can meet personal passion, professional interests, institutional mission/objectives, and community needs and disparities [1]. Advisors and chapter leaders can maximize success through frequent, open communication; understanding each other's vision, goals, interests, and responsibilities; strategic planning; monitoring progress; and aiming for agreed-upon core deliverables.

The Weight of Being an Advisor

Beyond serving chapter members, LMSA advisors **must** also manage their own professional success within the environment of a medical school. Medical schools have a social mission to graduate a diverse physician workforce; however, graduating and maximizing the potential of trainees are not synonymous. LMSA advisors, many of who are congruent in LHS+ identity, possess the aptitude to serve as credible role models, mentors, and champions, and can help trainees reach their full potential. However, for many advisors, based on their contract and the medical school culture, this level of activity and investment towards LHS+ medical students may be characterized as a "minority tax" rather than Full-Time Equivalent (FTE) or promotion capital [2]. Dependent on their faculty track, their chair's expectations, and appointment and promotion guidelines, their LMSA-related work may or may not be routinely documented and substantially valued. Advisors must proactively reflect on how their LMSA activities align with their contractual responsibilities and discuss with their departmental Chair or medical school Dean how the work is mutually valuable and credited.

The Role of Advisor as Defined by LMSA Bylaws and Constitution

LHS+ medical student organizations have been championed and led by students. Although advisors have always been present and have helped guide the movement, their defined roles and responsibilities have slowly emerged in the distinct LMSA National and various regional constitutions and bylaws. Furthermore, across constitutions and bylaws, there has been considerable variation in positions (and titles) for faculty/physicians, associated responsibilities, and extent of influence. FPAC advisors must be physicians, healthcare professionals, and/or established faculty or staff at a medical school accredited by the United States - (U.S.) based Liaison Committee on Medical Education (LCME) or the American Osteopathic Association's Commission on Osteopathic College Accreditation (AOA COCA). The LMSA National Constitution specifies that a chapter must have "A signed attestation by at least ONE (1) faculty member or senior administrator…to serve as the Chapter Advisor (4.3.2)".

In terms of advisory groups, LMSA's National constitution and bylaws allow for a Corporate Advisory Council, whereas LMSA West, LMSA Midwest, and LMSA Southwest have Advisory Boards [3–6]. LMSA National and LMSA West documents allow for the appointment of an Executive Director [4, 7]. Advisors have had some recognition in LMSA governing documents but not in the totality of what they have been called or expected to do by chapters, regional or national entities.

Illuminating and Defining the Role of Faculty/Physician Advisors

In the Fall of 2017, Co-Executive Director J.P. Sánchez, MD, MPH, and LMSA National President Eric Molina met to consider 'low-hanging' approaches to addressing the concept

of 'minority tax' for LMSA advisors. Of particular concern was the negative impact the 'minority tax' would have on the current pool and future pool of Hispanic/Latino-identified LMSA advisors; in 2021, 5.9% of faculty at allopathic medical schools identified as Hispanic/Latino [8] and in 2016–2017 1.7% of faculty at osteopathic medical schools identified as Hispanic/Latino [9]. Hispanic/Latino and other underrepresented in medicine (UiM) faculty, overwhelmed by the 'minority tax', may inadvertently discourage LHS+ students from entering academia and limit the future pool of LMSA advisors [10]. In response, LMSA National Co-Executive Director Dr. Sánchez drafted a proposal (10/2017) and Eric Molina obtained approval by the LMSA National Board for a detailed description of the responsibilities of chapter advisors and of a new National Physician Advisory Council (PAC), elections of individuals to PAC, and structured metrics for the evaluation of advisors. In 2018, to recognize non-physician advisors the name was changed to Faculty/Physician Advisory Council.

Based on the approved proposal, chapter-level faculty/physician advisors, in advising the LMSA chapters, were responsible for:

1. The development, implementation, and evaluation of an annual strategic plan that aligns with the mission and strategic plan of LMSA National;
2. Discussing ongoing and emerging Latino/Hispanic related health issues;
3. Helping chapters be engaged in LMSA National and Regional activities; and
4. Helping chapters determine the personal and professional interests of their members and work towards cultivating the next generation of Latino leaders

In addition, chapter-level faculty advisors were expected to:

1. Attend the LMSA regional or national conference;
2. Participate in the LMSA National Faculty orientation (offered via webinar quarterly or at the LMSA National Conference); and
3. Meet with LMSA Chapter Leaders monthly

Fig. 9.1 LMSA FPAC
National Coordinators
and Director

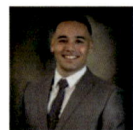 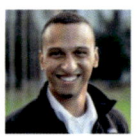 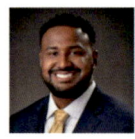

Louis Francisco Morales-
Shnaider, MSc, BS, OSC

Donald Rodriguez, PhD, MD
Candidate

Deion Ellis, MD, MMS

A National FPAC was organized to advise the LMSA National Board on organizational challenges (e.g. legal or financial issues), current challenges in health care related issues (e.g. enhancing care for undocumented populations), and best practices in cultivating the personal and professional development of LMSA members (e.g. the impact of AOA).

Based on the approved proposal, National FPAC members were to:

1. Provide written updates on current trends and challenges, and best practices in cultivating the personal and professional development of LMSA members to the executive LMSA National board
2. Serve as advisor to at least one member of the LMSA national board
3. Raise $1000 of capital for LMSA National (achieved through registration fees, purchasing tables at conference events, donating to scholarships, etc.)
4. Participate in 75% of 8 meetings per year (conference call or in person)
5. Co-present 1 faculty advisor training (for webinars or at the national conference)
6. Assist with the development of the faculty advisor evaluation letters

In 2019, to better support the activities of the LMSA FPAC, in particular, in improving the response rates for the annual directory of LMSA chapter advisors, submission of chapter strategic plans, and evaluation of chapter advisors, Dr. Sanchez asked for each current and future National FPAC member to donate $1250 to support the first paid staff member in the history of LMSA. In April 2020, Louis Francisco Morales-Shnaider, MSc, BS, OSC, President, Latino Medical School Association, University of Colorado Graduate School was hired as the first Part-Time Coordinator to support the work of the FPAC (Fig. 9.1). Louis was followed by Donald Rodriguez, PhD, MD Candidate at Pritzker College of Medicine between July 2021–April 2022 who also served in a part-time role. The success of the National Center for LMSA Leadership and Advancement in fundraising allowed Deion Ellis MD, MMS to become the first full-time staff member in May 2022 for LMSA FPAC.

Election of FPAC Members

Similar to the structure of the LMSA National Executive Board, the initial plan of National FPAC was to have representatives from across the country, with expertise to support LMSA leaders and members. FPAC was set to have up to 10 members with 2 individuals from each region (1 recommended by chapter presidents and 1 recommended by faculty advisors). Nominations were expected approximately 1–2 months prior to the LMSA National Conference. The final selection was based on approval by the Executive Director(s) and the National LMSA President. Terms were to be 1-year with subsequent terms of 1 year approved on a yearly basis after every LMSA National Conference (Table 9.1).

The Founding Council members (2017) were chosen because of their distinguished history in supporting Hispanic students. Dr. Homan-Sandoval brought historical expertise of NNLAMS and LMSA National as past Executive Director and past LMSA National Board Member; Associate Dean Lucio brought legal and diversity & inclusion expertise [11–13]; Associate Dean Martinez brought expertise in pre-medical pipeline/pathway programs

Table 9.1 Founding LMSA National FPAC members

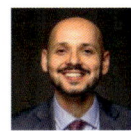

John Paul
Sánchez, MD,
MPH

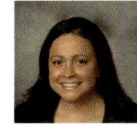

Elizabeth
Homan
Sandoval, MD,
MPH

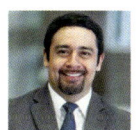

Francisco Lucio,
JD

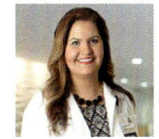

Denise Martinez,
MD

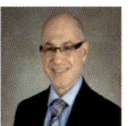

Pedro Mancias,
MD

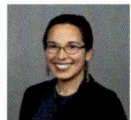

Sunny Nakae,
PhD, MSW

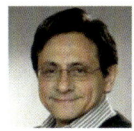

Hector Rasgado-
Flores, PhD

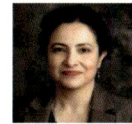

Monica Vela,
MD

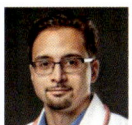

Orlando Sola,
MD, MPH

and diversity and inclusion [14, 15]; Associate Dean Nakae brought expertise in admissions and support for DACA students [16–27]; Dr. Sola brought expertise of health policy as the founder of the LMSA Health Policy Summit [28–30]; Associate Dean Vela brought expertise in Hispanic health, cultural competency and faculty development [25, 31–34]; and Dr. Sánchez brought expertise in diversifying academic medicine, in particular pre-faculty development through Building the Next Generation of Academic Physicians (BNGAP Inc.) [1, 10, 15, 21, 22, 24, 28, 30, 34–43]. In 2020, two new Board Members joined – Dr. Hector Rasgado-Flores, who brought expertise in research, and basic sciences. and student success [44–47] and Dr. Pedro Mancias, who brought senior leadership experience (e.g. endowed full professor and fellowship director) and greater engagement of the south [43].

Giving Credit Where Credit Is Deserved

To maintain and support advisor engagement and strengthen a network of LHS+ leaders, an evaluation system was created to document and validate their contributions. On an annual basis, chapter leaders have been expected to evaluate their advisors and national student leaders have been expected to evaluate their advisory council. The LMSA National President and National Executive Director (or designee) provide the Faculty/Physician National and Regional Advisors and the Chapter Advisors with a letter describing their level and quality of advisement to their LMSA chapter, regional leaders, or national leaders. The letter aims to help advisors improve their skill set through feedback from LMSA members. Ultimately this assists the advisors to succeed in their own personal and professional growth. The letter can be simply added to promotion portfolios and facilitate faculty or senior leadership promotion.

Metrics included on the evaluation form include:

1. Participation in faculty advisor orientation.
2. Level of participation in faculty advisor trainings (monthly webinars or during the national conference).
3. Chapter submission of a strategic plan.
4. Level of participation in regional or national activities (e.g. Regional or National Conference; LMSA Policy Summit).
5. Evaluation by chapter leadership based on the above criteria of faculty advisor responsibilities (using a Likert scale and free text).

Characteristics of LMSA Chapter Advisors

Since 2018, the FPAC has worked to create a directory of chapter advisors to build a stronger national network of support for LMSA members, to enhance communication among advisors, and facilitate advisor training and promotion. In December 2019, a survey was conducted among advisors to collect contact information to support a directory and identify advisors' personal and professional characteristics information to better support congruence for members. Between December 2019 and May 2020, data was collected **from at least one advisor** for 71% (96/136) of the LMSA chapters. The data collected was voluntary and limited by the responsiveness of the chapters' advisors.

Among the 96 chapters, that had at least one advisor respond to the survey, 66 reported one advisor, 20 had two, 8 had three, 1 had four, and 1 had five advisors - for a total of 139 advisors; 66 had at least one advisor with an MD or DO degree; and 70 had at least one advisor who identified as LHS+. **A goal of the FPAC is that 100% of chapters have at least one advisor who is MD or DO degree bearing and 100% of chapters have at least one advisor that is Hispanic-identified.**

Among the 139 advisors, 127 completed the survey and provided personal and professional information. Of the 127 advisors, 65 (52%) were men and 62 (48%) were women. In terms of sexual orientation, 105 identified as straight, 7 as gay, 4 as bisexual and 11 did not respond to the question.

Figure 9.2 shows the ethnicity and race reported by the advisors. Not surprising, the majority 92/127 (72%) were Hispanic, followed by 20 (16%) African-American/Black, 14 (11%) White, 4 (3%) Asian and 3 (2%) American Indian.

Of the 92 advisors identifying as LHS+, the five most prevalent nationalities were: Mexican - 36, Puerto Rican - 13, U.S. - 11, Colombian - 7, and Peruvian - 7, Ecuadorian – 4, Dominican – 4, Argentine - 3, Brazilian – 3, Cuban – 3, Salvadorean – 3, Chilean - 2, Panamanian – 2, Spanish – 2, Venezuelan – 2, Bolivian – 1, Uruguayan – 1, and Guatemalan – 1. This question was framed to assess ancestry and not birthplace.

45 of the 127 advisors were alumni of LMSA or one of the preceding regional groups that formed LMSA National (e.g. NBLHO, BHO, LMSA West, CMSA, LaRAMA, HAMSA, TAMSA, etc.). Among the 45 alumni, 42 were involved on the chapter level, 25 on the regional level, and 22 on the national level.

Figure 9.3 shows the number of years served by chapter advisors. The largest proportion 47 (37%) had served 2–4 years, followed by 27 (21%) serving <1 year, 16 (13%) serving 5–9 years, 15 (12%) serving 1 year, and 10 (8%) serving 10 or more years. Nearly one-third had served 1 year or less, an important group to mentor for longitudinal involvement.

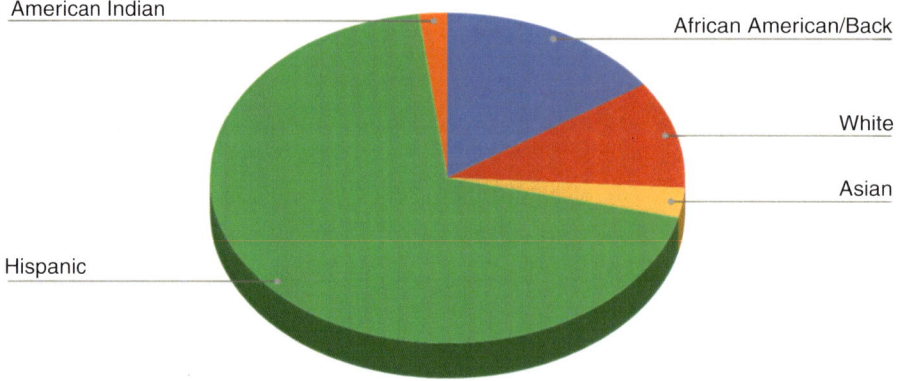

Fig. 9.2 Ethnicity and race of LMSA chapter advisors, 2020. (©LMSA)

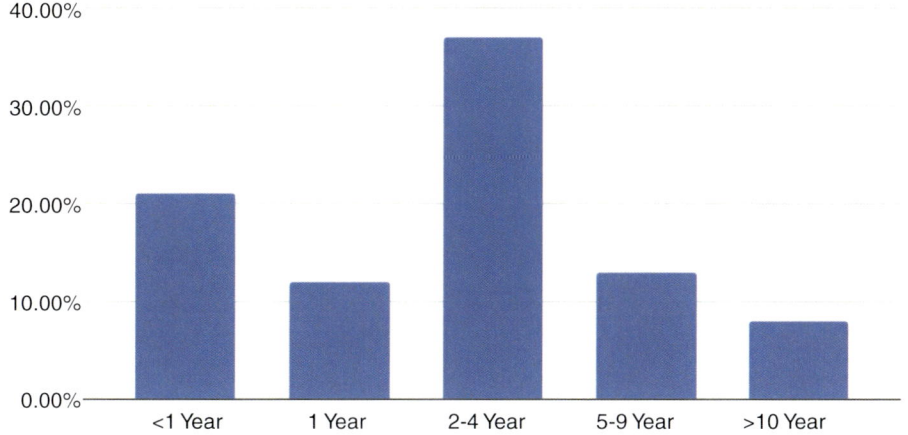

Fig. 9.3 Length of Time Serving as Chapter Advisor (©LMSA)

Table 9.2 Advisor Administrative/Non-Clinical/Clinical Affiliation and Top Ten Practice Areas of Intent reported by Graduates of Allopathic Medical Schools, 2019

Administrative	Non-clinical	Clinical	AAMC GQ[a]
12 Diversity and Inclusion	5 Public Health/Health Promotion	28 Internal Medicine	Internal Medicine
4 Medical Education	3 Humanities	20 Family Medicine	Pediatrics
2 Academic Affairs	2 Biochemistry	16 Pediatrics	Emergency Medicine
2 Student Affairs	2 Biomedical Sciences	6 Obstetrics and Gynecology	Family Medicine
1 Clinical Skills	2 Foundational Basic Sciences	5 Psychiatry/Behavioral Medicine	Obstetrics and Gynecology
1 Global Engagement	1 Engineering	2 Pathology	General Surgery
	1 Physiology	2 Clinical Sciences	Anesthesiology
	1 Chemistry	2 Surgery	Psychiatry
		1 Foundational Medical Sciences	Radiology
		1 ENT	Orthopedics

[a] The AAMC Graduation Questionnaire completed by graduating fourth medical students of LCME accredited allopathic medical schools asks "When thinking about your career, what is your intended area of practice?" [48]

Of the 127 advisors, 104 were faculty. In terms of rank, 7 were adjunct/volunteer, 7 instructor level, 37 assistant professors, 35 associate professors, and 18 full professors. In terms of tracks, 59 were on the educator track, 29 on the clinical track, 8 on the research track, 6 grouped as other, and 4 reported being administrators. In considering how many years advisors have before being ready for submission of their promotion credentials, 40 responded that it would be a period of 1 to 2 years, 19 reported 3–4 years, and 20 reported 5 or more years. Based on these proportions there is an ongoing need for FPAC to provide on-going, longitudinal support and professional development to ensure advisors succeed in the promotion process.

Table 9.2 highlights the affiliation (e.g. administrative, non-clinical and clinical) of advisors. Despite the wide variety of clinical departments represented, there were no advisors from the departments of emergency medicine, anesthesiology, radiology, or orthopedics; specialties shown to be in the top ten practice areas of the intent of all graduates of allopathic medical schools in 2019.

When asked "What are the benefits of serving as an LMSA advisor?" the most common themes were supporting the academic, personal, and/or professional development of members (25 respondents); mentoring trainees (21); networking with students and colleagues (17); learning about the unique challenges for LHS+ students in the MD/DO pipeline and/or health issues of LHS+ communities (7); personal fulfillment from serving the LHS+ community (6); increasing LHS+ diversity in the medical workforce (6); and leadership development of trainees (3).

In 2022 the survey was re-launched to attain updated information, as well as account for the growth in the number of LMSA chapter advisors. The re-launching of the survey resulted in new and updated data for over 200 advisors across the nation. This was done in conjunction with a survey for all LMSA alumni, which combined with the advisor respondents, increased the LMSA Alumni and Advisor Directory to nearly 500 individuals.

LMSA is fortunate to have attracted a talented, driven and diverse group of advisors eager to serve their communities. The great majority of these mentors are still in the relatively early stages of their careers. As they serve LMSA members, FPAC is responsible for enhancing their professional development and academic advancement.

LMSA FPAC Accomplishments, 2017–2022

Since 2017, FPAC has created novel scaffolding for LHS+ faculty/physicians to serve as chapter-, regional-, and national-level leadership and programming to develop them personally and professionally. Opportunities have included leadership roles on the regional and national levels which supports their promotion potential; training on promising and best practices to support LHS+ and other minoritized pre-medical and medical students holistically; instruction on and how to convert their work to scholarship as a means of reducing taxation and building capital. The hiring of the first (and subsequent) LMSA FPAC consultant and eventual full-time staff member as FPAC Coordinators has helped to build and maintain communication and achieve objectives among a national network of advisors.

Part of the vision of LMSA has been to create unity among students, advisors, healthcare professionals and alumni with the goal of promoting the recruitment, retention, and promotion of LHS+ identified individuals in clinical and academic medicine. As part of this vision, it has been imperative to ensure our advisors are prepared and trained, on an annual basis, to effectively guide future physicians and leaders of medicine. Interestingly, there are few standardized programs to enhance the knowledge, skills, and competence of advisors. One nationally recognized standardized program is the AAMC Careers in Medicine Program (CiM) [49]. Through CiM, advisors can receive training to help trainees (a) assess their interests, values, personality, and skills to choose specialties that best fit their attributes; (b) learn about characteristics of various specialties; and (c) land the most favorable residency [49]. As such, CiM focuses on specialty choice and does not offer expansive information on overall career opportunities. Moreover, it does not tailor content for diverse groups who have remained underrepresented in highly competitive specialties. Without proper training, advisors may miss opportunities to distinctly enhance LHS+ medical students' assets (e.g. build medical Spanish proficiency) and reduce deficits (e.g. build their limited professional network). With the evolution of FPAC, current LMSA members have submitted written complaints to National LMSA FPAC of experiencing microaggressions, discrimination, and sexual advances from LMSA and non-LMSA advisors and witnessing inappropriate conduct by advisors (e.g. excessive intoxication). Students have also commented about non-faculty advisors, especially of other partner organizations, lacking an understanding of LMSA history, policies, and procedures and knowledge and skills to help guide them about up-to-date medical education challenges and changes (e.g. racial/ethnic inequities with AOA designation; Step 1 scoring changed to Pass/Fail).

To address the lack of training for LMSA Advisors Dr. Sanchez created the LMSA Advisor Orientation and Training in 2017. The programming was first implemented at the 2017 LMSA National Conference at the Donald Zucker School of Medicine. The purpose of the training has been to bring together former and current advisors to (1) build a sense of an advisor community; (2) review with them the history, vision, and strategic plan of LMSA National; and (3) reflect and learn how to address on-going and emerging issues in promoting Latino representation in the medical and academic medicine workforces. From 2017 onward, to further promote professional development and scholarly productivity, advisors were encouraged to submit abstracts to be considered for workshop presentations during the training. This has provided advisors with an opportunity to present a workshop on a national level, which can support their academic promotion. Additionally, the training has served as an opportunity for advisors of junior rank to meet senior-rank advisors who can advise them on the promotion process or write them a letter of recommendation for their promotion package.

Core curricular content has included Orientation to LMSA and Prior Year Accomplishments (e.g. Review organizational history, structure, constitution, election procedures, and updated procedures); Faculty/Physician Advisory Council Structure, Function, Strategic Plan; Hispanic/Latino Students Needs and Assets and AAMC Resources; Effective Mentoring and Advising of LMSA Chapters; LMSA Opportunities: Achieving Scholarship and Promotion.

Invited topics have typically included new innovations in promoting Hispanic presence in the medical or academic medicine workforces, such as:

- "Office for Diversity and Inclusion: Engagement and Leadership Opportunities for Medical Students, Residents, Fellows" The workshop promoted Hispanic trainees' effectiveness in leading change within medical schools by becoming better acquainted with office policies and procedures. Presented by Cheryl Brewster, EdD, Herbert Wertheim College of Medicine [15].
- "Teaching Medical Students Cultural Humility by Creating Mentoring Programs in Partnership with the Hispanic Community". The workshop highlighted how LMSA members can complete scholarly work through community engagement activities. Presented by Claudio Cortes, DVM, PhD, Oakland University William Beaumont School of Medicine.
- "Jump Start Your Academic Career through Educational Scholarship: Publishing in AAMC MedEdPORTAL and Academic Medicine" The workshop encouraged advisors to publish their work in peer-reviewed journals to support promotion. Presented by Grace Huang MD, Editor in Chief, MedEdPORTAL, Dean, Faculty Affairs, Harvard Medical School.
- "Hispanic Applicants and Matriculants and Legal Concerns" The workshop summarized the prior and current legal challenges faced by Hispanic students in applying and matriculating to medical school, with a focus on Deferred Action for Childhood Arrivals (DACA) and undocumented status. Presented by Sunny Nakae PhD, MSW, and Francisco Lucio JD [12].
- "Getting Promoted as a Hispanic Faculty Member: Instructor/Assistant to Associate and Associate to Full Professor" The workshop detailed the current representation of Hispanics in academia and facilitators and challenges for Hispanics in the promotion process. Monica Vela, MD, FACP.

In 2021, Donald Rodriguez created a new catchy acronym for the program - LISTOS (LMSA Instruction, Support, Training & Orientation Session for Advisors). LMSA offers two LISTOS seminars annually, each seminar provides updated data points and often new sessions. As continuous training, improvement, and growth are necessary for LMSA's success, all those serving in an advisory capacity to LMSA students are expected to attend at least one LISTOS seminar each year to remain in good standing with the organization. As NHMA, HSHPS and other partner organizations have striven to have access and advise LMSA pre-medical and medical students, their members are expected to also complete this training on annual basis. Since its inception, LISTOS has averaged 200 advisors in attendance annually.

National Center for LMSA Leadership and Advancement

In 2021 FPAC launched the National Center for LMSA Leadership and Advancement to respond to the paucity of LHS+-identified faculty and senior administrative leaders. For example, in 2021, there was only one LHS+ identified Dean of an accredited allopathic or osteopathic medical school on the mainland USA, Interim Dean Juan C. Cendán MD of Herbert Wertheim College of Medicine. Pedro "Joe" Greer, Jr. MD, Dean was selected to lead Roseman University College of Medicine in seeking accreditation by the LCME. The four medical schools in Puerto Rico were led by LHS+-identified Deans (Olga Rodríguez de Arzola MD, Dean, Ponce Health Sciences University School of Medicine Ponce, Puerto Rico; Yocasta Brugal MD, Dean, San Juan Bautista, School of Medicine, Caguas, Puerto Rico; José A. Capriles-Quirós, M.D., M.H.S.A., Dean of the School of Medicine, Universidad Central Del Caribe; and Agustín Rodríguez González MD, Dean, University of Puerto Rico, School of Medicine, San Juan, Puerto Rico.)

The purpose of the center has been to provide LMSA faculty/physicians with the knowledge and skills to: (a) successfully support the academic, personal, and professional development needs of LMSA members and non-LMSA diverse trainees; (b) enhance discussion of Latina/o/x/e, Hispanic, or of Spanish Origin+ (LHS+) health-related discussions on their campus (e.g. equity, inclusion, bias); (c) understand how to utilize their LMSA work for promotion purposes and; (d) understand how to develop themselves to serve as senior leaders at academic health centers (e.g. Chairs, Dean, Chancellors, etc.) The model for this new national center was based on the successful model of the BNGAP National Center for Pre-Faculty Development [50]. Similar to the BNGAP Center, the LMSA Center has been situated within a diversity-related national organization rather than an academic health center, reducing overhead costs and political manipulation by a host institution. It has been financially supported by institutional/organizational memberships rather than solely by periodic state, federal, or private grant funding. Institutions could select from several membership tiers; each tier with its own set of benefits and annual fee. It exists in a virtual space and supported primarily by volunteer or part-time faculty/learners and a Center Director to reduce overhead costs. However similar to other Centers across the country it has been structured to produce scholarship, both research and education, affording diverse faculty/learners a further opportunity to advance.

Center offerings have included:

1. Heightened visibility of Center members' efforts to promote LHS+ inclusion in medicine and academic medicine through the LMSA FPAC El Informe: A National Newsletter to Guide, Develop & Honor LMSA Advisors Newsletter, web-site, list-serv, Facebook and Twitter accounts Center members were highlighted among the larger LMSA community.
2. Heightened networking opportunities for their institutional members through the LMSA network the constituents of Center members have had the opportunity to meet successful diverse faculty and collaborate on service, educational, and research endeavors on a local, regional, or national level.
3. Academic Medicine Medical Spanish Fellowship to promote medical Spanish publications
   (a) This on-line 1–2 year fellowship introduces a medical student/resident/fellow/faculty member to opportunities to publish in medical education journals; components and best practices to submitting a project to MedEdPORTAL; and work in a team to submit a Medical Spanish project to MedEdPORTAL. The fellowship closely aligns with the new MedEdPORTAL Collection, Language-Appropriate Health Care and Medical Language Education Collection, led by Collection Editors Pilar Ortega, MD, MGM and Débora H. Silva, MD, FAAP, MEd and supported by MedEdPORTAL Editorial Board Member Anibelky Almanzar, MD, MA.
4. Sponsored registrations to LMSA Chapter Advisor Orientation and Update on Promising Practices (currently known as LISTOS: The LMSA Instruction, Support, Training & Orientation Session for Advisors)

(a) The CME-based one-day training helps chapter advisors and faculty mentors become knowledgeable and well prepared regarding LMSA history, policies, and practices to effectively guide LMSA members.

5. Sponsored registrations to LIDEReS: The LHS+ Identity, Development, Empowerment, and Resources Seminar

(a) The CME-based two-day seminar brings together faculty and physician advisors from across the United States and provides participants with inspirational and practical guidance and tools for pursuing career advancement in academic medicine. The seminar also helps participants develop key professional competencies that build self-efficacy, communication skills, and leadership while expanding their network of colleagues, role models, advisors, and champions.

6. El Informe: A National Newsletter to Guide, Develop & Honor LMSA Advisors

(a) Members are subscribed to receive a quarterly newsletter which includes LMSA FPAC activities, career and funding opportunities, upcoming events, and spotlights faculty members and trainees who are leaders of LHS+ health. The newsletter is disseminated to 3000+ diverse trainees, physicians, and faculty quarterly.

7. Access to nationally recognized speakers for Hispanic Heritage Month activities

(a) A distinguished Faculty/Physician Advisory Council (FPAC) or Chapter Member of the National Latino Medical Student Association Inc. (LMSA) presents a zoom-based Grand Rounds on Hispanic health, policies, and/or practices such as:

- Latina/o/x/e, Hispanic or of Spanish Origin+ (LHS+) Identified Student Leaders in Medicine: More Than 50 Years of Presence, Activism, and Leadership
- Best practices in the recruitment and matriculation of Hispanic trainees to medical school, residency, and fellowship programs (e.g. DACA, holistic review, Step 1 scoring change)
- Best practices in supporting the academic, personal and professional development of Hispanic medical stu-

dents, residents, and fellows
- Best practices in the recruitment, retention and promotion of Hispanic faculty
- Hispanic presence and engagement in medical school leadership.

In July 2021, there were 16 inaugural institutional members of the center (Table 9.3).

It was through the membership of these center members that the first full-time staff member was

Table 9.3 National Center Members

Center member	Year joined
A.T. Still University School of Osteopathic Medicine in Arizona	2021
California University of Science and Medicine, School of Medicine	2021
Cleveland Clinic	2021
Kaiser Permanente Bernard J. Tyson School of Medicine	2021
Keck School of Medicine of USC	2021
Louisiana State University New Orleans HSC School of Medicine	2021
Nova Southeastern University Dr. Kiran C. Patel College of Allopathic Medicine	2021
Rosalind Franklin University of Medicine and Sciences	2021
Temple University – Lewis Katz School of Medicine	2021
Texas Tech University Health Sciences Center El Paso	2021
Touro University Nevada College of Osteopathic Medicine	2021
University of Arizona – Health Sciences	2021
University of Arizona College of Medicine, Phoenix	2021
University of Iowa Carver College of Medicine	2021
University of New Mexico - Health Sciences Center	2021
UT Health San Antonio Joe R. & Teresa Lozano Long School of Medicine	2021
Yale School of Medicine	2021
American Association of Colleges of Osteopathic Medicine (AACOM)	2022
Baylor School of Medicine	2022
East Carolina University Brody School of Medicine	2022
Morehouse School of Medicine	2022
Rutgers New Jersey Medical School	2022
Stanford School of Medicine	2022
Universidad del Caribe School of Medicine	2022
University of Minnesota Medical School	2022

funded. Dr. Deion Ellis, a recent medical school graduate, was selected as the inaugural full-time Director of the National Center for LMSA Leadership & Advancement. Through his concerted efforts in this position, and by the start of the 2023 academic year, the center grew to include 22 medical institutions and organizations, including the American Association of Colleges of Osteopathic Medicine (AACOM).

Having Dr. Ellis as a staff member enhanced productivity and extended the outreach of LMSA initiatives. In addition, he expanded the online LMSA alumni directory; expanded the LMSA Specialty Sections; increased the number of LMSA chapters across the nation (allopathic and Osteopathic); coordinated the implementation of the 2nd annual trip to Puerto Rico for residency recruitment and Spanish curriculum exchange; helped to facilitate the creation, dissemination, and analysis of needs assessment data on the unique forms of discrimination faced by LHS+ identified medical students during the residency application process; and managed the planning of the Virtual LMSA 50th Anniversary Reunion. Since starting in his position, Dr. Ellis has contributed significantly to the advancement of LMSA National, LMSA FPAC and the National Center.

El Informe: A National Newsletter to Guide, Develop & Honor LMSA Advisors

Despite the investment of student advisors and faculty to ensuring LHS+ inclusion in medicine, there has been a historical lack of media outlets to guide their practices, provide on-going professional development, and honor their contributions and accomplishments. In 2021, National FPAC leaders, with the support of Donald Rodriguez, launched a new e-newsletter, El Informe, for the continued growth and edification of current and future faculty advisors. The e-newsletter has been developed on a quarterly basis (January, April, July and October) every year since its inception. Issues have highlighted alumni/faculty advisors' work, publications, promotions; institutional position opportunities/announcements; and general updates. Since its

inception Dr. Orlando Sola has served as a managing editor of El Informe.

Hispanic Heritage Month Lecture Series

Frequently, medical students and residents have raised concerns to LMSA leaders that there has been a lack of educational content on LHS+ health equity taught in college, medical school, and during residency. LHS+ identified learners have struggled to find LHS+ identified presenters and educators or non-LHS+ identified faculty/advisors with expertise in LHS+ health equity. Although this material has been sought for the standing UME and GME curriculum, student leaders and senior administrators have struggled to identify inspirational and knowledgeable speakers for Hispanic Heritage Month (HHM), which occurs between September 15th and October 15th of each calendar year, and uniquely galvanizes LHS+ community members. In response, the National Center for LMSA Leadership and Advancement has identified LMSA alumni and current faculty/physician advisors, and clarified their content expertise, to serve as distinguished HHM distinguished speakers for zoom-based Grand Rounds on LHS+ health, policies, and/or practices across the country. The majority of speakers have donated their honorarium to support the center. In 2021, five potential presentation topics were offered to institutions and by 2022 the directory had expanded to nearly 40 topics.

LMSA FPAC Specialty Sections

The LMSA FPAC Specialty Sections were created in 2021 to provide a space for LHS+ premedical, medical students, alumni, and FPAC (e.g. faculty and physicians), who are interested in the same specialty, to network and discuss personal, professional, and academic-related concerns and opportunities. The chairs selected were LHS+ identified faculty physicians that held the rank of Associate Professor or higher and/or served as a Department Chair. The Specialty Sections initially began with four specialties being represented in 2021–2022 but with the work of National and Regional FPAC, it was expanded to include 10 specialties for 2022–2023 (Table 9.4). During the winter of 2023, 4 additional specialty chairs were added (https://fpac.lmsa.net/lmsa-fpac-specialty-sections) including Rolando De Leon MD for Obstetrics and Gynecology; Orlando Ortiz MD, MBA for Radiology; Marcelino Rivera MD for Urology; and Shirley Sharp DO, MS, FACOFP for Family Medicine.

Table 9.4 Specialties included in specialty sections by year

Starting year	Specialty	Section chair
2021	Internal Medicine	Emilio Carrillo MD, MPH
2021	PM&R	Monica Verduzco-Gutierrez, MD
2021	Pediatrics	Fernando Mendoza, MD, MPH
2021	Surgery	Jorge Ortiz, MD

(continued)

Table 9.4 (continued)

Starting year	Specialty	Section chair
2022	Anesthesiology	 Ruben Azocar, MD, MHCH, FASA, FCCM
2022	Cell Biology Physiology	 Hector Rasgado-Flores, PhD, MSc
2022	Emergency Medicine	 Lisa Moreno-Walton, MD, MS, MSCR
2022	Neurology	 Reena Thomas, MD, PhD

Table 9.4 (continued)

Starting year	Specialty	Section chair
2022	Orthopedics	Selina Silva, MD
2022	Psychiatry & Behavioral Sciences	Francisco Moreno, MD

LIDEReS: The LHS+ Identity, Development, Empowerment, and Resources Seminar

The on-going underrepresentation of LHS+ identi-fied faculty in the higher faculty ranks (e.g. associ-ate professor, full professor, tenure) and in senior administrative positions (e.g. Assistant and Associate Deans, Dean of the Medical School) was the primary impetus for the development of LIDEReS. In 2021, only 5.9% of faculty in allo-pathic medical schools were Hispanic, Latino, or of Spanish Origin, with less LHS+ representation in the advanced ranks of the professoriate - 5.4% of associate professors, 4.3% of full professors, and only 5 medical school deans [51]. Similar trends exist for LHS+ faculty/senior administrators at osteopathic medical schools [9]. Although other professional development programs have existed for racial and ethnic minoritized faculty (e.g. AAMC Minority Faculty Leadership Development Seminar and AAMC Mid-Career Minority Faculty Leadership Seminar) and women (e.g. AAMC Early Career Women Faculty Leadership Development Seminar), there has never been a pro-fessional development program designed and implemented by LHS+ identified faculty/senior

administrative faculty for LHS+ identified resi-dents and fellows with an academic contract in hand and junior, mid-career, and senior faculty/senior administrators, to help them progress to the next professional opportunity [52, 53]. LIDEReS was launched in July 2021, to provide LHS+ iden-tified faculty members, physicians, senior staff members, advisors, and residents and fellows with a contract in hand, from across the United States, with inspirational and practical guidance and tools for pursuing career advancement in academic med-icine. The multi-day seminar has been hosted annually, helping hundreds of participants develop key professional competencies that build self-effi-cacy, communication skills, and leadership while expanding their network of colleagues, role mod-els, advisors, and champions. Since July 2021, there have been a total of 78 distinguished modera-tors and speakers and over 260 participants.

The inaugural LIDEReS served as the first forum for junior and senior LHS+ identified faculty and leaders to convene with AAMC President Skorton and discuss the historical, on-going, and emerging challenges of building LHS+ inclusion in medicine and academic medicine. During the session, entitled A National Perspective on LHS+ Leadership in US Medical Schools, several questions were posed about LHS+ senior leadership at the AAMC. Many had noted great pride in the leadership of Dr. David Acosta as the first ever LHS+ identified AAMC Chief Diversity and Inclusion Officer but were unaware of any other senior AAMC leaders of LHS+ identity. In addition, the participants raised concerns of the lack of LHS+ identified AAMC Board of Director (BOD) Members, a lack of prior BOD LHS+ identified members, and a lack of transparency of the selection process to serve as a board member. At the conclusion of the session Dr. Skorton invited participants to formally submit concerns and suggestions to him. On December 15, 2021, LMSA FPAC penned a letter to the AAMC as an invitation to collaborate to achieve LHS+ inclusion and equity in academic medicine and healthcare. The letter outlined 10 recommended action steps. The letter was signed by **53** distinguished LHS+ academic medicine faculty and leaders across the nation (Figs. 9.4 and 9.5).

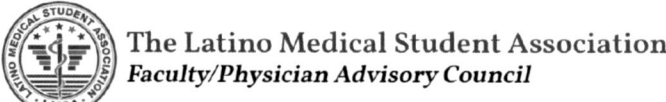

The Latino Medical Student Association
Faculty/Physician Advisory Council

December 15, 2021

Dear AAMC President and CEO Dr. Skorton:

Thank you again for your thoughtful participation in the Latina/o/x, Hispanic, or of Spanish Origin (LHS+)[1] Identity, Development, Empowerment, and Resources Seminar (LIDEReS) session "A National Perspective on LHS+ Leadership in US Medical Schools" held on July 30, 2021. LMSA Faculty and Physician Advisory Council (FPAC) members, who participated in the seminar, have met to respond to your inquiry as to how AAMC can enhance support of LHS+ communities at our academic medical centers.

The missions and objectives of the LMSA and AAMC are aligned; we both aspire to fix America's broken health care system for historically (and currently) marginalized communities. We both play a critical role in dismantling white supremacy and rebuilding inclusive communities in medicine and healthcare. LHS+ individuals represent almost 19% of the U.S. population, but only 7% of allopathic matriculants (alone) or 12.7% (alone and in combination with other races/ethnicities).[2] LHS+ students make up about 5.6% of osteopathic matriculants.[3] As trainees progress through UME and GME, these numbers decrease. These proportions are extremely concerning and have been for decades. We have consistently failed to increase representation despite extensive pipeline efforts. LHS+ representation, leadership, and support are critical if we are to produce a physician workforce capable of providing equitable and culturally responsive healthcare.

In terms of faculty, though approximately 5-6% are a part of the LHS+ community, only 2.3% are tenured professors, and to our knowledge there is only one <u>mainland</u> allopathic medical school dean, of a LCME-accredited medical school that identifies as part of the LHS+ community (e.g. Dr. Juan Cendan, interim Dean, Herbert Wertheim College of Medicine). All four deans of the LCME-accredited medical schools in Puerto Rico identify as part of the LHS+ community. Once again these proportions are extremely concerning to ensure that LHS+ voices and perspectives are present in informing the missions, strategic plans, and activities of the nation's leaders in medicine and healthcare.

LMSA has a network of thousands of physician alumni and current premedical and medical students who can inform, guide, and lead LHS+ inclusion efforts in partnership with the AAMC. In addition, we have collaborated with numerous LHS+ organizations who can further support LHS+ inclusion (e.g. National Hispanic Medical Association, Medical Organization of Latino Advancement, Hispanic Serving Health Professions Schools, MiMentor Alliance in Mentorship, etc.)

1

Fig. 9.4 Letter to the AAMC (©LMSA)

For 50 years the LMSA has subsidized support for historically white academic health centers and organizations who have continued their legacies of exclusion and neglect of LHS+, marginalized, and minoritized trainees. LMSA has created communities, safe spaces, mentor networks, and professional havens for LHS+ individuals with scant support from the AAMC and its member institutions. In alignment with the AAMC publication entitled "Addressing and Eliminating Racism at the AAMC and Beyond,"[4] we invite you to a dialogue about the following actionable steps to explicitly state and tangibly achieve LHS+ community inclusion and equity in academic medicine and healthcare:

1. Establish a council of LHS+ community representatives and stakeholders, consisting of members from within and external to AAMC, to advocate for, guide, and promote LHS+ initiatives and strategies at the AAMC. The council should report to the highest levels of leadership to give voice to the direction and priorities of the initiatives and ensure accountability.

2. Analyze the rich data, both quantitative and qualitative, on the state of LHS+ inclusion within the AAMC and pursue needed actions as part of the goals for fiscal year 2022 and beyond pertaining to recruitment; hiring; retention; professional and career development; staff advancement; and achieving a safe and inclusive environment for LHS+ communities.

3. Hold everyone at the AAMC responsible and accountable for continuous LHS+ inclusion and equity improvement through their DEI efforts, which include everyone's effort to address and eliminate ethnic and racial inequities in the workplace.

4. Edit the AAMC strategic plan to explicitly include LHS+ identity. For example, "We need to better understand how systemic barriers such as racism and *ethnoracism* and inconsistent access to quality education, beginning with pre-K, negatively affect diversity in academic medicine. And we must design bolder interventions to address the growing absence of Black men, the invisibility of American Indians and Alaska Natives in medical school, and *inattention and disregard to LHS+ inclusion* in the physician *and the academic workforces*, which are national crises."[5]

5. Celebrate the 50th Anniversary of LMSA by co-creating a document on LHS+ inclusion in Medicine and Academic Medicine; similar to the publications entitled - *Altering the Course of Black Males in Medicine* and *Reshaping the Journey: American Indians and Alaska Natives in Medicine*. This document should acknowledge the ongoing exclusion of LHS+ communities in medicine and academic medicine and contributing factors (e.g. lack of LHS+ communities on strategic planning documents; de-valuing of cultural assets such as Medical Spanish acquisition; lack of tailored leadership development for LHS+ communities; etc.)

6. Commit to an action plan to address the ongoing microaggressions and overt discrimination towards students who attend the 4 LCME-accredited medical schools in Puerto Rico, especially as they apply for residency and fellowship programs.

2

Fig. 9.4 (continued)

7. Regularly invite LMSA faculty, physician and student leaders to present to the AAMC Council of Deans and Board of Trustees on LHS+ communities in medicine and academic medicine and actions to enhance LHS+ inclusion.

8. Commit to dismantling the structural barriers that actively contribute to LHS+ exclusion in medicine such as the MCAT, spiraling costs of AMCAS and ERAS, and the lack of effective faculty development and mentorship at member institutions.

9. Apply the influence of the AAMC to encourage member schools to support local efforts aimed at increasing LHS+ representation in medicine, such as LMSA and LMSA+ chapters. These organizations play vital roles in accreditation and trainee support, yet are often underfunded and under supported, which contributes to the "minority tax" that jeopardizes the progress and achievement of LHS+ trainees. We ask you to consider that this is a majority subsidy - historically excluded groups are doing the work without the support of individuals who excluded them in the first place.

10. Join us at the 50th Anniversary of LMSA to further discuss the concerns of the LHS+ community and actionable steps to advance LHS+ inclusion in medicine and academic medicine. We are aware that the invite to meet with our community on Thursday March 3, 10-11:30am EST is not possible due to a prior commitment. Would you be willing to meet with our community on Friday, March 4 (50 minute discussion between 8am-6pm EST) or Saturday, March 5, (9:30-10:20am, 10:30-11:20am, 2:00-2:50pm, 3:00-3:50pm EST? If these days and times are not feasible, we would like to schedule some time to explore other times during the period of March 2-5, 2021.

We invite you to dialogue and partnership with us in this critical work. We are appreciative of your leadership and efforts to dismantle racism and ethnoracism in academic medicine and are working alongside you in the struggle. Thank you for the opportunity to submit these actionable steps, and we look forward to meeting to discuss our coordinated efforts to achieve LHS+ inclusion and equity in academic medicine and healthcare.

Gratefully,

John Paul Sánchez MD, MPH (He, Him, El), LMSA Executive Director, Executive Associate Vice Chancellor Health Sciences Center, Diversity, Equity and Inclusion (DEI), UNM Interim Executive Diversity Officer Professor with Tenure & Vice Chair DEI, Emergency Medicine Fellowship Director, Learning Environment Office University of New Mexico School of Medicine (UNM SOM)

Yvonne (Bonnie) Maldonado, MD Senior Associate Dean for Faculty Development and Diversity Taube Endowed Professor of Global Health and Infectious Diseases Professor of Pediatrics and of Epidemiology and Population Health Chief, Division of Pediatric Infectious Diseases Stanford University School of Medicine

3

Fig. 9.4 (continued)

Sunny Nakae, MSW, PhD, Senior Associate Dean for Equity, Inclusion, Diversity, and Partnership, Associate Professor of Medical Education, California University of Science and Medicine

Jessica Belmonte, University of New Mexico

Lorena Del Pillar Bonilla, MD, MS, Clinical Assistant Professor FIU, LMSA SE Regional Advisor

Carrie L. Byington, MD Executive Vice President University of California Health

Juan Emilio Carrillo, MD, MPH

Ricardo Correa, MD, EdD, FACP, FACE, University of Arizona College of Medicine-Phoenix

Leonor Corsino, MD, MHS

John Davis, PhD MD, Professor, Associate Dean for Curriculum, UCSF

Joel Dickerman, DO/Dean and Chief Academic Officer/ Kansas College of Osteopathic Medicine

Gino Farina, MD, Professor and Assistant Dean, Zucker School of Medicine at Hofstra/Northwell

Guadalupe Federico-Martinez, PhD, Assistant Dean, Faculty Affairs and Career Development; Associate Professor, Internal Medicine: University of Arizona College of Medicine-Phoenix

Cristina R. Fernandez, MD, MPH, Assistant Professor of Pediatrics, Columbia University Irving Medical Center

Jimena Franco, MD

Ana Gamero, PhD, Associate Professor, Temple University

Gabriel Garcia, Professor of Medicine (emeritus), Stanford University

Maria M. Garcia

Pedro Mancias, MD, Professor of Pediatrics, Assistant Dean ODI

Denise A. Martinez MD, Interim Associate Vice President and Associate Dean, University of Iowa Health Care, Carver College of Medicine

Fernando Mendoza, M.D., M.P.H., Emeritus Professor of Pediatrics and Associate Dean of Minority Advising and Programs, Stanford University, School of Medicine

Francisco A. Moreno, MD, Professor of Psychiatry, Associate Vice President University of Arizona Health Sciences Equity, Diversity and Inclusion

Lisa Moreno-Walton, MD, Louisiana State University Health Science Center New Orleans

Ana Núñez, MD FACP; Professor of Medicine, Vice Dean Diversity, Equity & Inclusion; University of Minnesota Medical School

Pilar Ortega, MD; Clinical Assistant Professor, University of Illinois College of Medicine

Hector Rasgado-Flores, MSc., PhD., Director of Diversity, Outreach and Success at Chicago Medical School/Rosalind Franklin University

Elena Rios, MD, MSPH, MACP, President & CEO, National Hispanic Medical Association

José E Rodríguez MD, FAAFP

Valerie Romero-Leggott, MD, LMSA Regional Advisor, She/Her/Ella
Vice Chancellor and Diversity, Equity & Inclusion Executive Officer
HSC Endowed Professorship for Equity in Health
Professor of Family & Community Medicine
Executive Director, UNM SOM Combined BA/MD Degree Program
PI, NM HCOP Academy

Nelson Sanchez, MD, Associate Professor of Medicine. Weill Cornell Medicine and Memorial Sloan Kettering Cancer Center

Orlando Sola MD, MPH

4

Fig. 9.4   (continued)

Joe GN Garcia, MD, Dr. Merlin K DuVal Endowed Professor of Medicine, University of Arizona

Jorge A Girotti, PhD, MHA - Research Assistant Professor-University of Illinois College of Medicine

José Luis González, MD, He/Him/Él Affiliate Member, Gehr Family Center for Health Systems Science & Innovation Associate Program Director Clinical Associate Professor of Medicine Keck Medicine of USC | LAC+USC Medical Center

Pedro "Joe" Greer Jr MD FACP FACG, Professor and Dean, Roseman University College of Medicine

Elizabeth Homan Sandoval, MD, MPH

Michelle J. Khan, MD, MPH, FACOG, Clinical Associate Professor, Dept of Obstetrics and Gynecology, Stanford University School of Medicine

Elizabeth T. Lee-Rey, MD, MPH

Suzanne Lopez, MD, Professor of Pediatrics, Vice Chair of Education, UTHealth Houston, McGovern Medical School

Giselle Y. López, MD, PhD, Assistant Professor, Duke University

Francisco Lucio, JD Associate Dean Equity, Diversity and Inclusion University of Arizona College of Medicine - Phoenix

Dr. Karina Madrigal, EdD MA

Julie Ann Sosa, MD MA FACS FSSO Leon Goldman, MD Distinguished Professor of Surgery and Chair, Department of Surgery, UCSF

Sylk Sotto-Santiago, EdD, MBA, MPS Vice-chair for Faculty Affairs, Development, and Diversity; Department of Medicine; Indiana University School of Medicine

Beatriz Tapia, Md EdD MPH

Reena Parada Thomas, MD, PhD, Associate Dean for Diversity in Medical Education, Stanford University

Peter Ureste, MD Assistant Clinical Professor of Psychiatry, University of California San Francisco

Celia Valenzuela, MD, Assistant Professor, Residency Program Director, Faculty Diversity Advisory Committee Chair

Monica Vela MD, FACP Professor of Medicine Department of Medicine Director, Hispanic Center of Excellence University of Illinois Center of Excellence

Larissa Velez, MD

Monica Verduzco-Gutierrez, MD, Professor & Chair, Rehabilitation Medicine, Long School of Medicine at UT Health San Antonio Jonathan Villena-Vargas, MD, Weill Cornell Medicine | New York Presbyterian

Algevis Wrench, Ph.D. Assistant Professor, Dr. Kiran C. Patel College of Allopathic Medicine (NSU MD), Nova Southeastern University

Arnold H. Zea, PhD. Associate Professor, LSUHSC-NO

Definition:

1. Latina/o/x, Hispanic or of Spanish Origin+ (LHS+), comparable to LGBTQ+, is an umbrella term reflective of communities with our common geographic (e.g. Caribbean; North, Central and

5

Fig. 9.4 (continued)

South America; and Spain) and Spanish language ancestry. It gives recognition to historical terms Latino, Latina, Hispanic, of Spanish Origin (e.g. used on standardized surveys), emerging generational/non-binary terms (e.g. Latinx), with the plus acknowledging other terms linked to national identity (e.g. Mexican, Chicana/o, Afro-Mexican, Mexican-American, Puerto Rican, Cubano, Honduran, etc.)

2. Association of American Medical Colleges. Table A-14.3: Race/Ethnicity Responses (Alone and In Combination) of Matriculants to U.S. MD-Granting Medical Schools, 2017-2018 through 2021-2022. https://www.aamc.org/media/8826/download?attachment Accessed on December 12, 2021.

3. 2020 AACOMAS Pro le Applicant and Matriculant Report https://www.aacom.org/docs/default-source/data-and-trends/2020-aacomas-applicant-matriculant-profile-summary-report.pdf?sfvrsn=d870497_22 Accessed on December 12, 2021

4. Addressing and Eliminating Racism at the AAMC and Beyond.
https://www.aamc.org/addressing-and-eliminating-racism-aamc-and-beyond Accessed on December 12, 2021

5. A Healthier Future for All. The AAMC Strategic Plan 2020.
https://strategicplan.aamc.org/AAMC-StrategicPlan-2020.pdf Accessed on December 12, 2021

6

Fig. 9.4 (continued)

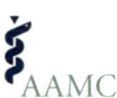

Association of
American Medical Colleges
655 K Street, NW, Suite 100, Washington, DC 20001-2399
T 202 828 0400
aamc.org

January 20, 2022

Dear LMSA Faculty and Physician Advisory Council:

Thank you for the thoughtful and insightful letter about the continued importance of elevating the voice and increasing the representation of LHS+ learners, faculty and leaders in academic medicine. It is critical for us to receive feedback from the community as we embark on our journey to become an anti-racist organization and persist in our equity, diversity and inclusion efforts to advance systems change.

Our missions are in direct alignment. For many years, our collaborations with LMSA and other LHS+ organizations have been critical to our work. We have benefited greatly from the contributions of the LHS+ faculty and leaders, many who have co-signed the letter, to develop new programs and initiatives, serve as faculty for our leadership development programs, and leaders in many of the AAMC affinity groups.

We have reviewed the recommendations as a leadership team and identified key thematic areas that may outline a path forward for AAMC, LMSA and other LHS+ organizations.

Enhance the LHS+ voice and engagement in academic medicine:
While our existing equity, diversity and inclusion efforts have always included the LHS+ community, the letter impressed upon us that as an organization we need to improve our communication and engagement strategies to better demonstrate that. The AAMC's efforts focused on "Addressing and Eliminating Racism at the AAMC and Beyond" is inclusive of the LHS+ community, and this is the ongoing work of the organization, not solely our Equity, Diversity and Inclusion team. We have also released the strategic plan action plans that have intentionally interwoven equity, diversity, inclusion and anti-racism that incorporates LHS+ community perspectives and needs. As we further develop our strategic planning processes, we will work with our leaders and staff to facilitate continued engagement of the LHS+ community and highlight examples of how the strategic plan will impact the LHS+ community.

Leveraging our data, we understand that there have been gains in LHS+ representation in academic medicine and that more needs to be done. A recent AAMC data snapshot also shows the importance of disaggregating data to recognize and address the diversity of the LHS+ community. Our most recent press release highlighted the increase in application, matriculation and enrollment of LHS+ students. In addition to LMSA, we have worked with HSHPS and NHMA to partner on various efforts focused on attracting and supporting LHS+ identified learners along the medical education continuum. With the ongoing engagement of LMSA and other LHS+ organizations, we aim to make this growth in applicants and enrollment a trend, not an anomaly.

LHS+ faculty and leadership development is also critical. We are excited about exploring the possibilities to better support our faculty and leaders. AAMC has longstanding faculty leadership development programs where the focus has been inclusive of LHS+ faculty. For over ten years, we have been a proud, active contributor to Building the Next Generation of Academic Physicians that has been a leader in engaging LHS+ medical students and residents to consider an academic career. More recently, we have appreciated the opportunity to partner with LMSA on the inaugural LIDERES program. However, we recognize that we must persist and also innovate to strengthen the LHS+ voice and representation in

Fig. 9.5 AAMC Response (©LMSA)

academic medicine. Building on the success of prior efforts, we welcome the opportunity to serve as a convener for a summit engaging diverse voices and organizations representing the LHS+ community to explore how we may build a collaborative and cohesive strategy focused on faculty and leadership.

Supporting the PR medical schools and their learners:
We recognize the significance of the medical schools in Puerto Rico to the US physician workforce. The AAMC leadership is familiar with the bias, discrimination and ignorance about the US citizenship status and LCME accreditation of the schools in Puerto Rico. Several years ago, the AAMC worked with the Deans in Puerto Rico to launch an information campaign via ERAS and our communications outlets to address and correct misperceptions and misinformation about their institutions and their medical students. This work led and supported by our former Chief Academic Officer, John Prescott, and Juan Amador, Director of Constituent Engagement occurred more than five years ago. We appreciate the letter raising our awareness of the need to reexamine the impact of these efforts. With Match Day approaching, we will explore the need for a new strategy informed by the Dean and leaders at the schools in Puerto Rico in collaboration with AAMC constituent groups, ERAS, ACGME, the COD, LMSA and other organizations.

Continued collaboration with LMSA
Our support for LMSA is unwavering. AAMC views LMSA as a significant partner in our efforts to advance equity, diversity, inclusion and anti-racism. We express deep appreciation for the responsiveness and ongoing engagement of LMSA leadership who have provided feedback on our programs and initiatives, served as speakers, and more recently participated in a restorative justice session with the Council of Deans. We value LMSA engagement in AAMC efforts. AAMC remains committed to supporting the National Policy Summit, engagement in conferences by presenting, exhibiting and providing financial sponsorship for the national conference, and other areas that are supportive of LMSA's mission.

We hope that you will see how we value and take seriously the recommendations. To strengthen and grow our collaborative efforts moving forward, we would like to start with a meeting with David Acosta, MD, Chief Diversity and Inclusion Officer, and the EDI leadership to develop concrete steps to enhance our engagement toward improved experiences and outcomes for the LHS+ community in medicine and the broader community.

Respectfully,

David J. Skorton, MD
President and CEO
Association of American Medical Colleges

Fig. 9.5 (continued)

On January 20, 2022, The AAMC responded with a letter from Dr. Skorton. Both letters were shared and discussed, through several meetings, with LMSA National student and faculty/administrative leaders and letter signatories. For some of the FPAC leaders the response was considered 'generic' and 'lacking commitment to real change' while others felt it was the beginning of many future conversations. The vast majority of discussants advocated for a larger coalition to consider and be responsive not only to the 10 recommended action steps outlined in the letter but to on-going issues. In May 2022, the first meeting of the LMSA FPAC Collaborator Council was held with leaders of American Association of Colleges of Osteopathic Medicine (AACOM) (President Robert Cain), Association of American Medical Colleges (AAMC) (Dr. Norma Poll-Hunter and Dr. David Acosta), Accreditation Council for Graduate Medical Education (ACGME) (Dr. William McDade), American Medical Association (AMA) (Mr. Craig Johnson), American Osteopathic Association (AOA) (President Kevin Klauer), National Hispanic Medical Association (NHMA) (Dr. Elena Rios), and LMSA National/LMSA FPAC. The Council was created for LHS+ community representatives and stakeholders, consisting of members from within and external to these organizations, to advocate for, guide, and promote LHS+ initiatives and strategies at these organizations. Since its inception, members of this group have met bi-annually to collaborate on LHS + -identified students', faculty and physicians' concerns.

The 50th Anniversary of the first LMSA chapter afforded a unique opportunity to maintain attention on LHS+ inclusion in medicine/academic medicine and bring together organizational leaders to discuss the 10 recommendations. In addition to student led programming, FPAC organized three educational tracks – LIDEReS, LISTOS, and Alumni/Professional Track. As a part of the LIDEReS seminar organizational leaders including David Acosta MD, Robert Cain DO, and Bobby Mukkamala, MD (Chair of the AMA Board of Trustees) were in attendance. In addition, for the first time at the LMSA National Conference, LHS+ identified authors participated in a book signing and provided free copies to attendees.

LMSA 50th Anniversary

Cincuenta Años de Comunidad: Fostering Service, Health Equity, and Leadership (All Images and artwork property of LMSA) (©LMSA)

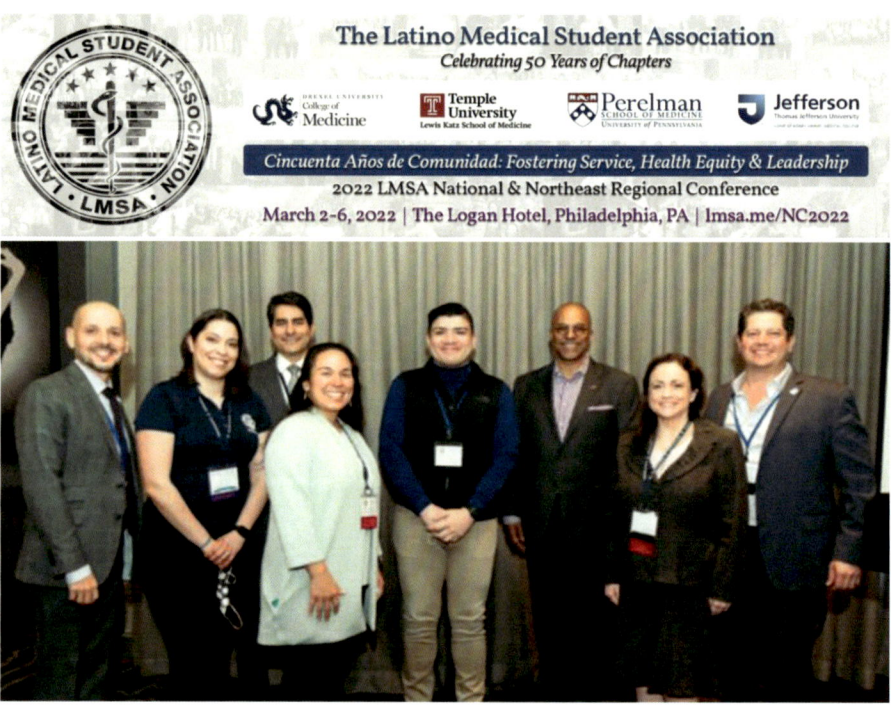

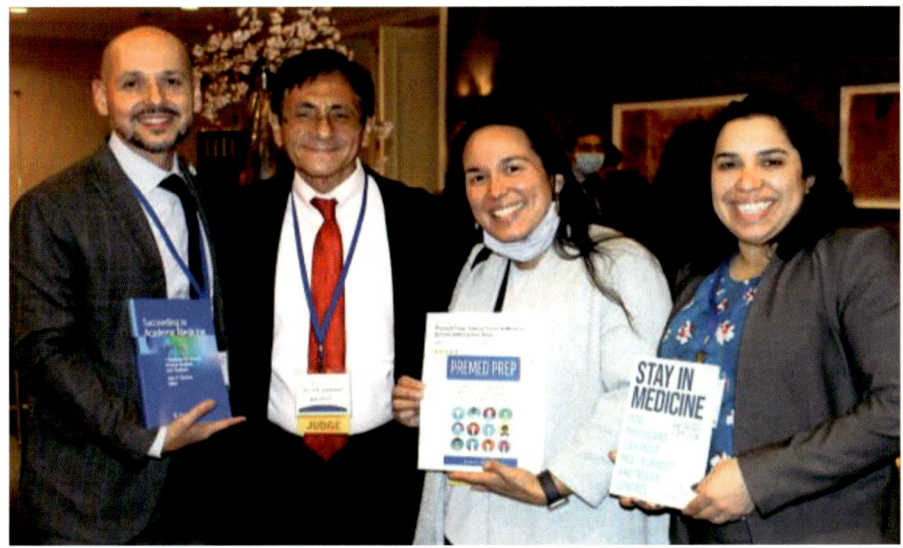

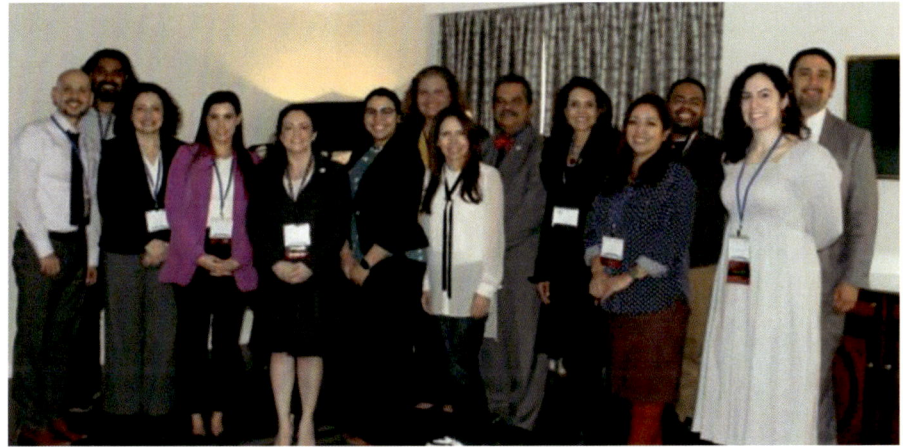

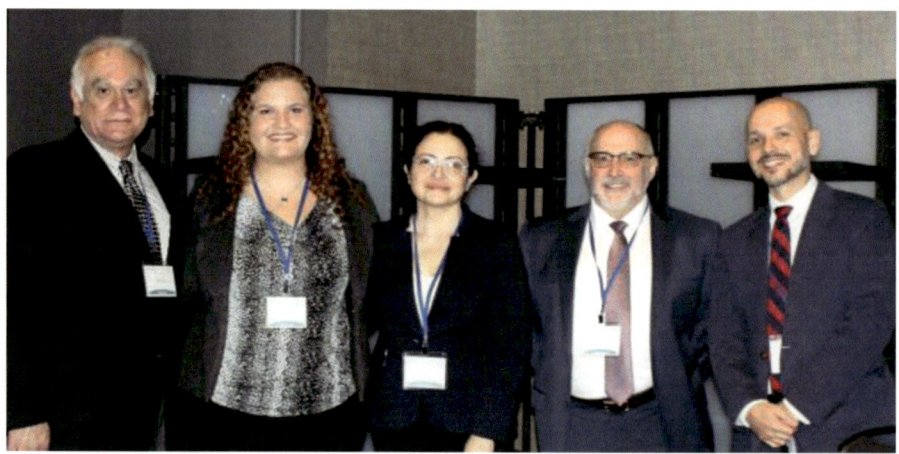

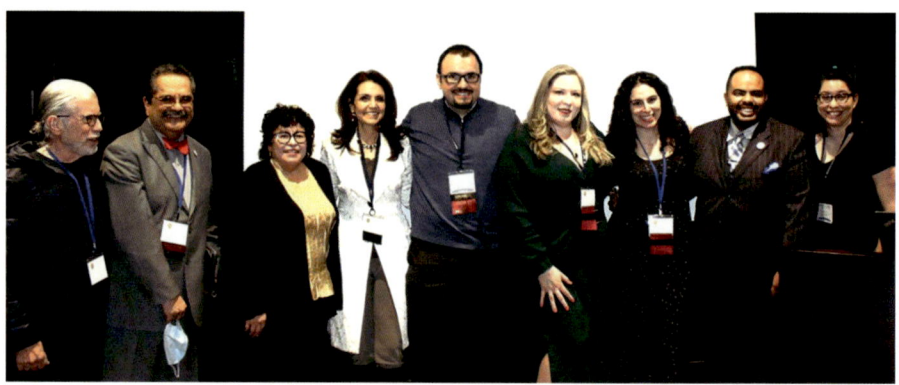

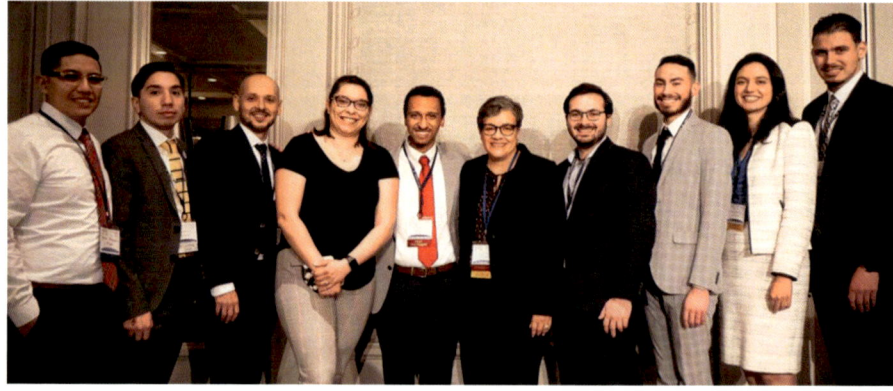

Recommendation 6. Commit to an action plan to address the ongoing microaggressions and overt discrimination towards students who attend the 4 LCME-accredited medical schools in Puerto Rico, especially as they apply for residency and fellowship programs.

After the 50th Anniversary, FPAC and the Collaborator Council attention shifted to work on the 10 recommendations especially recommendation 6 after the AAMC emailed the following correspondence to community members:

- The four medical schools in Puerto Rico are fully accredited by the Liaison Committee on Medical Education (LCME). Residents of Puerto Rico are U.S. citizens who carry U.S. passports, and graduates from these medical schools are graduates of a U.S. medical school, not international graduates.
  – AAMC Announcements and Information – May 9, 2022

For many in the LHS+ community an email alone, especially similar to prior emails, would inadequately address the on-going problem. For many students, alumni, faculty, and administrators it was neglectful, during calls for anti-racism/anti-ethnoracism, for LHS+ identified matriculants of the LCME-accredited medical schools on the U.S. mainland and in Puerto Rico to be mislabeled as "international", "non-U.S. citizens" or "non-English speakers" and endure an inequitable burden as they apply for residency positions and strive to become physicians for our U.S. population.

In response, members of the Collaborator Council, LMSA National student leaders, and the Deans of the four medical schools in Puerto Rico met to design and implement a needs assessment to quantify and further illustrate the frequency and burden of discrimination faced by LHS+ identified medical students when applying to residency programs, especially students matriculated at the four LCME-accredited medical schools in Puerto Rico.

The needs assessment was disseminated between July 19 and August 22, 2022. A snapshot of the data is seen below:

After the data was collected, several webinars were hosted to share the results as well as a press release disseminated broadly across the nation. Subsequently, additional presentations were given to the Accreditation Council for Graduate Medical Education (ACGME) DEI Officer Forum, The AACOM Dean's Forum and Retreat, several residency programs and GME offices. A follow-up study has been planned for February–March 2023.

Advancing Inclusion and Equity for the Osteopathic Community

Osteoapthic and allopathic students, faculty, physicians and administrators are equally valuable in advancing LHS+ health equity. As of December 2022, approximately 25% of LMSA student members and 20% of FPAC members have identified as a part of the osteopathic community. Only one LMSA National President, Lucas Warton, DO Candidate at Philadelphia College of Osteopathic. Medicine, has been from an osteopathic medical school. With osteopathic medical students representing nearly 1 in 4 medical students, it was critical for FPAC to enhance outreach to osteopathic medical school leadership. In the summer of 2022, LMSA FPAC and LMSA National entered into formal agreements with the American Osteopathic Association (AOA) and the American Association of Colleges of Osteopathic Medicine (AACOM) through the leadership of AOA President Dr. Kevin Klauer and AACOM President & CEO Dr. Robert Cain.

NEEDS ASSESSMENT RESULTS FROM CURRENT LHS+ IDENTIFIED MEDICAL STUDENTS
When asked —"Did you **hear** from upper-class persons or medical school graduates that during the residency application process they ..."

Type of discrimination	Puerto Rico Medical Students (%) n-113	Mainland Medical Students (%) n- 37	p-vadue^
Received offensive questions or comments regarding their own English proficiency? (Yes)	48.7%	48.6%	NS
Received notification of application denial because they were considered an international medical student? (Yes)	51.4%	35.3%	NS
Received offensive questions or comments because they were considered an international medical student? (Yes)	56.3%	29.4%	<0.01
Received offensive questions or comments based on the medical school they attended? (Yes)	61.3%	54.3%	NS
Were asked if they were a U.S. Citizen? (Yes)	64.6%	48.6%	NS
Were asked to show documentation or proof of U.S. Citizenship? (Yes)	43.1%	19.4%	<0.05

^Chi-square analyses were conducted to compare dependent variables across independent variables, p<0 05. NS represents 'not significant'.

The AOA and AACOM have had representatives serving on the LMSA FPAC Collaborator Council. Since the beginning of the partnerships with AOA and AACOM, as of December 2022, LMSA has increased the overall percentage of chapters at osteopathic medical schools from 36% to 77%. Through engagement with AACOM, LMSA has come to learn of 2 LHS+ identified AOA Board of Trustees (Dr. Sonia Rivera-Martinez and Dr. David Garza) who are vested in supporting greater representation of LHS+ identified individuals across organizations.

Increasing LMSA Chapters at Allopathic and Osteopathic Institutions

In celebration of LMSA's 50th Anniversary, LMSA FPAC subsequently began an initiative to fulfill the words stated by Dr. Sanchez at the gala, "No LHS+ identified medical student, anywhere in the U.S., should feel alone in medical school. By the end of 2022, we must aim to have a LMSA chapter at every osteopathic and allopathic medical school". Since then, Center Director Dr. Ellis worked in conjunction with LMSA National President Roxie Gonzales, LMSA National CDO Santos Acosta, and all the LMSA Regional Co-Directors (Larissa De Souza, Kimberly Flores, Claudia Torres, Jordan Juarez, Christopher Vazquez, Darisel Ventura Rodriguez, Sierra Sossamon, Luis Valdez, Robert Olmeda-Barrientos and Vanessa Nuñez) to achieve the goal of 100% of osteopathic and allopathic medical schools with a LMSA chapter. For schools unable to mobilize a new chapter by the end of 2022, LMSA worked to link students and faculty with a neighboring medical school with an LMSA chapter. A neighboring chapter can serve as a sponsor for LHS+ students without a chapter and provide support and inclusion so none of them feel isolated. The hope is that the additional neighboring support provides the guidance and resources necessary to have that institution start its own chapter in the near future. As of December 2022, 97% of allopathic medical schools had a LMSA chapter (up from 88% in June 2022), 2%

were connected with an established neighboring chapter, and 1% were in contact with LMSA FPAC to connect with a neighboring chapter. In terms of osteopathic medical schools, as of December 2022, 77% of had a LMSA chapter (up from 34% in June 2022) and 3% were connected with an established neighboring chapter.

Snapshot of LMSA FPAC Accomplishments

2017–2018
- 1st Advisor Orientation and Training
- Approval of FPAC

2018–2019
- 2nd Annual Advisor Orientation and Training
- Increase applicants for National Mentor of the Year and honor nominees
- Build directory of LMSA Chapter Advisor
- Provide guidance to LMSA National Executive Board on AOA response and Step 1 Pass/Fail response [34]

2019–2020
- 3rd Annual Advisor Orientation and Training
- Publish Content on Hispanic Health
- Respond to New ACGME Diversity Standard
- Recruit co-authors and contributors for new book on Latina/o/x/e, Hispanic or of Spanish Origin+ (LHS+) Identified Student Leaders in Medicine: More Than 50 Years of Presence, Activism, and Leadership

2020–2021
- 4th Annual Advisor Orientation and Training + Midyear session
- Expanded number of LMSA National FPAC Advisors
- Instituted National FPAC Advisor contribution of $1250 to hire FPAC Coordinator
- Created aligned regional advisory councils/boards
- Build alumni database
- Drafted book on Latina/o/x/e, Hispanic or of Spanish Origin+ (LHS+) Identified Student

Leaders in Medicine: More Than 50 Years of Presence, Activism, and Leadership

- Launched El Informe: A National Newsletter to Guide, Develop & Honor LMSA Advisors

2021–2022

- 5th Annual LISTOS (formerly known as Advisor Orientation & Training)
- LIDEReS Training
- Maintain alumni base
- Build specialty groups
- Launch National Center for LMSA Leadership & Advancement
- Raise capital for LMSA staff member(s) through celebration of 50th Anniversary of LMSA Chapters
- Revise book on Latina/o/x/e, Hispanic or of Spanish Origin+ (LHS+) Identified Student Leaders in Medicine: More Than 50 Years of Presence, Activism, and Leadership
- Continue Hispanic Heritage Month lecture series (with video recordings) for 2021

2022–2023

- 6th Annual LSITOS
- 2nd Annual LIDEReS Training
- Hired 1st full-time LMSA Staff Member
- Increased Institutional Members of the National Center for LMSA Leadership & Advancement
- Expanded Online Alumni Directory
- Expanded Specialty Sections
- 2nd Annual Trip to Puerto Rico for Residency Recruitment and Spanish Curriculum Exchange
- Created, Disseminated and Analyzed Data on the Unique Forms of Discrimination Faced by the Medical Students of Puerto Rico
- Continued Hispanic Heritage Month lecture series (with video recordings) for 2022
- Hosted LMSA 50th Anniversary
- Hosted LMSA 50th Anniversary Reunion - Planning for the Next 50 Years
- Revised and Published Book: Latina/o/x/e, Hispanic or of Spanish Origin+ (LHS+) Identified Student Leaders in Medicine: More

Than 50 years of Presence, Activism, and Leadership

- Drafted LIDEReS Book
- Increased Percentage of Medical Institutions with an LMSA Chapter to 95% (Allopathic & Osteopathic Combined)
- Launched Collaborative Group Comprised of AACOM, AAMC, ACGME, AMA, AOA, HSHPS, NHMA, LMSA National and LMSA FPAC
- Supporting Endowed Awards for LHS+ Identified Academic Medicine Leaders (Valerie-Romero Leggott MD, Diversity, Equity, and Inclusion Excellence Award, Health Sciences Center, University of New Mexico; Nilda Soto MSEd, Diversity, Equity, and Inclusion Excellence Award, Albert Einstein College of Medicine; Nelson Felix Sánchez, MD LGBTQ+ Excellence Award at Weill Cornell Medicine)
- Launch LMSA FPAC LHS+ Health Equity Medical Education Project
- Launch LMSA FPAC Medical School Fund Campaign for the first mainland bilingual, bicultural medical school

Looking Ahead

With the LHS+ population representing the largest non-white racial/ethnic group in the U.S., the current proportion of LHS+ faculty is insufficient to advise current LHS+ medical students and prepare the entire workforce to address unique LHS+ health issues and disparities. FPAC will be well positioned to recruit, train, and support LHS+ physicians and faculty as they assume leadership roles on the local/institutional, regional or national level. In doing so, LHS+ physicians and faculty can be supported to break through the LHS+ glass ceiling and assume senior administrative positions within academic medicine, as Residency Directors, Deans, Chairs, and other positions. LHS+ medical students will then have a larger cohort of congruent role models, mentors, and champions to support their development.

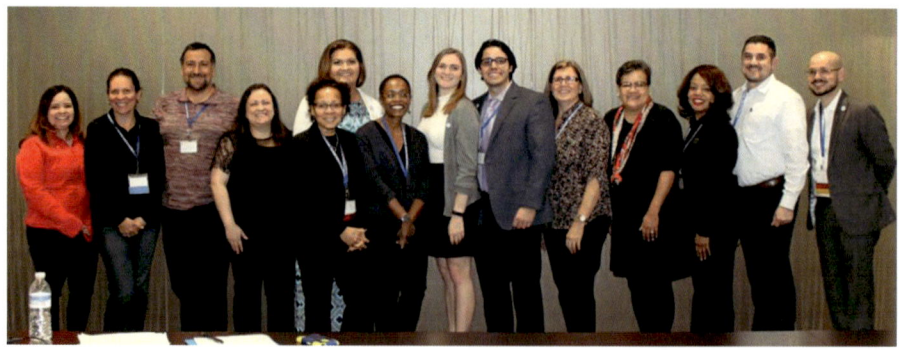

1st Annual LMSA National Orientation and Advisor Training, 2017 (©LMSA)

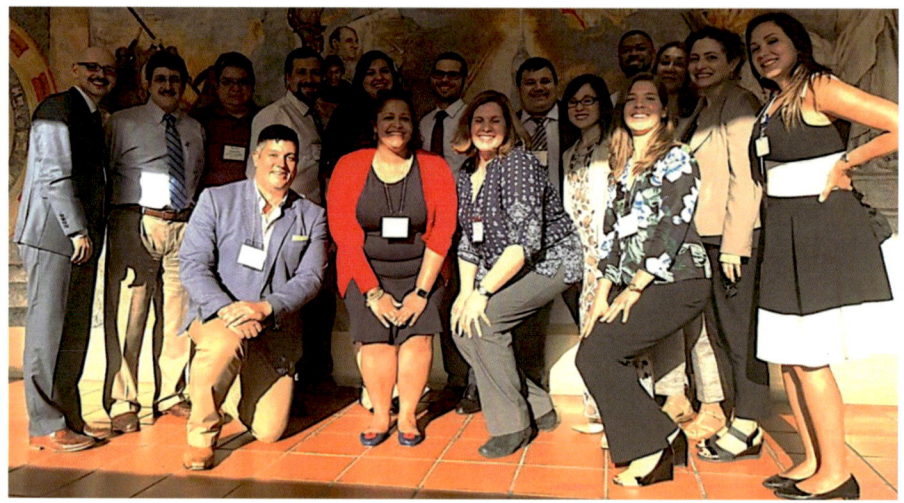

2nd Annual LMSA National Orientation and Advisor Training, 2018 (©LMSA)

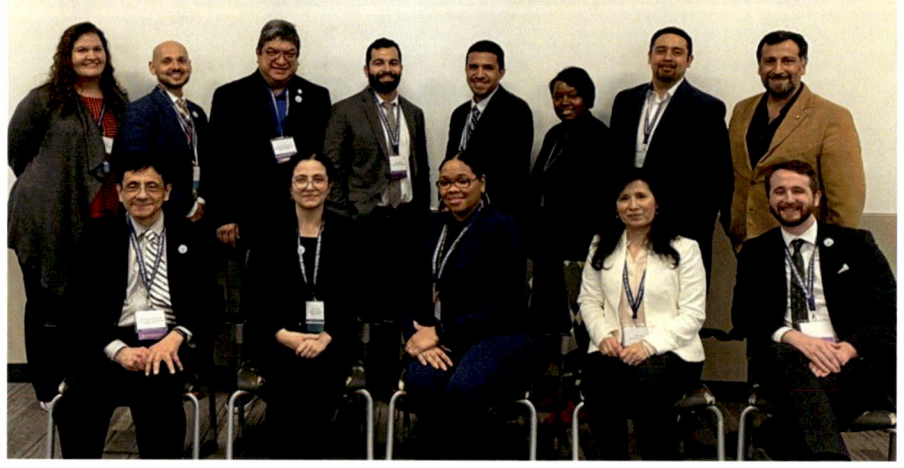

4th Annual LMSA National Orientation and Advisor Training, 2020 (©LMSA)

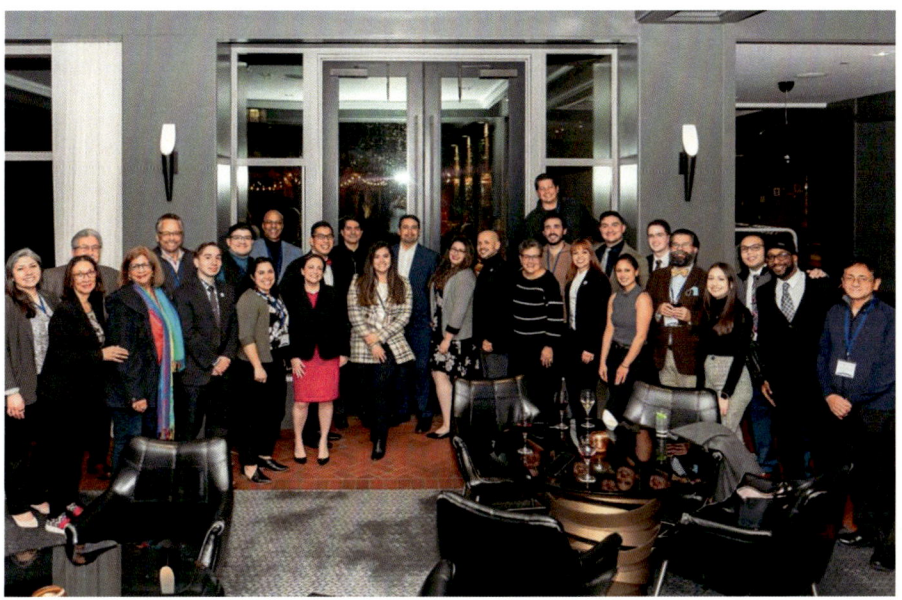

LISTOS, 2022 (Philadelphia, PA) (©LMSA)

References

1. Nakae S, Soto-Greene M, Williams R, Guzman D, Sánchez JP. Helping trainees develop scholarship in academic medicine from community service. MedEdPORTAL. 2017;13:10659. https://www.mededportal.org/publication/10659/

2. Rodríguez JE, Campbell KM, Pololi LH. Addressing disparities in academic medicine: what of the minority tax? BMC Med Educ. 2015;15(1):1–5.

3. LMSA Archives. LMSA Midwest Constitution and Bylaws. https://docs.google.com/document/d/1EF-lVXR5Fl4b63zFQ_z5pZUXL03Fb5mrxOfWP-5mACMI/edit. Accessed 1 Jan 2023.

4. LMSA Archives. LMSA West Constitution and Bylaws https://drive.google.com/file/d/1kIAynd1DbMjiB1f0pk0yrwRcyDm22BXC/view?usp=share_link. Accessed 1 Jan 2023.

5. LMSA Archives. LMSA Northeast Constitution and Bylaws https://docs.google.com/document/d/1XvS88rIPPWfGVA0p1VrUL8RB2vKRCP1dvr7Ay6fzuBY/edit?usp=sharing. Accessed 1 Jan 2023.

6. LMSA Archives. Southwest Constitutions and Bylaws https://drive.google.com/file/d/0B93uV_CMmb_lSEpwVlczM-1doQVZ0RzRhZXUyTm9BLXQ3OEFr/view?usp=sharing&resourcekey=0-E2Kks3qzToBJ6rFls3t8A. Accessed 1 Jan 2023.

7. LMSA Archives. LMSA National Constitution https://docs.google.com/document/d/1XvS88rIPPWfGVA0p1VrUL8RB2vKRCP1dvr7Ay6fzuBY/edit?usp=share_link. Accessed 1 Jan 2023.

8. AAMC 2022. Table 8. U.S. Medical School Faculty by Gender and Race/Ethnicity, 2021. https://www.aamc.org/media/9711/download. Accessed 10 Jan 2023.

9. AACOM. 2016-17 Osteopathic Medical College Faculty by Race/Ethnicity. https://www.aacom.org/docs/default-source/archive-data-and-trends/2016-17-osteopathic-medical-college-faculty-by-race-ethnicity.pdf?sfvrsn=1b12597_10. Accessed 10 Jan 2023.

10. Sánchez JP, Peters L, Lee-Rey E, Strelnick H, Garrison G, Zhang K, Spencer D, Ortega G, Yehia B, Berlin A, Castillo-Page L. Racial and ethnic minority medical students' perceptions of and interest in careers in academic medicine. Acad Med. 2013;88(9):1299–307.

11. Vij N, Singleton I, Bisht R, Lucio F, Poon S, Belthur MV. Ethnic and sex diversity in academic orthopaedic surgery: a cross-sectional study. J Am Acad Orthop Surg Glob Res Rev. 2022;6(3):e2.100321. https://doi.org/10.5435/JAAOSGlobal-D-21-00321.

12. Lucio F. COVID-19 and Latinx disparities: highlighting the need for medical schools to consider accepting DACA recipients. Acad Med. 2022;97(6):812–7. https://doi.org/10.1097/ACM.0000000000004576. Epub 2022 May 19

13. Singleton IM, Poon SC, Bisht RU, Vij N, Lucio F, Belthur MV. Diversity and inclusion in an orthopaedic surgical society: a longitudinal study. J Pediatr Orthop. 2021; https://doi.org/10.1097/BPO.0000000000001851. Epub ahead of print

14. Termini CM, McReynolds MR, Rutaganira FU, Roby RS, Hinton AO Jr, Carter CS, Huang SC, Vue Z, Martinez D, Shuler HD, Taylor BL. Mentoring during uncertain times. Trends Biochem Sci. 2021;46(5):345–8.

15. Castillo ND, Piserchio JP, Brewster C, Martinez D, Sánchez JP. Office of diversity, equity, and inclusion: engagement and leadership opportunities for trainees. MedEdPORTAL. 2022;18:11282.

16. Nakae S, Rojas Marquez D, Di Bartolo IM, Rodriguez R. Considerations for residency programs regarding accepting undocumented students who are DACA recipients. Acad Med. 2017;92(11):1549–54.

17. Nakae S, Porfeli EJ, Davis D, Grabowski CJ, Harrison LE, Amiri L, Ross W. Enrollment management in undergraduate medical school admissions: a complementary framework to holistic review for increasing diversity in medicine. Acad Med. 2021;96(4):501–6.

18. Nakae S, Subica AM. Academic redlining in medicine. J Natl Med Assoc. 2021;113(5):587–94.

19. Nakae S, Palermo AG, Sun M, Byakod R, La T. Bias breakers: continuous practice for admissions and selection committees. MedEdPORTAL. 2022;18:11285.

20. Mason HR, Ata A, Nguyen M, Nakae S, Chakraverty D, Eggan B, Martinez S, Jeffe DB. First-generation and continuing-generation college graduates' application, acceptance, and matriculation to US medical schools: a national cohort study. Med Educ Online. 2022;27(1):2010291.

21. Nakae S, Haywood Y, Love LJ, Kothari P, Saldaña F, Sánchez JP. Office of student affairs: engagement and leadership opportunities for medical students, residents, and fellows. MedEdPORTAL. 2021;17:11093.

22. Nakae S, Kothari P, Johnson K, Figueroa E, Sánchez JP. Office of admissions: engagement and leadership opportunities for trainees. MedEdPORTAL. 2020;16:11018.

23. Garcia A, Lapidus A, De Witt ML, Jawiche J, Lopez MM, Nakae S, Mason H. Deferred action for childhood arrivals (DACA): maximizing impacts in medical education and health care. MedEdPORTAL. 2022;18:11279.

24. Nakae S, Parrish WP, Sánchez JP. Office of admissions: engagement and leadership opportunities for medical students. Acad Med. 2022;97(3):471.

25. Woodruff JN, McDade WA, Nakae S, Vela MB. COVID-19 has exacerbated inequities that hamper physician workforce diversification. JAMA Netw Open. 2022;5(10):–e2238566.

26. Nakae S, Rojas Marquez D, Ortiz Y, Chen ACR. Critical praxis with undocumented students in medical education. critical praxis in student affairs: social justice in action. Sterling: Stylus Publishing, LLC; 2022.

27. Nakae, Sunny. Chapter 4 design: structural equity practices in medical school admissions. In: Poon, OiYan and Bastedo, Michael (eds.). Rethinking college admissions: research-based practice and policy. Cambridge, MA: Harvard Education Press; 2022.

28. Sánchez JP, Sola O, Ramallo J, Sánchez NF, Dominguez K, Romero-Leggott V. Hispanic medical organizations' support for LGBT health Issues. LGBT Health. 2014;1(3):161–4.

29. Solá O, Marquez C. Integrating social determinants of health into clinical training during the COVID-19 pandemic. PRiMER. 2020;4:28.

30. Sola O, Kothari P, Mason HRC, Onumah CM, Sánchez JP. The crossroads of health policy and academic medicine: an early introduction to health policy skills to facilitate change. MedEdPORTAL. 2019;15:10827.

31. Vela M, Erondu A, Smith N, Woodruff J, Chin M. Eliminating explicit and implicit biases in health care: evidence and research needs. Annu Rev Public Health. 2022;43 https://doi.org/10.1146/annurev-publhealth-052620-103528.

32. Appah-Sampong A, Zakrison T, Vela M, Saunders M, Zhang L, Dorsey C. Evaluating the thematic nature of microaggression among racial and ethnic minority surgeons. J Am Coll Surg. 2022;235:210–6. https://doi.org/10.1097/XCS.0000000000000249.

33. Vela M, Lypson M, McDade W. Diversity, equity, and inclusion officer position available: proceed with caution. J Grad Med Educ. 2021;13:771–3. https://doi.org/10.4300/JGME-D-21-00576.1.

34. McDade W, Vela M, Sánchez JP. Anticipating the Impact of Step 1 Pass/Fail Decision on Underrepresented in Medicine (UiM) Students. Acad Med 2020 Sep;95(9):1318–21.

35. Silva Díaz D, Garcia G, Clare C, Su J, Friedman E, Williams R, Vazquez J, Sánchez JP. Taking Care of the Puerto Rican Patient: Historical Perspectives, Health Status, and Health Care Access. MedEdPORTAL 2020. https://www.mededportal.org/doi/full/10.15766/mep_2374-8265.10984.

36. Paredes Molina CS, Spencer DJ, Morcuende M, Sanchez JP. An introduction to research work, scholarship, and paving a way to a career in academic medicine. MedEdPORTAL. 2018;14:10686.

37. Guilliames C, Sule H, Perez H, Hubbi B, Sánchez JP. Providing trainees with an introduction and decision-making framework for pursuing an academic residency position. MedEdPORTAL. 2018;14:10667.

38. Callahan EJ, Banks M, Medina J, Disbrow K, Soto-Greene M, Sánchez JP. Providing diverse trainees an early and transparent introduction to academic appointment and promotion processes. MedEdPORTAL. 2017;13:10661.

39. Sánchez JP, Poll N, Acosta D. Advancing the latino physician workforce-population trends, persistent challenges, and new directions. Acad Med. 2015;90(7):849–53.

40. Yehia B, Cronholm P, Wilson N, Palmer S, Sisson S, Guilliames C, Poll-Hunter N, Sánchez JP. Mentorship and pursuit of academic medicine careers: a mixed methods study of residents from diverse backgrounds. BMC Med Educ. 2014;14:26.

41. Sánchez JP, Peters L, Lee-Rey E, Strelnick H, Garrison G, Zhang K, Spencer D, Ortega G, Yehia B,

Berlin A, Castillo-Page L. Racial and ethnic minority medical students' perceptions of academic medicine careers. Acad Med. 2013;88(9):1299–307.

42. Sánchez JP, Castillo-Page L, Spencer D, Yehia B, Peters L, Kaye-Freeman B, Lee-Rey E. Building the next generation of academic physicians initiative: why, who, how and "what are we missing?". Acad Med. 2011;86(8):928–31.

43. Fernández CR, Silva D, Mancias P, Roldan EO, Sánchez JP. Hispanic identity and its inclusion in the race discrimination discourse in the united states. Acad Med. 2021;96(6):788–91. https://doi.org/10.1097/ACM.0000000000003904.

44. Anderson AJ, Sanchez B, Reyna C, Rasgado-Flores H. It just weights in the back of your mind: microaggressions in science. J Women Minor Sci Eng. 2019;26(1):1–30. https://doi.org/10.1615/JWomenMinorScienEng.2020029197.

45. Rasgado-Flores H, Fernandez C, Gonzalez RG Succeeding along the research track as an underrepresented in medicine faculty. Workshop, LMSA LIDEReS, 2021, Philadelphia, PA.

46. Mroczkowski A, Sánchez B, Flores L, De Los Reyes W, Ruiz J, Rasgado-Flores H. How mentors contribute to Latinx youth's social capital in the sciences. J Adolesc Res. 2021;37(1):128–61. https://doi.org/10.1177/074355842098545.

47. Rasgado-Flores H, Pomarico Y, Rasgado CP, Sumoza P. Cultural considerations for healthcare treatment of Latinos in the United States. In: Olivier MMG, Croteau-Chonka CC, editors. Global health and volunteering beyond borders. Cham: Springer; 2019. p. 231–42.

48. AAMC Graduation Questionnaire 2019, Question 29. https://www.aamc.org/system/files/2019-08/2019-gq-all-schools-summary-report.pdf. Accessed 6 June 2020.

49. Career in Medicine, Association of American Medical Colleges (AAMC). https://www.aamc.org/cim/. Accessed 24 May 2020.

50. Building the Next Generation of Academic Physicians Inc. www.bngap.org. Accessed 10 Jan 2023.

51. AAMC 2022. Table 15: U.S. Medical School Faculty by Gender, Race/Ethnicity, Rank, and Tenure Status, 2021. Source: AAMC Faculty Roster, December 31, 2021 snapshot, as of December 31, 2021. https://www.aamc.org/media/9746/download. Accessed 10 Jan 2023.

52. AAMC. Minority Faculty Leadership Development Seminar. https://www.aamc.org/career-development/leadership-development/minfac. Accessed 20 Jan 2023.

53. AAMC. Frequently Asked Questions about the Seminar: Early-Career Seminar for Women Faculty. https://www.aamc.org/professional-development/leadership-development/ewims/faq. Accessed 20 Jan 2023.

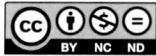

Maria Santos, Debora Silva, and Fidencio Saldana

LHS+ Identity: A Growing Identity Among Medical Students

As the demographics of medical students have changed throughout the last century, the OSA have had to adjust their practices to ensure equitable advising for the next generation of the physician workforce. The pre-2003 AAMC definition of underrepresented students included only Mexican Americans, Native Americans, and mainland Puerto Ricans [1]. Today, this definition has broadened including medical students from almost every country in North and South America. This broadened definition responds to the changing demography of LHS+ individuals in the US. At this moment, not only is there geographic diversity, but LHS+ families have also been in the United States for varying lengths of time. Some have been in the United States for multiple generations, while some are recent immigrants. There is also diversity in parental educational attainment and socioeconomic status, as well as intersectionality with other identities. There is no stereotypical student, or a one size fits all approach to the LHS+ student. The student affairs professional must recognize this and be agile and willing to explore the needs of their students.

Domains of Expertise: Offices of Student Affairs

> **Student Wellness and Mental Health:** Build, promote, and manage programs, policies, and interventions to enable student wellness and mental health. Collaborate across the academic health center and the broader community to recognize and counsel students as necessary to sustain optimal health, wellness, and performance [2].

Medical student burnout is an ongoing challenge facing our workforce today, and many of these students will go on to experience physician burnout or even suicidal ideology [3]. Still, not all students will respond to the same intervention [4]. A meta-analysis by Rotenstein et al. estimates the prevalence of depression or depressive symptoms among medical students as 27.2% and that of suicidal ideation as 11.1% [5]. Programs are encouraged to "collaborate across the academic health center and the broader community to recognize and counsel students as necessary to sustain optimal health, wellness, and performance." [5]

M. Santos (✉)
Family Medicine, Duke Family Medicine and
Community Health, Durham, NC, USA
e-mail: maria.santos217@duke.edu

D. Silva
Department of Pediatrics, School of Medicine,
University of Puerto Rico, San Juan, PR, USA

F. Saldana
Harvard Medical School, Boston, MA, USA

© The Author(s) 2024
J. P. Sánchez, D. Rodriguez (eds.), *Latino, Hispanic, or of Spanish Origin+
Identified Student Leaders in Medicine*, Sustainable Development Goals
Series, https://doi.org/10.1007/978-3-031-35020-7_10

Professional organizations such as the American Medical Association (AMA) and the Association of American Medical Colleges (AAMC) have focused efforts and developed programs on medical students wellbeing. [6, 7] Individual medical schools have developed programs ranging from student-driven initiates to approaching wellness through curricular changes. [8, 9]

There are several stressors that Hispanic medical students face in comparison to their peers. For instance, these students are more likely to have experienced high levels of acculturation stress early on in their lives, which is highly associated with depression in Hispanics [10]. Although this has not been well studied in the medical school population, it is a known phenomenon among college students [11]. Many in the Hispanic community also face increased pressures from familism, or familialismo, a centralist focus/duty to the family and family members such as—providing financial support, being a caregiver, or continuing to be present for the family despite the demands of being a student [12]. These can lead to internalized struggles or perhaps hesitancy asking for help from those outside of this family unit [13]. Lastly, institutionalized racism, such as inequitable educational or economic opportunities, and discrimination, as well as the recent anti-immigrant sentiment, may be another added stressor carried through medical training [14]. Minority students have found their race/ethnicity had adversely affected their medical school experience citing ethno-racial discrimination, ethno-racial prejudice, feelings of isolation, and different cultural expectations as causes. Students reporting such experiences were more likely to have burnout and depressive symptoms [4].

Wellness programs should be designed with these specific needs in mind to identify unique resources and avenues to explore the idea of mental health and wellness of LHS+ medical students. More research looking at the LHS+ physician and medical student workforce and the unique barriers to "wellness" and "mental health" will be crucial to develop these programs. Additionally, the OSA should hire faculty and staff that are well-versed in how to address these with novel interventions and approaches aimed at addressing the obstacles LHS+ medical students face in achieving wellness and mental health as a LHS+ medical student.

> **Student Professional & Career Development:** Empower and guide students in setting and advancing their achievement of effective, individual-driven career and professional goals. Provide students resources and a supportive community of advisors, mentors, and staff to promote their development and transition from medical school to residency training [2].

A key element of the OSA is ushering a student through their professional identity formation as they decide what type of medicine they would like to practice, as well as the environment they would like to practice in—community practice, academic medicine, health policy, etc. The AAMC Careers in Medicine (CiM) program is a national resource that can lead a student through this process as an adjunct to the individual programs developed at each medical school [15]. A crucial part of this identity formation requires medical students to see physicians that look like them as role models to envision themselves in the various clinical and faculty positions.

As previously stated, the LHS+ population is fast-growing, therefore, the LHS+ workforce will need to grow. Thus, here needs to be more investment in recruiting and maintaining LHS+ students in academic settings [16]. As an example, the representation of LHS+ physicians is lacking across specialties, with the lowest representation in ophthalmology, radiology, radiation oncology, and otolaryngology. [17–20] Unfortunately, programs such as the CiM provides little content tailored to students underrepresented in medicine. The CiM information is primarily focused on specialty choice and less so on having students develop a fuller appreciation of career options, such as faculty or senior administrative positions, government, or business. This is particularly relevant when you consider that LHS+ are not only underrepresented in certain medical specialties, but also in academic medicine. In 2020, among medical school faculty, solely 5.9% are of Latino, Hispanic, or of Spanish identity, and this is inclusive of the medical school faculty from the four medical schools in Puerto Rico [21].

Increasing LHS+ medical student awareness and interest in academic medicine careers can eventually yield a higher proportion of HS+ faculty and leaders who can staff or support the OSA responsibilities. Programs such as Building the Next Generation of Academic Physician (BNGAP Inc., www.bngap.org), a national organization focused on diverse medical students and resident awareness and interest in academia, provides the resources to explore further and potentially embark on an academic medicine career. [22] The Latino Medical Student Association and BNGAP have developed curricula to raise Hispanic trainees' awareness of, interest in, and preparedness for academic careers, including engagement and leadership opportunities with the Office of Student Affairs [23].

Beyond medical school, there is little research showing strategies to promote a successful transition from medical school to residency training that is unique to the LHS+ population. One could speculate, however, that by including LHS+ faculty in the conversation throughout the transition into the residency, these students will be better equipped and supported to join the physician workforce while celebrating their unique identity.

> **Student Academic progression:** Build, promote, and leverage resources, policies, programs, and interventions to enable *successful academic progression for all students.* Collaborate across the academic health center and the broader community to help students proactively address and mitigate risks and issues necessary to optimize their educational experience and growth [2].

Academic advising is also a key component of the OSA. Medical students will enter medical school with different degrees of exposure to the basic sciences, and many may be first-generation college students. Medical school academic support varies throughout the country. Some will provide pre-matriculation programs that target students underrepresented in medicine (UiM) [24–27].

One aspect of academic progression is that of standardized exams. UiM students consistently score lower on standardized exams compared to white and Asian students [28]. Experts widely accept that these differences are due to the consequences of structural racism, stereotype threat, and inequities in education, housing, and household income [28, 29]. On the whole, UiM students have more limited financial means. They are thereby unfairly disadvantaged compared to others who can afford the expensive test preparation services and mentoring that are beneficial to test-takers [30, 31]. Cumulatively, these factors may adversely influence UiM students' performance on high-stakes examinations such as the Medical College Admission Test and the USMLE Step 1. This unfairly limits their chances of matriculating into medical school or gaining acceptance to a residency program in a preferred specialty.

Another area worth exploring is the variability in clinical grades, depending on your ethno-racial identity. Clinical grading disparities have been studied and show favor for white students when compared to underrepresented minorities. Differences have been found in the quality of narrative evaluations associated with UiM status [32]. Also, there are disparities in clinical grading and medical school letters of evaluation [33]. The objective and subjective value or effect of LHS+ medical students' clinical evaluations when they are tasked or voluntarily agree to use their medical Spanish or cultural proficiency to care for LHS+ patients is unknown. More work needs to be done to hone in on the root causes of and address the disparity.

> **Student Diversity and Inclusion:** Position diversity as a key driver of educational excellence, a diverse physician workforce, and ultimately equitable health care for all. Advocate for and foster an inclusive, engaging environment to optimize student performance and experience [2].

Once LHS+ students are recruited into medical school, having an inclusive and engaging environment to support their academic, professional, and personal development is crucial. It is not only important to showcase diversity and inclusion in the recruitment process, but also that it is an integral part of student life upon matriculation to medical school. Medical schools seek to accomplish this in a variety of ways, including specialized programming and through offices of student diversity and inclusion.

Offices of student diversity may be under the OSA or separate entities. Their purpose is multifold and includes the recruitment and retention of students that are underrepresented in medicine. These offices are typically staffed by faculty that are UiM and provide support for underrepresented students. Specific programming by diversity offices, as well as the medical school in general, can celebrate the unique skill set and experiences of LHS+ medical students and physicians in a variety of ways such as: organizing LHS+ faculty speaker events, teaching the history of LHS+ in medicine, or perhaps a social media campaign during Hispanic Heritage Month. While these examples are not all-inclusive, they present the opportunity for programs to be advocates and allies to LHS+ medical students, and thus, enhance their medical training experience.

> **Student Financial Assistance:** Provide medical students, applicants, and graduates with sufficient financial aid and effective debt management counseling, education, and resources. Establish mechanisms and recognize opportunities to enable students to minimize medical education debt [2].

The cost of medical school continues to rise every year and can be more than $100,000 for tuition alone [34]. The need for financial assistance is needed for two main reasons. First, tuition rates continue to increase every year, and second, Hispanic medical students are more likely to come from lower socioeconomic status than their white counterparts. The majority of Hispanic medical students come from households with a combined gross income of less than $50,000 per year than their white and Black or African American peers [35]. For the 2019–2020 school year, the average cost for 1 year of medical school was $37,556 for residents and $61,858 for non-residents at public medical schools. Not surprisingly, private medical schools' costs were even higher at $60,665 for a resident and $62,230 for a non-resident [35]. Thus, Hispanics pursuing medical education will require funding from loans that will inevitably lead to long term debt. Additionally, another group that requires unique assistance are DACA (Deferred Action for Childhood Arrivals) students. These students are not eligible for federal funding and have limited options for financing their medical education.

LHS+ students not only face significant barriers in affording the application fees for medical school, but face additional burdens affording the increasing costs of medical education. The OSA should provide appropriate counseling and debt management resources that are unique to the LHS+ medical student population. Additionally, the data around these resources (minimizing medical education debt) needs to be documented

and shared to standardize the best approach to help this student population in financing their education. There are a variety of financing options, and schools should hire financial counselors that are well versed in guiding LHS+ students through debt management.

> **Medical School Recruitment & Admission:** Develop and execute effective, data-driven pipeline programs and admission policies, processes, and practices to ensure a broadly diverse and well-rounded student body that advances the mission of the medical school [2].

The significance of this area is evident in the definition outlining the purpose of an inclusive and engaging environment—to optimize student performance and experience. There has been some improvement in the recruitment of a more diverse workforce over the last century. However, the rate at which LHS+ medical student enrollment has grown is not sufficient enough to compare to the growth that the LHS+ population has experienced on the national level. Hispanics are now the largest non-white racial or ethnic group in America (approximately 19%) [36], yet only 12% of allopathic medical students and 5.8% of physicians are Hispanic [37]. There needs to be monumental changes to the recruitment of LHS+ medical students. Even more alarming, the percentage of allopathic LHS+ medical students has only changed from 4.9% in 1980 to only 12.0% in 2022, reflecting the need for improved recruitment and retention strategies. As mentioned previously in this chapter, the future physician workforce will need to address the unique challenges that LHS+ communities experience. It will require investing in physicians with similar lived experience. There needs to be a more significant push and investment in pathway programs that will ultimately increase the number of LHS+ applicants so that more can enroll in medical school. Additionally, the recruitment efforts need to expand beyond the college years to cover primary education and exposure to the medical field.

> **Student Records Management:** Interpret, communicate, and act in accordance with the laws, regulations, and school standards for maintaining the academic records of students. Establish and oversee processes to ensure the ongoing integrity, security, and fulfillment of information needs [2].

The OSA work closely with the Offices of the Registrar on student records management. These offices maintain student records, process course registration, provide documentation to support application and licensure processes, and maintain course catalogs. Also, they develop plans and policies that protect student privacy. As stewards of student data these offices ensure the enforcement of guidelines under the Family Educational Rights and Privacy Act (FERPA) which is the Federal law that protects the privacy of student education records. FERPA protects student records offices from divulging information such as DACA or other immigration status.

> **Unit Operations Management:** Establish, execute, and allocate resources necessary to support strategic and programmatic goals and priorities and overall direction of student affairs. Lead efforts to maintain ongoing alignment of services and programs with the dynamic needs of students and the mission of the school [2].

The concept of unit operations management brings together the idea of organizing all medical offices that provide student services establish a learning environment conducive to the success of all learners. In regards to the LHS+ student, it involves gathering identifying barriers and developing best practices. All departments, and the school as a whole, must be held accountable to pre-established metrics of success. As strategic plans are designed, issues of diversity and inclusion should be a priority.

Conclusion

Like so many times before, medical school education will need to adjust to the ever changing landscape of a more diverse student population. As we advance into a new diverse physician workforce, we must understand how to support this workforce throughout the stages of training. The eight areas of expertise outline a clear direction for the OSA and Deans to embark on as we move towards a new generation of physicians. Given LHS+ individuals are the largest ethnic/racial minority, the OSA must begin to address the unique experience of LHS+ students and acknowledge the unique experiences that each UiM group experiences throughout

medical training. As the offices devoted to overseeing and enhancing the medical student experience, prioritizing research, and innovation in the LHS+ medical student experience is crucial as we move into the next decade.

References

1. Underrepresented in Medicine Definition. https://www.aamc.org/what-we-do/mission-areas/diversity-inclusion/underrepresented-in-medicine. Accessed 5 January 2023.
2. GSA Performance Framework. AAMC 2016. https://www.aamc.org/system/files/2019-08/gsaframework-overview.pdf. Accessed 5 January 2023.
3. Ishak W, Nikravesh R, Lederer S, Perry R, Ogunyemi D, Bernstein C. Burnout in medical students: a systematic review. Clin Teach. 2013;10(4):242–5.
4. Dyrbye LN, Thomas MR, Massie FS, et al. Burnout and suicidal ideation among U.S. medical students. Ann Intern Med. 2008;149:334–41.
5. Rotenstein LS, Ramos MA, Torre M, et al. Prevalence of depression, depressive symptoms, and suicidal ideation among medical students: a systematic review and meta-analysis. JAMA. 2016;316(21):2214–36.
6. Medical Student Well-being. AMA 2020. https://students-residents.aamc.org/attending-medical-school/medical-school-survival-tips/medical-student-well-being/
7. Medical Student Well-being. AMA 2020. https://www.ama-assn.org/topics/medical-student-well-being
8. Zackoff M, Sastre E, Scott Rodgers S. Vanderbilt wellness program: model and implementation guide. MedEdPORTAL. 2012; https://doi.org/10.15766/mep_2374-8265.9111.
9. Slavin SJ, Schindler DL, Chibnall JT. Medical student mental health 3.0: improving student wellness through curricular changes. Acad Med. 2014;89(4):573–7.
10. Cervantes RC, Gattamorta KA, Berger-Cardoso J. Examining difference in immigration stress, acculturation stress and mental health outcomes in six Hispanic/Latino nativity and regional groups. J Immigrant Minor Health. 2019;21:14–20.
11. French SE, Chavez NR. The relationship of ethnicity-related stressors and Latino ethnic identity to well-being. Hisp J Behav Sci. 2010;32(4):410–28.
12. Sy SR, Romero J. Family responsibilities among Latina college students from immigrant families. J Hisp High Educ. 2008;7(3):212–27.
13. Campos B, Schetter CD, Abdou CM, Hobel CJ, Glynn LM, Sandman CA. Familialism, social support, and stress: positive implications for pregnant Latinas. Cultur Divers Ethnic Minor Psychol. 2008;14(2):155–62.
14. Phelan SM, Burke SE, Cunningham BA, et al. The effects of racism in medical education on students' decisions to practice in underserved or minority communities. Acad Med. 2019;94(8):1178–89.

15. Careers in Medicine, AAMC. https://www.aamc.org/cim/

16. Sánchez JP, et al. Advancing the Latino physician workforce-population trends, persistent challenges, and new directions. Acad Med. 2015;90(7):849–53.

17. Xierali IM, Nivet MA, Pandya AG. U.S. Dermatology department faculty diversity trends by sex and underrepresented-in-medicine status, 1970 to 2018. JAMA Dermatol. 2020;156(3):280–287.

18. Parmeshwar N, Stuart ER, Reid CM, Oviedo P, Gosman AA. Diversity in plastic surgery: trends in minority representation among applicants and residents. Plast Reconstr Surg. 2019;143(3):940–9.

19. Abelson JS, Symer MM, Yeo HL, et al. Surgical time out: our counts are still short on racial diversity in academic surgery. Am J Surg. 2018;215(4):542–8.

20. Deville C, Hwang WT, Burgos R, Chapman CH, Both S, Thomas CR Jr. Diversity in graduate medical education in the United States by Race, Ethnicity, and Sex, 2012 [published correction appears in JAMA Intern Med. 2015;175(10):1729]. JAMA Intern Med.

21. Association of American Medical Colleges. Table 3: U.S. Medical School Faculty by Rank and Race/Ethnicity, 2020. https://www.aamc.org/media/8906/download. Accessed 5 January 2023.

22. Building the Next Generation of Academic Physicians. http://bngap.org

23. Nakae et al. Office of Student Affairs: Engagement and Leadership Opportunities for Medical Students, Residents, and Fellows. MedEdPORTAL. February 5, 2021. https://www.mededportal.org/doi/full/10.15766/mep_2374-8265.11093

24. Frierson HT Jr. Impact of an intervention program on minority medical students' National Board Part I performance. J Natl Med Assoc. 1984;76(12):1185–90.

25. Kosobuski AW, Whitney A, Skildum A, Prunuske A. Development of an interdisciplinary prematriculation program designed to promote medical students' self efficacy. Med Educ Online. 2017;22(1):1272835.

26. Keith L, Hollar D. A social and academic enrichment program promotes medical school matriculation and graduation for disadvantaged students. Educ Health (Abingdon). 2012;25(1):55–63.

27. Lindner I, Sacks D, Sheakley M, et al. A pre-matriculation learning program that enables medical students with low prerequisite scores to succeed. Med Teach. 2013;35(10):872–3.

28. Low D, et al. Racial/ethnic disparities in clinical grading in medical school. Teach Learn Med. 2019;31(5):487−96.

29. Johnson JC, et al. Extending the pipeline for minority physicians: a comprehensive program for minority faculty development. Acad Med. 1998;73(3):237–44. https://doi.org/10.1097/00001888-199803000-00011.

30. Lucey CR, Saguil A. The consequences of structural racism on MCAT scores and medical school admissions: the past is prologue. Acad Med. 2020;95(3):351–6.

31. Cohen JJ. The consequences of premature abandonment of affirmative action in medical school admissions. JAMA. 2003;289(9):1143–9.

32. Rojek AE, Khanna R, Yim JWL, et al. Differences in narrative language in evaluations of medical students by gender and under-represented minority status. J Gen Intern Med. 2019;34(5):684–91.

33. Low D, Pollack SW, Liao ZC, et al. Racial/ethnic disparities in clinical grading in medical school. Teach Learn Med. 2019;31(5):487–96.

34. Tuition and Student Fees Reports https://www.aamc.org/data-reports/reporting-tools/report/tuition-and-student-fees-reports. Accessed 5 January 2023.

35. Current Trends in Medical Education. https://www.aamcdiversityfactsandfigures2016.org/report-section/section-3/#figure-30

36. United States Census Quick Facts. https://www.census.gov/quickfacts/fact/table/US/RHI725221. Accessed 5 January 2023.

37. Association of American Medical Colleges 2022 MSQ All Schools Summary Report (Excel) Table 1. Demographic Data. https://www.aamc.org/data-reports/students-residents/report/matriculating-student-questionnaire-msq

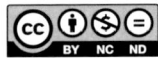

The Role of Medical Education Offices in Preparing the Physician Workforce to Care for LHS+ Individuals

Pilar Ortega, Edgar Figueroa, José E. Rodríguez, and Débora Silva

Introduction

LHS+ medical students and faculty have changed the landscape of U.S. medical education—both through collective organizational representation and individual leadership. Providing culturally and linguistically competent care to the growing U.S. LHS+ population requires more beyond increased representation of LHS+ individuals in the physician workforce [1]. While this is an undoubtedly critical step, the physician workforce, including LHS+ physicians and others interested in the care of LHS+ communities, must also receive educational opportunities that adequately prepare them to care for this vulnerable population.

Medical education must evolve to reflect the needs of the patient population to ensure that physicians are prepared to equitably care for their communities [2]. While LHS+ identified and other underrepresented minority physicians are more likely to practice in underserved communities [3, 4], the skills needed to do so are not innate abilities but rather competencies that must be taught, assessed, and sustained over the course of medical education [5]. Some evidence indicates that physicians from minority communities are more familiar with underserved communities, thus facilitating their skills training and their likelihood to serve underserved communities [6]. These skills include the ability to recognize population health disparities, to provide language-appropriate care, to identify cultural or linguistic miscommunication or misunderstandings, and to understand the social risk factors that may present unique barriers to LHS+ access to care. Furthermore, there is evidence that a medical school environment in which students are exposed to negative, explicit ethno-racial attitudes negatively affects medical student intent to practice in underserved communities [7]. Conversely, inclusion of positive experiences to learn to address racial, ethnic, and linguistic issues in health may increase physician workforce preparedness and willingness to care for vulnerable populations [8]. In this chapter, we will discuss the integration of three pivotal areas of LHS+ influence in medical education: LHS+ health and health disparities, cultural competency, and medical Spanish education.

P. Ortega (✉)
Department of Medical Education, Department of Emergency Medicine, University of Illinois College of Medicine at Chicago, Chicago, IL, USA
e-mail: portega@acgme.org

E. Figueroa
Weill Cornell Medical College, New York, NY, USA

J. E. Rodríguez
University of Utah Health, Salt Lake City, UT, USA

D. Silva
Department of Pediatrics, School of Medicine, University of Puerto Rico, San Juan, PR, USA

© The Author(s) 2024
J. P. Sánchez, D. Rodriguez (eds.), *Latino, Hispanic, or of Spanish Origin+ Identified Student Leaders in Medicine*, Sustainable Development Goals Series, https://doi.org/10.1007/978-3-031-35020-7_11

LHS+ Health, Health Disparities, and Cultural Competency in Medical Education

LHS+ health issues are defined as diseases or health conditions that disproportionately affect the U.S. LHS+ population. The National Institute on Minority Health and Health Disparities (NIMHD) has recently proposed definitions for the terms "minority health" and "health disparities," which are often used interchangeably but have distinct meanings [9]. Extrapolating from the definition of minority health, Hispanic health can be defined as "the health characteristics and attributes of [the Hispanic ethnic group] who are socially disadvantaged due in part by being subject to potential discriminatory acts." [9] NIMHD's proposed definition of a health disparity is "a health difference that adversely affects defined disadvantaged populations, based on one or more health outcomes." [9] In the context of medical education, the significance of these distinct definitions is that educational interventions should be adjusted to include knowledge and skills related to minority health and health disparities. In particular, health topics covered in medical education should include attention to health disparities with regards to specific outcomes: differences in the prevalence of disease, including onset and progression in a minority population; premature or excessive mortality; global burden of disease; health behaviors; and self-reported daily functioning or symptom management [9]. As a further differentiation between minority health and health disparities, Hispanic health and culture present advantages and potentially protective factors (e.g., Hispanic paradox) for certain diseases; these may potentially be leveraged to improve population health [10].

The process for integrating LHS+ health and health disparities, or more broadly, minority health and health disparities, into medical education has been gradual. In 2000, the Liaison Committee on Medical Education (LCME) issued curriculum content standard 7.6, requiring that medical schools include curricula that teach "cultural competence and health care disparities." [11] Cultural competence has been defined by the Association of American Medical Colleges (AAMC) as "a set of congruent behaviors, knowledge, attitudes, and policies that come together in a system, organization, or among professionals that enables effective work in cross-cultural situations" and applied to patient-centered health care practice [12, 13]. Moreover, communication skills education (standard 7.8) is considered another required element of LCME curriculum content standards [11]. Interpersonal and communication skills are also recognized as one of the six core graduate medical education competencies by the Accreditation Council for Graduate Medical Education (ACGME) [14]. Thus, allopathic medical schools are required to teach cultural competence, health care disparities, and medical communication skills to form competent physicians. Although these standards for medical graduates should be intentionally integrated into—rather than "added-on" to—medical school curricula [13], efforts to address and integrate these competencies are highly variable. Often, their integration lacks structure or evidence (due to lack of prior study), and may not be consistently or sufficiently adapted to the dynamic changes in the racial, ethnic, and linguistic attributes of the U.S. population. According to a recent report of clinical learning environments in graduate medical education, "education and training on health care disparities and cultural competency was largely generic, and often did not address the specific populations served by the institution"—prompting a call to action to further define the expectations for medical schools and residency programs in effectively teaching relevant, patient- and population-centered health care disparities and cultural competency knowledge and skills [15]. In 2017, the ACGME formally established teaching health care disparities as a needed "pathway to excellence," describing that residents, fellows and faculty members should be educated on reducing health care disparities (Clinical Learning Environment Review Health Care Quality Pathway 5) [16].

Hispanic Centers of Excellence (HCOEs) established at some U.S. medical schools have played an important role in the recruitment, financial, and scholarly support of LHS+ medical students and faculty. In some cases, HCOEs offered enrichment programs to pre-health students as early in the medical education pipeline as high school. Other HCOE programs extended through medical school, residency, and faculty careers, supporting research of relevance to Hispanic health, education, and career advancement [17, 18]. However, limited funding for Centers of Excellence has presented a challenge to sustaining such enrichment programs geared at increasing the representation and advancement of groups historically underrepresented in medicine (URM). Moreover, the potential impact of these programs and the representation of LHS+identifying individuals in medicine may not be accurately captured by data that prioritizes race but not necessarily other identifiers pertaining to ethnicity, nationality/ancestry, or language. Individuals who identify as LHS+ may identify with any race; may represent many distinct nationalities and ancestries, including combinations of multiple nationalities and racial profiles; and may have varying language proficiencies. As a result, there is a paucity of data regarding important factors that may influence access to care for Hispanic individuals, making Hispanic health research particularly challenging [19]. This is also true for Hispanic medical students and physicians, who may self-identify in diverse ways and may have different levels of language proficiencies in Spanish and varying cultural experiences, despite often being assumed to be bilingual and multicultural [20].

The rich diversity of the LHS+ physician workforce is one of the reasons that organizations, such as the Latino Medical Student Association (LMSA), have a critical role in unifying medical students and physicians in enacting needed changes in medical education. A call-to-action has been proposed to address Hispanic health and health disparities at all levels of medical education, including pre-health pipeline programs [21], medical school [18, 19], graduate medical education [22], medical practice [23], and continuing medical education [24].

In a less formal capacity, the presence of LHS+ students and faculty in the medical education classroom has had a critical, though underrecognized, role in addressing health issues and disparities in medical education. Anecdotal examples include, but are not limited to:

- The Latina medical student who raises her hand during endocrinology pathophysiology class to ask a question about why the incidence of diabetes is greater in her family's neighborhood compared to a predominantly white neighborhood three blocks away;
- The Latino physician faculty member who sits on the curriculum review committee and whose presence and voice are a constant reminder to the administration to include courses that address race, ethnicity, language, and social determinants of health into the institution's formal medical school curriculum; and
- The bilingual medical student who is overburdened with requests from her attendings or senior residents to help by interpreting for yet another Spanish-speaking patient on their inpatient service.

Not only is there evidence that medical students are often asked to serve as linguistic ambassadors and interpreters for patients without first assessing their communication skills [25], but data also suggest that unprepared and untrained interpreters such as students may carry significant psychological burdens for serving in these roles [26]. Student voices that have demanded medical education reform that addresses the needs of underserved communities have long-represented an important driver for institutional change [27].

LHS+ students and faculty have relied upon organizations such as LMSA to provide mutual support and to advocate for resolutions towards equity-driven medical education for all medical students. The publication of literature on medical education strategies to address LHS+ health and health disparities has been comparatively limited. In 2016, a systematic review identified a paucity of literature focusing on Hispanic health and education despite the Hispanic/Latino population representing the largest ethnic minority in the U.S. [28] More recently, the body of academic literature presenting data from the lens of

Hispanic health and health disparities has grown; much of this growth stems from the emergence of disease-specific literature reviewing outcomes of Hispanic patients with diabetes [29, 30], cancer [31], asthma [32], and psychiatric disorders [33], among others. Additionally, as Hispanic students and faculty sometimes work in underserved communities and assume primary care roles, often in a volunteer or service-learning capacity, curricula developed and implemented through collaboration with community-based organizations or student-run free clinics provide another avenue for cultural competency and health care disparities education [34]. However, literature specifically addressing medical education focused on Hispanic health, health disparities, and Hispanic-related cultural competency and humility is still lacking.

At the time of the writing of this chapter, searches using Google Scholar and the U.S. National Library of Medicine resources PubMed and MEDLINE demonstrated a paucity of articles related to the development, implementation, and evaluation of medical school curricula related to LHS+ health. Of articles that met search criteria (Hispanic health medical education, Latino/Latina/Latinx health medical education, minority health medical education), only three articles were identified that explored a medical school curriculum focused on Hispanic culture and health. Two articles describe teaching skills through the partnership between an academic center and community center; reports on the "Health Scholars Program" [35] and the "Hispanic Cultural Competence Project" [36] describe how academic-community partnerships can allow students to learn and apply knowledge about culture and social determinants of health in a LHS+ community. Another article describes the historical perspective, health status, and care of the Puerto Rican patient [37]. This latter publication was generated through a call to action to LHS+ trainees and faculty by J.P. Sánchez, MD, MPH, Executive Director of LMSA National and founding Associate Editor of the MedEdPORTAL collection on Diversity, Inclusion and Health Equity. Dr. Sánchez actively called for submissions describing the health status and experiences

of communities of Spanish-speaking ancestry (e.g., Mexican, Spanish, Cuban, Peruvian, etc.). One article was not focused on a medical education audience but presents a Hispanic-focused educational intervention focused on caregivers for Latino elders [38]. Of note, articles specifically addressing medical education curricula pertaining to medical Spanish education are not reported in this search of Hispanic cultural competency curricula and will be reviewed in the next section of this chapter. Additional literature discusses cultural competency education in medical school but only peripherally addresses Hispanic health [39–45]; such work may also yield opportunities to replicate and expand curricula in the context of care for the LHS+ population.

U.S. medical schools in Puerto Rico (PR) provide a unique medical education experience because the great majority of their students and faculty are Hispanic, along with 98.9% of Puerto Rico's population [46]. PR's four LCME-accredited medical schools (University of Puerto Rico School of Medicine, Ponce Health Sciences University School of Medicine, Universidad Central del Caribe School of Medicine and San Juan Bautista School of Medicine) collectively graduate approximately 230 LHS+ students per year [47]. In addition, PR has 45 specialty residency programs and 30 subspecialty programs accredited by the ACGME, with a total of 965 medical residents and fellows in the 2019–2020 academic year [48]. Since the vast majority of PR clinical encounters involve Spanish-speaking LHS+ patients, medical education in PR medical schools and residency programs is necessarily bilingual and requires knowledge of LHS+ health issues. Graduates from PR programs are proficient in both English and Spanish, since they must meet the same requirements as all U.S. medical students to pass standardized licensing examinations in English, but must practice clinical medicine in Spanish. Further, since the PR medical schools graduate so many LHS+ students, PR medical schools have been an important source of LHS+ residents throughout the U.S. Moreover, PR medical schools engage in research related to health care disparities. Some examples include research partnerships with other U.S. medical schools and research centers [49, 50], Master's programs in clinical and translational research [51], and community-based participatory research [52]. While the PR medical schools' contributions to diversity and community health have been recognized by the AAMC [53, 54], no published literature to date describes these medical schools' unique curricular characteristics that could be used to inform other programs' curricula pertaining to LHS+ health.

In the absence of medical education literature, it is important to search curricula content of other disciplines. Some published medical education curricula with a focus on global health may have important utility for locally addressing minority health [34]. For cultural competency education specifically, a majority of the cultural competency curricular literature has been published by their allied health professions but not in medical education for physicians [55]. There is a significant need to academically evaluate and publish effective curricula for cultural competency education related to LHS+ health in medical school settings. Additionally, it will be important for future LHS+ cultural competency educational interventions to be studied with respect to their effectiveness in educational settings [56, 57], as well as their downstream effect on health outcomes and health disparities [58].

Medical Spanish in Medical Education

The development of medical Spanish education within U.S. medical schools has been primarily driven by medical student demand and frequently facilitated through student leadership in LMSA [59]. Medical students who identify as Hispanic are significantly more likely to report higher proficiencies in Spanish compared to the general medical student population, according to Electronic Residency Application System (ERAS) data [60]. Specifically, over 95% of Latino residency applicants in 2013 reported at least intermediate Spanish language skills compared to 53.2% of all applicants, and 84.5% Latinos reported native/functionally native profi-

ciency [60]. This data reinforces the pre-existing linguistic communication skills that Hispanic candidates bring to medical school and residency. These skills, however, must be developed, enriched, assessed, and certified in order to ensure patient safety [61] and to properly recognize the values of medical bilingualism. Despite lack of formal medical Spanish education or assessment, many students, resident physicians, and practicing physicians with self-reported bilingual abilities—or who are assumed by superiors to have bilingual skills based on factors such as last name, skin color, or Hispanic self-identity—are placed in the position of using their limited skills in patient care [25, 61]. Such encounters may endanger patient safety due to risk of miscommunication [5, 61, 62].

Medical Spanish experts, including medical education experts, physicians, and language professors have recently developed a growing body of literature on best practice guidelines regarding medical Spanish education in medical schools [63–65]. Best practice recommendations agree on the need to focus on medical students with existing intermediate or greater Spanish skills; the importance of longitudinal, progressive skills acquisition; and the need for skills assessment and training in interpreter use for all medical students regardless of Spanish skill level. Examples of medical Spanish medical school curricula that have been published include: one medical Spanish course with objective structured clinical examinations [66], two web-based modules or vignettes [67, 68], a student-run Spanish program [69], a proposed method for certifying medical students as trained interpreters [70], a medical Spanish clinical conversational skills course for medical students [71], and a description of three medical Spanish programs at three medical schools and discussion of best practices in medical Spanish [2].

Among best practices in medical Spanish education, regional varieties of Spanish and other factors that affect the linguistic diversity of LHS+ individuals must be acknowledged in efforts to teach linguistic competency for medical students. For example, U.S. cities and regions may vary in the nationality or ancestry of origin of their local

LHS+ populations, and regional variations in language may affect patient and provider communication due to differences in word choice, accent, pronunciation, and cultural beliefs [72]. Additionally, many U.S. immigrants from Latin America may report a primary language that is not Spanish [73]; indigenous languages such as Maya, Nahuatl, Zapoteco, Mixteco, K'iche', Q'eqchi', and Mam are spoken in some regions of the U.S. Awareness of the dynamic linguistic attributes of patient populations should be used to inform and enhance medical education language and communications curricula.

National LMSA resolutions have supported the growth and development of medical Spanish educational opportunities at U.S. medical schools [74]. Many LMSA chapters are further involved in a national collaborative group known as the Medical Spanish Taskforce (MST), which was initiated following an expert panel meeting—the Medical Spanish Summit—in March 2018 [65]. The MST is a volunteer interdisciplinary team of medical Spanish experts, including participants with professional background in medicine, linguistics, second language education, health policy, medical education, and interpreting/translation, among others. Through the MST, collaborators from medical schools across the U.S. contribute to the advancement of evidence-based medical Spanish education and are currently evaluating a national standardized curriculum for medical Spanish education.

While medical Spanish courses in medical school address an important need in building the Spanish language-concordant physician workforce, efforts in linguistic competency education for physicians should not end there. Researching clinical outcomes of language concordance in medical communication is a critical step to documenting the effectiveness of medical Spanish educational efforts. Language concordance research to date indeed demonstrates improved patient outcomes for patients with non-English language preference when patients and physicians speak the same language [75]. Language skills in medical communication should be a continued area of assessment, one that should include documentation of physician language proficien-

cies beyond medical school, and one in which bilingual LHS+ physicians have a significant vested interest in order to address the growing Spanish-speaking physician deficit [76].

Conclusions

As the LHS+ population in the U.S. continues to grow, LHS+ leaders and educators must continue to advocate for and actively promote thoughtful integration by medical schools of curricular components covering LHS+ health issues, health disparities faced by LHS+ communities, cultural competency, and medical Spanish. Sustaining programs that implement strategies to teach and address these facets of LHS+ healthcare will require formal integration into the operations of undergraduate and graduate medical education institutions. Moreover, the maintenance and expansion of such programs depend on the production of peer-review research demonstrating that LHS+-focused curricular efforts help institutions improve patient outcomes, achieve public health priorities, enhance learner competencies and performance outcomes, and meet licensing and accreditation requirements of agencies such as the LCME and the ACGME. Next steps needed in medical education implementation and research include introducing improved assessment and documentation of medical student and physician language proficiencies, enhanced structure to LHS+-specific cultural competency and health disparities curricula, and increased opportunities for interdisciplinary and interinstitutional collaborations to standardize and evaluate best practices in medical education programs that respond to the health needs in the LHS+ community.

Looking forward, medical education must use the lessons learned over the past hundred years to catalyze sustainable change in medical education that promotes LHS+-focused health education. First, medical education core content should formally incorporate health issues and health care disparities present in diverse U.S. patient populations, specifically including LHS+ groups. Health care disparities and cultural competency courses should not be solely addressed through add-on or extracurricular enrichment activities but rather as a core element in medical education content, which should be dynamically reviewed to appropriately address changes in population demographics. Secondly, integrated LHS+ health curricula should be rigorously evaluated using medical education research methodology, and validated educational strategies should be published and shared for more widespread accessibility and implementation. The experience of PR's medical schools may represent an important example of curricular integration that should be further evaluated and published. Thirdly, the incorporation of cultural and linguistic competencies in medical education should promote and incentivize professional multilingualism and patient-centered communication skills, including the formal structuring of medical Spanish educational programs, competencies, and assessment, as well as the academic publication of peer-reviewed Spanish-English bilingual medical education materials. Finally, the continued creation and growth of LHS+ identified organizational networks such as LMSA and the promotion, support, and retention of LHS+ individuals in medical education leadership roles will remain critical to maintaining forward momentum to enhance LHS+-responsive medical education.

References

1. Fernández A, Pérez-Stable EJ. ¿Doctor, habla Español? Increasing the supply and quality of language-concordant physicians for Spanish-speaking patients. J Gen Intern Med. 2015;30(10):1394–6. https://doi.org/10.1007/s11606-015-3436-x.

2. Ortega P, Pérez N, Robles B, Turmelle Y, Acosta D. Strategies for teaching linguistic preparedness for physicians: medical Spanish and global linguistic competence in undergraduate medical education. Health Equity. 2019, July 1;3(1):312–8. https://doi.org/10.1089/heq.2019.0029.

3. Rodríguez JE, Campbell KM, Pololi LH. Addressing disparities in academic medicine: What of the minority tax? BMC Med Educ. 2015;15:6.

4. Neill T, Irwin G, Owings CS, Cathcart-Rake W. Rural Kansas family physician satisfaction with caring for Spanish-speaking only patients. Kans J Med. 2017;10:1–15.

5. Diamond LC, Jacobs EA. Let's not contribute to disparities: the best methods for teaching clinicians how to overcome language barriers to health care. J Gen Intern Med. 2010;25(2):189–93. https://doi.org/10.1007/s11606-009-1201-8.

6. Marrast LM, Zallman L, Woolhandler S, Bor DH, McCormick D. Minority physicians' role in the care of underserved patients: Diversifying the physician workforce may be key in addressing health disparities. JAMA Intern Med. 2013;174(2):289–91.

7. Phelan SM, Burke SE, Cunningham BA. The effects of racism in medical education on students' decisions to practice in underserved or minority communities. Acad Med. 2019;94(8):1178–89. https://doi.org/10.1097/ACM.0000000000002719.

8. O'Connell TF, Ham SA, Hart TG, Curlin FA, Yoon JD. A national longitudinal survey of medical students' intentions to practice among the underserved. Acad Med. 2018;3(1):90–7. https://doi.org/10.1097/ACM.0000000000001816.

9. Duran DG, Pérez-Stable EJ. Novel approaches to advance minority health and health disparities research. Am J Public Health. 2019;109(S1):S8–S10. https://doi.org/10.2105/AJPH.2018.304931.

10. The Lancet Editorial Board. The Hispanic paradox. Lancet. 2015;385(9981):1918. https://doi.org/10.1016/S0140-6736(15)60945-X.

11. Liaison Committee on Medical Education. Functions and structure of a medical school: Standards for accreditation of medical education programs leading to the MD degree; 2020. http://lcme.org/publications

12. Cross TL. Towards a culturally competent system of care: a monograph on effective services for minority children. National Center for Cultural Competence: Georgetown University; 1989.

13. Association of American Medical Colleges. Cultural competence education; 2005. https://www.aamc.org/system/files/c/2/54338-culturalcomped.pdf

14. Accreditation Council for Graduate Medical Education. ACGME core competencies; 2023. https://www.ecfmg.org/echo/acgme-core-competencies.html

15. Wagner R, Koh N, Bagian JP, Weiss KB. CLER 2016 national report of findings. Issue Brief #4: Health Care Disparities. Accreditation Council for Graduate Medical Education, Chicago, Illinois USA; 2016. ISBN-13: 978-1-945365-07-2.

16. CLER Evaluation Committee. CLER pathways to excellence: Expectations for an optimal clinical learning environment to achieve safe and high quality patient care (health care quality pathway 5), Version 1.1; 2017. Accreditation Council for Graduation Medical Education.

17. Martínez GA. Medical Spanish for heritage learners: a prescription to improve the health of Spanish-speaking communities. In: Building communities and making connections. Cambridge: Cambridge Scholars Publishing; 2010.

18. Ghaddar S, Ronnau J, Saladin SP, Martínez G. Innovative approaches to promote a culturally competent, diverse health care workforce in an

196

P. Ortega et al.

institution serving Hispanic students. Acad Med. 2013;88(12):1870–6.

19. Ortega P. Spanish language concordance in U.S. medical care: a multifaceted challenge and call to action. Acad Med. 2018;93(9):1276–80. https://doi.org/10.1097/ACM.0000000000002307.

20. Diamond LC, Tuot DS, Karliner LS. The use of Spanish language skills by physicians and nurses: policy implications for teaching and testing. J Gen Intern Med. 2012;27(1):117–23.

21. Ortega P, Park YS, Rodriguez AJ, Girotti JA. Evaluation of a Spanish health topics course for undergraduate pre-health Latino students. Cureus J Med Sci. 2019;11(10):e5825. https://doi.org/10.7759/cureus.5825.

22. Maldonado, M.E., Fried, E.D., DuBose, T.D, Nelson, C. & Breida, M. (2014). The role that graduate medical education must play in ensuring health equity and eliminating health care disparities. Ann Am Thorac Soc, 11(4), 603–607. doi:https://doi.org/10.1513/AnnalsATS.201402-068PS.

23. Nesbitt S, Palomarez RE. Review: Increasing awareness and education on health disparities for health care providers. Ethn Dis. 2016;26(2):181–90. https://doi.org/10.18865/ed.26.2.181.

24. Like RC. Educating clinicians about cultural competence and disparities in health and health care. J Contin Educ Heal Prof. 2011;31(3):196–206. https://doi.org/10.1002/chp.20127.

25. Vela MB, Fritz C, Press VG, Girotti J. Medical students' experiences and perspectives on interpreting for LEP patients at two U.S. medical schools. J Racial Ethn Health Disparities. 2016;3:245–9.

26. Showstack R. Patients don't have language barriers; the healthcare system does. Emerg Med J. 2019;36(10):580–1. https://doi.org/10.1136/emermed-2019-208929.

27. Poma PA. Hispanic cultural influences on medical practice. J Natl Med Assoc. 1983;75(10):941–6.

28. Price JH, Khubchandani J. Health education research and practice literature on Hispanic health issues. Health Promot Pract. 2016;17(2):172–6. https://doi.org/10.1177/1524839915626675.

29. Aguayo-Mazzucato C, Diaque P, Hernandez S, Rosas S, Kostic A, Caballero AE. Understanding the growing epidemic of type 2 diabetes in the Hispanic population living in the United States. Diabetes Metab Res Rev. 2019;35(2) https://doi.org/10.1002/dmrr.3097.

30. Parker MM, Fernández A, Moffet HH, Grant RW, Torreblanca A, Karter AJ. Association of patient-physician language concordance and glycemic control for limited-English proficiency Latinos with type 2 diabetes. JAMA Intern Med. 2017;177(3):380–7. https://doi.org/10.1001/jamainternmed.2016.8648.

31. Moreno PI, Yanez B, Schuetz SJ. Cancer fatalism and adherence to national cancer screening guidelines: Results from the Hispanic Community Health Study/Study of Latinos (HCHS/SOL). Cancer Epidemiol. 2019;60:39–45. https://doi.org/10.1016/j.canep.2019.03.003.

32. Baek J, Huang K, Conner L, Tapangan N, Xu X, Carrillo G. Effects of the home-based educational intervention on health outcomes among primarily Hispanic children with asthma: a quasi-experimental study. BMC Public Health. 2019;19(1) https://doi.org/10.1186/s12889-019-7272-5.

33. Alarcón RD, Parekh A, Wainberg ML, Duarte CS, Araya R, Oquendo MA. Hispanic immigrants in the USA: social and mental health perspectives. Lancet Psychiatry. 2016;3(9):860–70. https://doi.org/10.1016/S2215-0366(16)30101-8.

34. Webber S, Butteris SM, Houser L, Coller K, Coller RJ. Asset-based community development as a strategy for developing local global health curricula. Acad Pediatr. 2018;18(5):496–501. https://doi.org/10.1016/j.acap.2018.02.001.

35. O'Brien MJ, Garland JM, Murphy KM, Shuman SJ, Whitaker RC, Larson SC. Training medical students in the social determinants of health: The Health Scholars Program at Puentes de Salud. Adv Med Educ Pract. 2014;5:307–14. https://doi.org/10.2147/AMEP.S67480.

36. Nora LM, Daugherty SR, Mattis-Peterson A, Stevenson L, Goodman LJ. Improving cross-cultural skills of medical students through medical school-community partnerships. West J Med. 1994;161(2):144–7.

37. Silva DH, García G, Clare C. Taking care of the Puerto Rican patient: Historical perspectives, health status, and health care access. MedEdPORTAL. 2020;16:10984.

38. Cruz-Oliver, D.M., Ellis, K., Sánchez-Reilly, S. (2016). Caregivers like me: an education intervention for family caregivers of Latino elders at end-of-life. MedEdPORTAL, 12, 10448. doi.org/10.15766/mep_2374-8265.10448.

39. Tervalon M. Components of culture in health for medical students' education. Acad Med. 2003;78(6):570–6. https://doi.org/10.1097/00001888-200306000-00005.

40. Neff J, Holmes SM, Knight KR. Structural competency: curriculum for medical students, residents, and interprofessional teams on the structural factors that produce health disparities. MedEdPORTAL. 2020;16:10888. https://doi.org/10.15766/mep_2374-8265.10888.

41. DallaPiazza M, Padilla-Register M, Dwarakanath M, Obamedo E, Hill J, Soto-Greene ML. Exploring racism and health: an intensive interactive session for medical students. MedEdPORTAL. 2018;14:10783. https://doi.org/10.15766/mep_2374-8265.10783.

42. Perdomo J, Tolliver D, Hsu H. Health equity rounds: an interdisciplinary case conference to address implicit bias and structural racism for faculty and trainees. MedEdPORTAL. 2019;15:10858. https://doi.org/10.15766/mep_2374-8265.10858.

43. Chow CJ, Case GA, Matias CE. Tools for discussing identity and privilege among medical students, trainees, and faculty. MedEdPORTAL. 2019;15:10864. https://doi.org/10.15766/mep_2374-8265.10864.

44. Yoon MH, Blatt BC, Greenberg LW. Medical students' professional development as educators revealed through reflections on their teaching following a students-as-teachers course. Teach Learn Med. 2017;29(4):411–9. https://doi.org/10.1080/10401334.2017.1302801.

45. Simpson SA, Long JA. Medical student-run health clinics: important contributors to patient care and medical education. J Gen Intern Med. 2007;22:352–6. https://doi.org/10.1007/s11606-006-0073-4.

46. U.S. census bureau quickfacts: Puerto Rico. Census Bureau QuickFacts; 2020, April 29. https://www.census.gov/quickfacts/PR.

47. Association of American Medical Colleges. Diversity in Medicine: Facts and Figures 2019: Table 7. U.S. medical schools with 200 or more Hispanic or Latino graduates (alone or in combination), 2009–2010 through 2018–2019; 2019, August 19. https://www.aamc.org/data-reports/workforce/data/table-7-us-medical-schools-200-or-more-hispanic-or-latino-graduates-alone-or-combination-2009-2010.

48. Accreditation Council for Graduate Medical Education. Graduate medical education totals by state | Academic year 2019-2020 | United States; 2020. https://apps.acgme.org/ads/Public/Reports/Report/13

49. Appleyard C, Antonia S, Sullivan D. Building a long distance training program to enhance clinical cancer research capacity in Puerto Rico. Rev Recent Clin Trials. 2015;9(4):254–62. https://doi.org/10.2174/1574887110666150127110721.

50. Estapé-Garrastazu ES, Noboa-Ramos C, Jesús-Ojeda LD, Pedro-Serbiá ZD, Acosta-Pérez E, Camacho-Feliciano DM. Clinical and translational research capacity building needs in minority medical and health science Hispanic institutions. Clin Transl Sci. 2014;7(5):406–12. https://doi.org/10.1111/cts.12165.

51. Estape E, Segarra B, Baez A, Huertas A, Diaz C, Frontera W. Shaping a new generation of Hispanic clinical and translational researchers addressing minority health and health disparities. P R Health Sci J. 2011;30(4):167–75.

52. García-Rivera EJ, Pacheco P, Colón M. Building bridges to address health disparities in Puerto Rico: the "Salud Para Piñones" project. P R Health Sci J. 2017;36(2):92–100.

53. Association of American Medical Colleges. 2018 Spencer Foreman Award for Outstanding Community Service; 2018. https://www.aamc.org/what-we-do/aamc-awards/spencer-foreman/2018-university-of-puerto-rico-som

54. Howley EK. AAMC award winners honored. Association of American Medical Colleges; 2019. https://www.aamc.org/news-insights/2019-aamc-award-winners-honored

55. Abrishami D. The need for cultural competency in health care. Radiol Technol. 2018;89(5):441–8.

56. Betancourt JR. Cross-cultural medical education: conceptual approaches and frameworks for evaluation. Acad Med. 2003;78(6):560–9. https://doi.org/10.1097/00001888-200306000-00004.

57. Deliz JR, Fears FF, Jones KE, Tobat J, Char D, Ross WR. Cultural competency interventions during medical school: a scoping review and narrative synthesis. J Gen Intern Med. 2020;35(2):568–77. https://doi.org/10.1007/s11606-019-05417-5.

58. Butler M, McCreedy E, Schwer N. Improving cultural competence to reduce health disparities. Agency for Healthcare Research and Quality (US); 2016.

59. Morales R, Rodríguez L, Singh A. National survey of medical Spanish curriculum in U.S. medical schools. J Gen Intern Med. 2015;30(10):434–9.

60. Diamond L, Grbic D, Genoff M, Gonzalez J, Sharaf R, Mikesell C, Gany F. Non–English-language proficiency of applicants to US residency programs. JAMA. 2014;312(22):2405–7.

61. Flores G, Mendoza FS. ¿Dolor aquí? ¿Fiebre?: A little knowledge requires caution. Arch Pediatr Adolesc Med. 2002;56(7):638–40.

62. Regenstein M, Andres E, Wynia MK. Appropriate use of non-English language skills in clinical care. JAMA. 2013;309(2):145–6.

63. Reuland DS, Frasier PY, Slatt LM, Alemán MA. A longitudinal medical Spanish program at one US medical school. J Gen Intern Med. 2008;23(7):1033–7.

64. Hardin KJ, Hardin DM. Medical Spanish programs in the United States: a critical review of published studies and a proposal of best practices. Teach Learn Med. 2013;25(4):306–11.

65. Ortega P, Diamond L, Alemán MA, Fatás-Cabeza J, Magaña D, Pazo V, Pérez N, Girotti JA, Ríos E. Medical Spanish standardization in U.S. medical schools: consensus statement from a multidisciplinary expert panel. Acad Med. 2020;95(1):22–31.

66. Ortega P, Park YS, Girotti JA. Evaluation of a medical Spanish elective for senior medical students: improving outcomes through OSCE assessments. Med Sci Educ. 2017;27(2):329–37. https://doi.org/10.1007/s40670-017-0405-5.

67. Cesari WA, Brescia WF, Harricharan Singh K, Oni A, Cheema A, Coffman C, Creek A, Torres C, Mencio M, Clayton S, Weaver C, Weaver J. Medical Spanish. MedEdPORTAL. 2012;8 https://doi.org/10.15766/mep_2374-8265.9171.

68. Rampal A, Wang C, Kalisvaart J. Pediatric medical Spanish vignettes. MedEdPORTAL. 2009;5:5110. https://www.mededportal.org/publication/5110

69. Dawson AL, Patti B. Spanish acquisition begets enhanced service (S.A.B.E.S.): a beginning-level medical Spanish curriculum. MedEdPORTAL. 2011;7:9057. https://www.mededportal.org/publication/9057

70. O'Rourke K, Gruener G, Quinones D, Stratta E, Howell J. Spanish bilingual medical student certification. MedEdPORTAL. 2013;9:9400. https://www.mededportal.org/publication/9400

71. Pérez N. Student acceptance of clinical conversational Spanish in medical curriculum. Cogent Med. 2018;5(1):1475691.

72. Ortega P, Prada J. Words matter: translanguaging in medical communication skills training. Perspect

Med Educ. 2020;9:251–5. https://doi.org/10.1007/s40037-020-00595-z.

73. Flood D, Rohloff P. Indigenous languages and global health. Lancet Global Health. 2018;6(2):e134–5. https://doi.org/10.1016/S2214-109X(17)30493-X.

74. Latino Medical Student Association. Resolution: medical Spanish curriculum in medical schools; 2016. https://lmsa.net/policy/wp-content/uploads/2016/10/ReferenceCommitteeReport.pdf

75. Diamond L, Izquierdo K, Canfield D, Matsoukas K, Gany F. A systematic review of the impact of patient-physician non-English language concordance on quality of care and outcomes. J Gen Intern Med. 2019;34(8):1591–606. https://doi.org/10.1007/s11606-019-04847-5.

76. García ME, Bindman AB, Coffman J. Language-concordant primary care physicians for a diverse population: the view from California. Health Equity. 2019;3(1):343–9. https://doi.org/10.1089/heq.2019.0035.

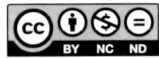

LHS+ Individuals in Graduate Medical Education

12

Glenn E. García Jr and Larissa Velez

Nota bene: This book uses "LHS+", however, the data may use "Hispanic", "Latino," "Latina," "Latinx," "Latine", "Latin American," "Spanish Origin" or lump these groups into a larger category with African Americans and Native Americans. Here, "Underrepresented Racial Minority" (URM) is used in reference to folks in the aforementioned larger category. Other nomenclatures exist, but the data used in this chapter primarily used the term URM.

Oddly, it is easier to end a discussion on the state of LHS+ in Graduate Medical Education (GME) than to begin one. A literature review will reveal a myriad of terms, endpoints, and solutions, but where does the story begin? A sociologist may begin with the SAT, universities, and GPAs. Historians would look at immigration and population movements. As GME does not exist in a vacuum, both starting points have equal merit. The preceding chapters are as important as these pages to understand the full picture, and we pick up where our colleagues have left off—medical school or Undergraduate Medical Education (UME).

According to the Accreditation Council on Graduate Medical Education (ACGME), in the 2018–2019 year, LHS+ individuals consist of 5.3% of residents and fellows [1]. The AAMC reports that in 2019 11.0% of US medical school matriculants identified as LHS+ [1, 2]. More concerning are specialty areas where the percentage of LHS+ individuals is critically low, such as radiology, orthopedic surgery, and otolaryngology [3]. Some tout Latin American graduates as a potential solution, but the data is scarce. The Educational Commission for Foreign Medical Graduates does not release regular reporting on the racial and ethnic composition of internationally trained physicians aspiring to enter residencies and fellowships. A 2008 study reported that ECFMG-certified Foreign Medical Graduates (FMG's) are more likely to be LHS+ (about 8%) than graduating U.S. seniors and about 1 in 5 of those LHS+ FMG's are U.S. citizens [4]. The data admittedly appears promising. The caveat is that ECFMG certification does not guarantee a residency position, and the ACGME does not have published data for the race and ethnicity of the IMG's in GME. Therefore, we cannot tell if LHS+ FMG's are linguistically bound to Puerto Rico's GME programs or even how many of them make it to residency programs. In other words, all we can do is postulate on their potential impact based upon 15–20-year-old data. Thus, constrained by the data, our focus will be on graduates from LCME-accredited institutions.

G. E. García Jr (✉)
HCA Healthcare/USF Morsani College of Medicine
GME: Bayonet Point Hospital, Hudson, FL, USA
e-mail: glenn@glenngarciamd.com

L. Velez
UT Southwestern Medical Center, Dallas, TX, USA

© The Author(s) 2024
J. P. Sánchez, D. Rodriguez (eds.), *Latino, Hispanic, or of Spanish Origin+ Identified Student Leaders in Medicine*, Sustainable Development Goals Series, https://doi.org/10.1007/978-3-031-35020-7_12

The path to GME invariably starts with the choice of medical school. More prestigious medical schools can be an asset, especially for students who are pursuing GME training in specialties where programs are scarce and extremely competitive. US News and World Report ranks medical schools by primary care and by research output. Medical students get ranked not only by quartiles based on test performance but also by taking a series of national standardized tests. The first one is the United States Medical Licensing Examination (USMLE's) Step 1 examination. This is where the first true "weeding out" process for GME begins. A score of 270 opens the doors to the most coveted and lucrative specialties, while a score below 200 can shut candidates out. Considering LHS+ and underrepresented racial minority (URM) students' USMLE Step 1 score lags behind their peers, this potentially translates into fewer career opportunities [5]. Failure of passing USMLE Step 1, though not very common, is higher also for LHS+ and URMs. A study has shown that failure to pass Step 1 on the first attempt leads to a higher likelihood of training in primary care specialties; intent to practice in underserved areas, and taking more than 4 years to graduate from medical school [6]. In this study, the relative risk of not passing Step 1 on the first attempt was 7.4 for LHS+ individuals. Therefore, LHS+ individuals and other URM students are being excluded from GME programs before we assess their clinical skills and knowledge. As Step 1 score reporting changes to pass/fail in January 2022, the National Board of Medical Examiners (NBME) hopes to decrease GME's reliance on Step 1 scores as a quality metric for candidates [7].

As the focus shifts away from Step 1, a student's performance on clinical rotations (clerkships) becomes more prominent; for LHS+ individuals, this may still represent a disadvantage. Studies have shown that LHS+ and URM students are less likely to receive Honors grades than their peers [8]. Clerkship grades are partially subjective and vary between institutions, so the evaluation comments are supposed to serve as a clearer indication of the candidate's professional and clinical identity. On clerkship evaluations, LHS+ students are less likely than non-URM peers to be described as "superior" or "integral." [8] Unfortunately, LHS+ and URM students are more likely to have more negatively coded descriptors used in both their clinical evaluations and the Medical School Performance Evaluation—a comprehensive evaluation prepared by the school to send as part of a student's residency application [9, 10]. Understandably, many reviewers fall into the trap of associating those adjectives to lower clinical skills or knowledge level. However, these words are in a pool of over 70% of descriptors more common to non-URMs that have no relation to clerkship performance [8]. Unless we accept the notion that student competency is related to LHS+ ethnicity and/or race, we must recognize that clerkship grades and evaluations are potentially biased and cannot be relied upon as purely objective measures of LHS+ and other URM students' clinical performance.

Beyond recognizing USMLE and clerkship grades as biased, institutional leaders should consider the question "How ought GME Program Directors best assess the LHS+ medical student?" The answer is to do so the same way we should evaluate all candidates—holistically. Holistic reviews give a balanced consideration of academic metrics, experiences, competencies and attributes [11]. It aims to assess applicants based on their unique backgrounds. The process is applied equitably across the entire applicant pool. At all times, the organization's mission and vision are kept aligned with this holistic review, with the goal of finding applicants who will meaningfully contribute to the institution's mission. Table 12.1 describes in more detail some of the elements in the holistic review process.

The holistic review expands the set of criteria by which applicants are reviewed. In standard reviews, excessive relevance is given to objective metrics of academic excellence, such as Alpha Omega Alpha (AOA), the medical student honor society, or Gold Humanism Society recognition. For example, AOA status is highly valued by many residency programs. URM students are underrepresented in AOA Chapters across the

Table 12.1 Elements of the Holistic Review Process

Area	Examples
Experiences "the path"	• Educational background • Leadership roles • Life experiences • Healthcare Experiences • Community service • Volunteerism • Research Experience • Professional associations • Experience with Diverse populations • World/Societal context
Attributes "current skills, abilities, and personal qualities"	• Interest in specialty • Leadership • Cultural competence • Proficiency in second language • Professional stature • Intellectual curiosity • Team player • Integrity • Ethnicity • Gender identity • Socioeconomic status
Competencies "the core competencies and the milestones" "how they apply their skills, knowledge, and abilities"	• Patient Care • Medical Knowledge • Practice-based learning and Improvement • Professionalism • System-based learning • Interpersonal and Communication skills
Academic and Scholarly Metrics	• MSPE • Letters of evaluation/recommendation (grades, honors, ranking) • GPA • Publications • Presentations • Grants • Licensing Examination scores • Combined or additional degrees (MBA, MPH, PhD) • Awards • Recognitions • Scholarships

Adapted from https://www.aamc.org/services/member-capacity-building/holistic-review

nation [12, 13]. As outstanding academic performance is the foremost criterion for AOA membership [14], racial and ethnic grading disparities present an unintended dilemma. URM students are less likely to receive a grade of Honors for clerkships (a common component of AOA membership criteria) [8], but the USMLE examinations have been viewed as an opportunity to even the score. Outside the top quartile of USMLE Step 1 scores, LHS+ students are less likely to be inducted into AOA than their White colleagues [12]. Even setting aside the debate of racial and ethnic bias in standardized testing, we still see inequality. Therefore, until AOA membership selection is holistically reformed, its use as an applicant screening criterion disadvantages URM students—who already have difficulty getting through the screening process [15]. In at least one specialty-specific survey, URM minority students were interviewed in fewer programs than their non-URM counterparts (15 vs 20) [16]. The study did not differentiate between interviews offered vs interviews attended, but it still shows a significant difference in the number of programs where an URM candidate has the opportunity to interview.

The issues LHS+ individuals face with GME recruitment do not end with the application screening process and the interview invitations but continue into the ranking of applicants. Many in academic medicine are aware of "fit"—referring to how well a candidate would mesh with the current culture of a program. If a program lacks diversity, then placing added value on candidates who match that profile serves only to perpetuate the lack of diversity [17]. Of course, the assumption is that the reader values or (at the very least) is intrigued by the concept of diversifying GME. Though one might think that program directors value diversity when ranking candidates, half of the surveyed program directors do not view a candidate's URM status as at least "somewhat important." [18] This is but a small part of the undervaluing of areas in which LHS+ applicants excel. About 70% of program directors did not value bilingualism during resident recruitment [18], which is one of the benefits of LHS+ diversity. Even if LHS+ candidates have more leadership and volunteer experiences than their URM counterparts, those attributes are less important to program directors and, thus, unlikely to help them match [19]. Authors have noted that URM candidates will often have more structured research experiences than non-URM candidates; however, non-URM candidates were more likely to publish—another example of how LHS+ candidates can end up undervalued [20]. Preventing structural components that undervalue URM candidates is key to the components of the ACGME standard on diversity:

> The program, in partnership with its Sponsoring Institution, must engage in practices that focus on mission-driven, ongoing, systematic recruitment and retention of a diverse and inclusive workforce of residents, fellows (if present), faculty members, senior administrative staff members, and other relevant members of its academic community [21].

The ACGME requires programs to go beyond diversity fairs. The reality is that GME programs must change how they educate residents to accommodate a more diverse program. Relying on old teaching methods ignores the needs of these new trainees and likely contributes to the misconception that LHS+ applicants may not be as strong as their colleagues. There are no traditionally LHS+ medical schools in the continental United States; however, successful training models can be found at historically Black medical schools. Morehouse School of Medicine used a familial teaching environment to increase student engagement leading to the MCAT underpredicting URM students' USMLE Step 1 scores; the important discovery is that the close faculty-trainee relationship was the key to the latter's success [22]. In other words, by changing the institution's approach to the culture of medical education, the faculty facilitated trainees' success. Medicine has discussed culturally competent care, but the time has come to discuss culturally competent medical education.

LHS+ trainees are asked to assimilate to the culture of medicine, without developing their cultural identities in medicine. The United States is home to the second-largest Spanish-speaking population in the world [23]. Yet, only one LCME-accredited medical school (outside of Puerto Rico) requires medical Spanish for graduation [24]. Language is but one of many cultural contributions LHS+ trainees contribute to a program and patients across the United States. Understanding nuances in patients' cultural belief systems can be the difference between an unnecessary Psychiatry consultation and pausing to listen and address patients' concerns. Although the mainland United States is beginning to address Medical Spanish and other LHS+ cultural contributions, there are LCME-accredited models for our institutions to emulate.

Puerto Rico, a colony of the United States, has four LCME-accredited medical schools that combine to graduate about 300 students each year [25]. Each school serves as an example of a homogenous faculty and student body of LHS+ individuals. Research, service, and innovations are conducted within the patient population's culture; thus, learning from Puerto Rican medical schools, residencies, and fellowships is integral as mainland U.S. schools endeavor to culturally develop LHS+ physicians. One of the benefits of rotating at the LCME-accredited schools in Puerto Rico (in addition to a high-quality, hands-on clinical education) is the ability for LHS+ students in the mainland to hone Spanish as an academic language—as opposed to a social language used at home [26]. In turn, greater partnerships with Puerto Rican schools can dispel the misunderstanding amongst residency programs that these U.S. MD students are foreign medical graduates [27]. These candidates present an unique opportunity to diversify a program while training physicians more likely to work in one of the most medically underserved areas in the United States [28]. Additionally, Puerto Rico suffers from a deficit of subspecialists—partially due to the loss of physicians to higher wages in the U.S. and the lack of fellowship programs on the island [28]. Thus, the training of Puerto Rican students and residents can help to decrease healthcare disparities in both the United States and Puerto Rico.

Programs have developed some effective models for marketing, recruiting and matching LHS+ individuals and other URM applicants [29]. There are two ways to categorize the strategies presented in the literature: active or passive. Active recruitment primarily utilizes finances and/or man-hours to recruit. While, passive recruitment primarily utilizes a change in how candidates are selected for interview and ranking.

Models vary widely; however, intentionality and unconscious bias training are ubiquitous.

Unconscious bias training is key to mitigating the subjective nature of GME recruitment and to subsequently identifying qualified LHS+ candidates. This is essential for passive recruitment models, which depend on a paradigm shift. McGovern Medical School at UTHealth's Internal Medicine Residency matriculated more URM candidates (without increasing URM applicants) through a passive recruitment model [11]. Their model began by highlighting the diversity of Houston, TX; the program's commitment to diversity; and had URM faculty interact with candidates. Then, the program tweaked the interview questions from the familiar "tell me about yourself" to standardized questions that were aimed at identifying their most important and desirable characteristics (e.g., teamwork, problem-solving, and adaptation to change). Finally, the program redesigned interview criteria to be inclusive of areas in which URM candidates excel – commitment to underserved communities, leadership roles, Spanish fluency—all which are representative of the Houston population (about two-thirds of Houston, TX identifies as Black or Hispanic) [30]. Finally, the program decreased the emphasis on the USMLE scores. The success of this program proved the path to diversity need not depend on large funding sources or outreach to more LHS+ individuals. The key, as always, is to value the talent present in candidate pools. This model may not work for everyone. Passive models are great for programs who have a diverse talent pool but lack diversity in their house-staff. The paradigm shift will open the door for LHS+ individuals and other URM applicants who have already been knocking.

For programs who struggle to attract URM applicants or programs that have a limited applicant pool, an extra investment is necessary. Active recruitment modalities allow programs to find and attract applicants who otherwise may not have considered training with them. Denver Health Residency in Emergency Medicine followed guidelines published by the Council of Residency Directors in Emergency Medicine – which were developed in response to EM's diver-

sity falling behind other specialties with regards to diversity. There were three recommended interventions:

- Scholarship-based Externship Programs
- Funded Second-look Events
- Involvement of URM faculty during recruitment

These interventions resulted in an increased number of applications from URM candidates and the number of URM matriculants [31]. The costs associated with active recruitment will depend on the program and the institution. Collaboration between departments and applying for grants through organizations, such as the Hispanic Centers for Excellence, can help alleviate the financial burden of active recruitment. Additionally, there are novel ways to conduct active recruitment at lower costs. The Ohio State University's Cardiovascular Medicine Fellowship Program ran active recruitment by leveraging an URM faculty member's Grand Rounds invitations at diverse residency programs to identify and court URM residents. The URM faculty member also committed to mentor the residents as fellows. The rest of their recruitment was passive; however, the authors noted an increase in URM applicants and matriculants [32]. A program's ability to execute this form of active recruitment would be dependent upon the presence of a willing URM faculty, which may more than likely be scarce. Engaging in virtual mentoring of medical students is another way to do active recruitment at a low cost. Many national organizations have programs for virtual advising and virtual mentoring. Finally, no opportunity should go unused. When program faculty are participating in regional and national meetings, they should participate in any recruitment activities, such as residency and fellowship fairs. Students should do the same and pay attention for specialty-specific activities happening on campus or in their cities; making sure to attend and network at local meetings when possible. Table 12.2 describes some important activities for LHS+ students during medical school that can help maximize their chances of a successful match.

Table 12.2 Actions and activities to succeed in applying to GME programs

- Find your support network of family and friends
- Learn to take care of yourself, physically, mentally, and spiritually
- Seek out mentors, advisors, and sponsors
- Engage in specialty-specific student interest groups
- Utilize and engage with diversity groups in your medical school, national organizations, or area of specialty
- Participate in opportunities that will enhance your career: summer research electives, paid scholarships, etc.
- Engage in community service in a way that is meaningful to you
- Do your research when applying to programs: look at websites; ask alumni and students in classes above you; look at institutional and program statements about diversity and inclusion; reach out to current residents and faculty
- Research the city and community the program serves and see if they align with what you value

Adapted from: https://www.cordem.org/globalassets/files/student-resources/applying-guide%2D%2D-underrepresented-applicant.pdf

Given the dearth of LHS+ trainees in GME, it is imperative to ensure that a concerted effort is made to retain those we have and get them into fellowships or, more importantly, careers in academic medicine. The retention of trainees is tied to the career satisfaction and the experience of being a minority. The data reveal high rates of attrition amongst Hispanic residents [33]. When correlated with research revealing that being as Hispanic is associated with an increase relative risk of dissatisfaction with specialty [34], several questions arise. There are no published investigations into whether or not Hispanics have matched into their desired specialty or have changed the specialty to which they intended to apply while in medical school. If this is due to poor match outcomes or applicant screening, then it is a tragedy. Given data that URM residents perform no differently from their non-URM colleagues in objective clinical assessments [35], issues in recruitment may have unnecessarily (and unintentionally) negatively impacted the careers of LHS+ physicians.

Premature departures from a training program are costly. Recruitment is a huge investment, and the loss of a trainee results in additional work-loads for other residents and a lower program morale and poor career outcomes for the dismissed resident. These factors, which limit inclusivity, are accompanied by other potential contributors to attrition. Hispanics and other URM residents report experiencing microaggressions and other racist incidents during training and being forced to serve as racial/ethnic ambassadors [36]. While workplace incidents are common across professions and backgrounds, Hispanic trainees may lack confidants who can share their burdens and serve as release valves. URM residents are less likely to use resident wellness services out of fear that the use of the services will not be fully confidential [37]. The solution to these issues is more inclusivity.

LHS+ students and residents are as capable as other trainees. When discussing challenges LHS+ individuals face, it is done in the context that they have graduated from LCME-accredited medical schools, passed the USMLE, and are fully acknowledged academically. Thus, the obstacles stem not from the applicant but from a system that organically evolved to accommodate a homogenous socioeconomic demographic. Formal medical education in the United States took off in the Gilded Age (late nineteenth Century) and transformed dramatically well into the mid twentieth Century [38]. During this time period (see Fig. 12.1 below), the U.S. government was at war with Native American tribes [39]; Jim Crow and segregation of African Americans were in full effect [40]; and Hispanics were being lynched and sterilized [41–43]. In other words, certain populations were conspicuously absent from the inception and evolution of medical education in the United States and are thus unsurprisingly underrepresented in the field created in their absence. Please note this is not a condemnation of medical education, but a call for reform to allow all Americans to thrive.

Residency and fellowship programs can take steps to help LHS+ residents excel during residency. The solutions to developing LHS+ residents come from the residents themselves. URM residents suggested in-person, practical trainings to address racism and microaggressions and for programs to work to eliminate the fear of

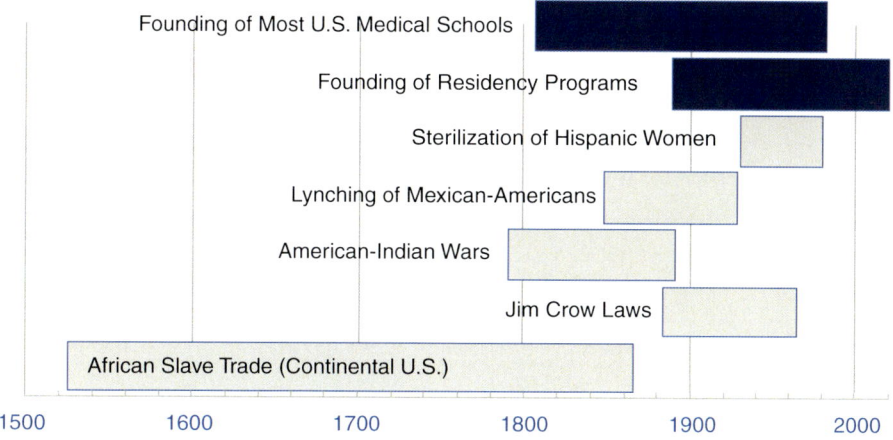

Fig. 12.1 Development of medical education in the context of concurrent U.S. historical events

reporting incidents [44]. Additionally, residents have enjoyed the opportunity to serve as mentors to URM students – which has shown to increase their interest in academic medicine [45]. Hispanic and other URM residents have an increase in satisfaction and interest in academic medicine when they have URM faculty mentors [46]. The importance of mentorship cannot be overstated throughout this process. The retention, satisfaction, and (most importantly) success of LHS+ residents all hinge upon mentorship.

Throughout this book, it's clear URM faculty hold diversity and inclusion together at every level. The issue is academia (and medicine as a whole) lacks a proportional amount of URM physicians to handle the load. Currently LHS+ inidividuals represent a disproportionately low 5.8% of all physicians and 6.3% of physicians in academia [47, 48]. Of LHS+ individualsphysicians with academic appointments, 65% hold non-tenured positions, 19% are Associate Professors, and 16% are Professors [49]. These paltry numbers are going to be the backbone of diversity and inclusion efforts that support the training of LHS+ physicians. Thus, the recruitment and retention of LHS+ academic physicians will be essential to all levels of LHS+ trainees.

Recommendations on how to recruit LHS+ faculty are scarce. The availability of published research into LHS+ recruitment decreases as the level increases from UME to GME to faculty appointments. Few institutions have imple-

mented programs to recruit LHS+ and URM physicians to their faculty; disappointingly, even fewer have tracked and published statistics regarding their URM faculty recruitment programs [50]. The jury is still out. Some programs have yielded success [50], while others have not [51]. The U.S. medical schools with URM faculty recruitment programs tended to be higher ranked and to have larger faculties; additionally, those that reported success instituted programs with mentoring, career development, social climate, and financial support components [50].

The reality is that it will take both time and money to recruit LHS+ faculty. Mentorship is important throughout anyone's career; however, LHS+ physicians will be aware of the stigmas associated with being an URM in academic medicine—especially the disparity in promotions to tenured positions and Associate Professor to Professor [20]. In the recruitment of LHS+ faculty, programs are working against decades of inequality. Even if Rome were built in a day, it was certainly not built for free. If institutions cannot shoulder the financial burden, then the federal government has an opportunity and an obligation to fund LHS+ faculty appointments, which have the additional public health benefit of attracting in more clinical study subjects from the LHS+ community [52].

Hope comes from within. Time and time again, the literature demonstrates that research and authorship in medical school and residency will mitigate promotional disparities [20]. In essence, having early career opportunities for mentorship and publishing will cultivate future generations of LHS+ academic physicians. Although medical schools and GME programs may lack formal programs to address the aforementioned revelation, LHS+ physicians and trainees are leading by example and uniting to close these gaps. In 1994, the National Hispanic Medical Association (NHMA) was founded as a dedicated network of Hispanic physicians to provide advocacy, education, leadership development, and networking [53]. In 2010, Building the Next Generation of Academic Physicians (BNGAP Inc.) was founded to increase diverse trainees' awareness of, interest in and preparedness for academic careers; a novel approach to increase diverse GME staff and leaders [54]. These professional societies are invaluable grassroots networks through which mentors and mentees can be identified. They may serve to identify solutions and serve as points of outreach, but there is no sole intervention to close the gaps. Diversity and inclusion will require efforts at all levels to achieve parity.

References

1. Data Resource Book Academic Year 2018-2019. PDF Accreditation Council for Graduate Medical Education; 2018. https://www.acgme.org/Portals/0/PFAssets/PublicationsBooks/2018-2019_ACGME_DATABOOK_DOCUMENT.pdf
2. AAMC. Matriculating Student Questionnaire. 2019. https://www.aamc.org/media/50081/download. Accessed on September 25, 2023.
3. Deville C, Hwang WT, Burgos R, Chapman CH, Both S, Thomas CR Jr. Diversity in graduate medical education in the United States by Race, Ethnicity, and Sex, 2012. JAMA Intern Med. 2015;175(10):1706–8. https://doi.org/10.1001/jamainternmed.2015.4324.
4. Norcini JJ, van Zanten M, Boulet JR. The contribution of international medical graduates to diversity in the U.S. physician workforce: graduate medical education. J Health Care Poor Underserved. 2008;19(2):493–9. https://doi.org/10.1353/hpu.0.0015.
5. Williams M, Kim EJ, Pappas K, et al. The impact of United States Medical Licensing Exam (USMLE) step 1 cutoff scores on recruitment of underrepresented minorities in medicine: a retrospective cross-sectional study. Health Sci Rep. 2020;3(2):e2161. https://doi.org/10.1002/hsr2.161.

6. McDougle L, Mavis BE, Jeffe DB, et al. Academic and professional career outcomes of medical school graduates who failed USMLE Step 1 on the first attempt. Adv Health Sci Educ Theory Pract. 2013;18(2):279–89. https://doi.org/10.1007/s10459-012-9371-2.
7. Change to pass/fail score reporting for Step 1. Federation of State Medical Boards and National Board of Medical Examiners®. June 1, 2020, https://usmle.org/incus/#decision
8. Rojek AE, Khanna R, Yim JWL, et al. Differences in narrative language in evaluations of medical students by gender and under-represented minority status. J Gen Intern Med. 2019;34(5):684–91. https://doi.org/10.1007/s11606-019-04889-9.
9. Ross DA, Boatright D, Nunez-Smith M, Jordan A, Chekroud A, Moore EZ. Differences in words used to describe racial and gender groups in Medical Student Performance Evaluations. PLoS One. 2017;12(8):e0181659. https://doi.org/10.1371/journal.pone.0181659.
10. Low D, Pollack SW, Liao ZC, et al. Racial/ethnic disparities in clinical grading in medical school. Teach Learn Med. 2019;31(5):487–96. https://doi.org/10.1080/10401334.2019.1597724.
11. Aibana O, Swails JL, Flores RJ, Love L. Bridging the gap: holistic review to increase diversity in graduate medical education. Acad Med. 2019;94(8):1137–41. https://doi.org/10.1097/ACM.0000000000002779.
12. Boatright D, Ross D, O'Connor P, Moore E, Nunez-Smith M. Racial disparities in medical student membership in the alpha omega alpha honor society. JAMA Intern Med. 2017;177(5):659–65. https://doi.org/10.1001/jamainternmed.2016.9623.
13. Gordon M. A Medical School Tradition Comes Under Fire for Racism. NPR; 2020. https://www.npr.org/sections/health-shots/2018/09/05/643298219/a-medical-school-tradition-comes-under-fire-for-racism
14. How Members Are Chosen. Alpha Omega Alpha; 2020. https://alphaomegaalpha.org/how.html
15. Teherani A, Harleman E, Hauer KE, Lucey C. Toward creating equity in awards received during medical school: strategic changes at one institution. Acad Med. 2020;95(5):724–9. https://doi.org/10.1097/ACM.0000000000003219.
16. Jarman BT, Kallies KJ, Joshi ART, et al. Underrepresented minorities are underrepresented among general surgery applicants selected to interview. J Surg Educ. 2019;76(6):e15–23. https://doi.org/10.1016/j.jsurg.2019.05.018.
17. Shappell E, Schnapp B. The F word: how "Fit" threatens the validity of resident recruitment. J Grad Med Educ. 2019;11(6):635–6. https://doi.org/10.4300/JGME-D-19-00400.1.
18. Angus SV, Williams CM, Stewart EA, Sweet M, Kisielewski M, Willett LL. Internal medicine residency program directors' screening practices and perceptions about recruitment challenges. Acad Med. 2020;95(4):582–9. https://doi.org/10.1097/ACM.0000000000003086.

19. Results of the 2018 NRMP Program Director Survey. National Resident Matching Program, Data Release and Research Committee; 2018. https://mk0nrmp3oyqui6wqfm.kinstacdn.com/wp-content/uploads/2018/07/NRMP-2018-Program-Director-Survey-for-WWW.pdf

20. Jeffe DB, Yan Y, Andriole DA. Do research activities during college, medical school, and residency mediate racial/ethnic disparities in full-time faculty appointments at U.S. Medical schools? Acad Med. 2012;87(11):1582–93. https://doi.org/10.1097/ACM.0b013e31826e3297.

21. McDade WA. Increasing graduate medical education diversity and inclusion. J Grad Med Educ. 2019;11(6):736–8. https://doi.org/10.4300/JGME-D-19-00760.1.

22. Elks ML, Herbert-Carter J, Smith M, Klement B, Knight BB, Anachebe NF. Shifting the curve: fostering academic success in a diverse student body. Acad Med. 2018;93(1):66–70. https://doi.org/10.1097/ACM.0000000000001783.

23. Hernández-Nieto R, Gutiérrez MC. Hispanic map of the United States 2017. Informes del Observatorio/Observatorio Rep. 2017; https://doi.org/10.15427/or035-11/2017en.

24. Paul L. Foster School of Medicine Homepage. Texas Tech University Health Sciences Center - El Paso; 2020. https://elpaso.ttuhsc.edu/som/

25. Data from: Table B-2.2: Total Graduates by U.S. Medical School and Sex, 2014–2015 through 2018–2019. 2019. Online.

26. Garcia GE Jr, Salcedo PA. Lost in transition: trainees' perspectives on their bilingual experiences in clinical medicine. Acad Med. 2018;93(6):821–2. https://doi.org/10.1097/ACM.0000000000002213.

27. Bias Faced by Med Students in Puerto Rico During Residency Process. Accessed 10 June 2020. https://www.youtube.com/watch?v=nwrVosNsJOw. Online.

28. Silva Diaz DHGJ GE, Clare C, Su J, Friedman E, Williams R, Vazquez J, Sanchez JP. Taking care of the Puerto Rican patient: historical perspectives, health status, and health care access. Workshop. Accepted for Publication by MedEdPortal; 2020.

29. Capers Q, McDougle L, Clinchot DM. Strategies for achieving diversity through medical school admissions. J Health Care Poor Underserved. 2018;29(1):9–18. https://doi.org/10.1353/hpu.2018.0002.

30. QuickFacts Houston city, Texas. July 1, 2019. https://www.census.gov/quickfacts/fact/table/houstoncity-texas/PST120219. Accessed 10 May 2020.

31. Tunson J, Boatright D, Oberfoell S, et al. Increasing resident diversity in an emergency medicine residency program: a pilot intervention with three principal strategies. Acad Med. 2016;91(7):958–61. https://doi.org/10.1097/ACM.0000000000000957.

32. Auseon AJ, Kolibash AJ Jr, Capers Q. Successful efforts to increase diversity in a cardiology fellowship training program. J Grad Med Educ. 2013;5(3):481–5. https://doi.org/10.4300/JGME-D-12-00307.1.

33. Lu DW, Hartman ND, Druck J, Mitzman J, Strout TD. Why residents quit: national rates of and reasons for attrition among emergency medicine physicians in training. West J Emerg Med. 2019;20(2):351–6. https://doi.org/10.5811/westjem.2018.11.40449.

34. Dyrbye LN, Burke SE, Hardeman RR, et al. Association of clinical specialty with symptoms of burnout and career choice regret among US resident physicians. JAMA. 2018;320(11):1114–30. https://doi.org/10.1001/jama.2018.12615.

35. Lypson ML, Ross PT, Hamstra SJ, Haftel HM, Gruppen LD, Colletti LM. Evidence for increasing diversity in graduate medical education: the competence of underrepresented minority residents measured by an intern objective structured clinical examination. J Grad Med Educ. 2010;2(3):354–9. https://doi.org/10.4300/JGME-D-10-00050.1.

36. Osseo-Asare A, Balasuriya L, Huot SJ, et al. Minority resident physicians' views on the role of race/ethnicity in their training experiences in the workplace. JAMA Netw Open. 2018;1(5):e182723. https://doi.org/10.1001/jamanetworkopen.2018.2723.

37. Ey S, Moffit M, Kinzie JM, Choi D, Girard DE. "If you build it, they will come": attitudes of medical residents and fellows about seeking services in a resident wellness program. J Grad Med Educ. 2013;5(3):486–92. https://doi.org/10.4300/JGME-D-12-00048.1.

38. Custers E, Cate OT. The history of medical education in Europe and the United States, with respect to time and proficiency. Acad Med. 2018;93(3S Competency-Based, Time-Variable Education in the Health Professions):S49–54. https://doi.org/10.1097/ACM.0000000000002079.

39. Indian Wars Campaigns. U.S. Army Center of Military History. Accessed 1 June 2020, https://history.army.mil/html/reference/army_flag/iw.html

40. Jim Crow Era. Georgetown Law Library. Updated Apr 1, 2020. Accessed June 1, 2020, https://guides.ll.georgetown.edu/civilrights

41. Carrigan WD, Webb C. The lynching of persons of Mexican origin or descent in the United States, 1848 to 1928. J Soc Hist. 2003;37(2):411–38. https://doi.org/10.1353/jsh.2003.0169.

42. Novak NL, Lira N, O'Connor KE, Harlow SD, Kardia SLR, Stern AM. Disproportionate sterilization of Latinos under California's Eugenic Sterilization Program, 1920-1945. Am J Public Health. 2018;108(5):611–3. https://doi.org/10.2105/AJPH.2018.304369.

43. Lopez I. Chapter 1: The birth control movement in Puerto Rico. In: Matters of Choice: Puerto Rican Women's Struggle for Reproductive Freedom. New Brunswick, NJ: Rutgers University Press; 2008.

44. Khan NR, Taylor CM 2nd, Rialon KL. Resident perspectives on the current state of diversity in graduate medical education. J Grad Med Educ. 2019;11(2):241–3. https://doi.org/10.4300/JGME-D-19-00062.1.

45. Youmans QR, Adrissi JA, Akhetuamhen A, et al. The STRIVE initiative: a resident-led mentorship frame-

work for underrepresented minority medical students. J Grad Med Educ. 2020;12(1):74–9. https://doi.org/10.4300/JGME-D-19-00461.2.

46. Yehia BR, Cronholm PF, Wilson N, et al. Mentorship and pursuit of academic medicine careers: a mixed methods study of residents from diverse backgrounds. BMC Med Educ. 2014;14:26. https://doi.org/10.1186/1472-6920-14-26.

47. Data from: Figure 18. Percentage of all active physicians by race/ethnicity, 2018. Diversity in Medicine: Facts and Figures 2019; 2020. Online.

48. Data from: Table 5: U.S. Medical School Faculty by Degree and Race/Ethnicity, 2019; 2020. Online.

49. Data from: Table 3: U.S. Medical School Faculty by Rank and Race/Ethnicity, 2019. 2019 US Medical School Faculty; 2020. Online.

50. Adanga E, Avakame E, Carthon MB, Guevara JP. An environmental scan of faculty diversity programs at U.S. medical schools. Acad Med. 2012;87(11):1540–7. https://doi.org/10.1097/ACM.0b013e31826cf4fb.

51. Washington DM, Paasche-Orlow MK, Liebschutz JM. Promoting progress or propagating problems: strategic plans and the advancement of academic faculty diversity in U.S. Medical Schools. J Natl Med Assoc. 2017;109(2):72–8. https://doi.org/10.1016/j.jnma.2016.10.001.

52. Sanchez JP, Poll-Hunter NI, Acosta D. Advancing the Latino physician workforce-population trends, persistent challenges, and new directions. Acad Med. 2015;90(7):849–53. https://doi.org/10.1097/ACM.0000000000000618.

53. Membership Benefits. National Hispanic Medical Association. https://www.nhmamd.org/membership/membership-benefits/

54. Building the Next Generation of Academic Physicians. BNGAP. https://www.bngap.org/

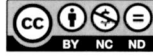

LHS+ Faculty Development and Advancement

Sylk Sotto-Santiago and Francisco Moreno

Background

In addition to limited representation, multiple reports document challenges in achievement of traditional metrics of academic performance, retention and success of minoritized faculty members [1]. Whereas, approximately 19% of Americans identify as Hispanic or Latino [2], the Association of American Medical Colleges (AAMC) reports that 5.9% of total faculty listed in their 2021 roster from allopathic medical schools were Hispanic, Latino, or of Spanish Origin, whether single or multiple race/ethnicity, compared to 62.3% White non-Hispanic faculty [3]. This disparity is more evident in the advanced ranks of the professoriate, whereby AAMC reports that Hispanic, Latino, or of Spanish Origin, whether single or multiple race/ethnicity, faculty represented 6.7% of instructors, 6.8% of assistant professors, 5.4% of associate professors, and 4.3% of full professors [4]. The American Association for Colleges of Osteopathic

Medicine (AACOM) report that 1.7% of total faculty listed in their 2016–2017 roster were LHS+ [5]. AACOM reports similar trends to AAMC whereby in 2016–2017 LHS+ faculty represented 3.5% of instructors, 4.9% of assistant professors, 2.5% of associate professors, and 1.5% of full professors [5]. The lack of LHS+ individuals is also evident on the medical school dean level whereby in December 2022 there were only 5 Hispanic identified Deans of a U.S. LCME accredited medical school; 1 on the mainland (Juan C. Cendan, M.D., Dean of Herbert Wertheim College of Medicine) and 4 on the island of Puerto Rico (Yocasta Brugal M.D., Dean, San Juan Bautista School of Medicine, Caguas, Puerto Rico; Jose Capriles M.D., Dean, Universidad Central del Caribe School of Medicine, Bayamón, Puerto Rico; Interim Dean Humberto M. Guiot, University of Puerto Rico School of Medicine San Juan, Puerto Rico; Olga Rodríguez de Arzola M.D., Dean, Ponce Health Sciences University School of Medicine Ponce, Puerto Rico). Among accredited osteopathic medical schools, there was only one LHS+ identified dean Italo R. Subbarao, DO, MBA of William Carey University, College of Osteopathic Medicine [6].

Studies on LHS+ faculty in academic medicine are limited, however extant work in higher education demonstrates that LHS+ faculty uniquely engage students, improve LHS+

S. Sotto-Santiago (✉)
Department of Medicine, Indiana University School of Medicine, Indianapolis, IN, USA
e-mail: ssotto@iu.edu

F. Moreno
The University of Arizona College of Medicine Tucson, University of Arizona Health Sciences, Office of Equity, Diversity, and Inclusion, Tucson, AZ, USA

© The Author(s) 2024
J. P. Sánchez, D. Rodriguez (eds.), *Latino, Hispanic, or of Spanish Origin+ Identified Student Leaders in Medicine*, Sustainable Development Goals Series, https://doi.org/10.1007/978-3-031-35020-7_13

students' higher education retention and degree completion rates, and conducting academic research on racial/ethnic communities [7].

LHS+ faculty are as productive as their White colleagues and found to be more involved in their departments or campuses than their White colleagues [8]. LHS+ faculty may be particularly subject to cultural taxation, as the number of LHS+ faculty has not kept pace with the growth of LHS+ student enrollment leading to additional stresses and burdens placed on this group, while productivity expectations are not reconsidered [8]. The low representation of LHS+ among the faculty, together with projected growth in demand among LHS+ students, suggests that there will be more future demands on the time of LHS+ faculty members serving as role models, advisors and champions [9]. Additional time spent on service activities and teaching and/or mentoring minoritized students may also result from LHS+ faculty members' strong sense of responsibility to serve their racial/ethnic communities, as other minoritized faculty often do.

As a minoritized group in medicine, similar studies documented that a promotion disparity exists between minoritized faculty in medicine and White faculty. Minoritized faculty are more frequently found in early career positions than leadership positions and promoted at lower rates, while lacking institutional and formalized mentorship [10, 11]. Minoritized faculty tend to be disproportionately positioned to engage in service work such as diversity and inclusion efforts, institutional, and clinical service activities [10, 11]. Moreover, they are rarely trained on how to document service-related work as scholarly work (e.g. peer-reviewed publications) or for promotion purposes. This commitment to service and promotion and tenure results in emotional burnout for many LHS+ faculty members [12]. Because salary is also dependent on academic rank, clinical and research efforts, even financial incentives contribute to pay-inequities [13].

While discrimination of LHS+ faculty can happen in several domains, significant narratives have centered on culture and credentials [14]. According to Verdugo scholars have shown that LHS+ faculty believe they are discriminated against due to appearance and accusations that their positions are a result of diversity initiatives [14]. Scholars have also demonstrated how cultural differences cause LHS+ faculty to feel excluded from available opportunities and abstain from participating. These perceptions produce barriers to engagement and credibility, precluding LHS+ faculty from being positive role models for LHS+ students [13, 14].

The low proportion of LHS+ faculty especially in visibly impactful positions, challenges the social and academic success of LHS+ students who are themselves minoritized (11.5% of incoming matriculants at allopathic medical schools and 6.8% of incoming matriculants at osteopathic medical schools in 2021) [15, 16]. Although it is important to acknowledge the generous contributions by non-LHS+ equity minded senior faculty who mentor and train LMSA students, residents, and early career LHS+ faculty, the gap in ethnic/cultural concordance between faculty members, trainees, and the communities we must serve is perceived as an obstacle affecting satisfaction and benefit from the relationship [17].

Concordance between patients and physicians may be of particular importance when working with less acculturated LHS+ communities given the linguistic, literacy, socioeconomic, and other cultural elements that impact wellness, health concepts, health seeking, and acceptance in this community [18]. Our chapter describes asset-based efforts to support faculty development, some of which may be applied to individuals along the continuum of academic development including efforts to encourage and prepare trainees along the aspiring pre-faculty pathway.

Socialization

Socialization is the process through which individuals acquire and incorporate understanding of the institution with shared attitudes, beliefs, values, and skills [19]. Socialization can positively affect LHS+ faculty retention and promotion, and student's introduction to the academy. Therefore, impacting the personal, professional and academic development of LHS+ students. The difference in experiences and belonging in academic medicine can be addressed through anticipatory socialization, strong mentoring networks, extensive networking opportunities, focused priorities, and intentional or goal-oriented work demands [19]. Literature on the socialization of URM individuals often includes the very important pre-faculty phases, yet the assessment of impact of socialization on faculty success is less well studied.

Various studies found that Latina/o doctoral students utilized family and community members as support systems, particularly for emotional support when navigating hostile environments [20–24] and revealed that LHS+ medical students do not have access to privileged knowledge that can only occur through faculty mentoring [25].

Multiple variables predict the career selection and success of medical school faculty such as: the aggregate of the individual's inspiration, preparation, experiences, and identity prior to joining the faculty ranks; commitment of the institution to the academic mission over common competing demands; availability of qualified and committed mentors and content experts; development of writing skills and habits for scientific audiences and granting agencies; access to project based research training-experience; leadership skills development; balanced portfolios of teaching, and service that are congruent to the content of the faculty member scholarship focus, and work-life balance; among others.

LHS+ faculty often have experiences and trajectories less concordant with traditional markers of advancement [26], however focused forms of support for pre-faculty and early career academics [27] which optimize asset-based development opportunities may be the best form of ensuring success [28].

LHS+ Faculty Development

Faculty and educational development focuses on the continuous improvement of individual's instructional and educational skills, including their professional and personal development opportunities that contribute to career advancement [29, 30] We have strong evidence that faculty development programs increase retention, productivity, and lead to tenure and promotion [31].

Successful faculty development programs include: effective mentoring panels; focused instruction on areas of excellence such as clinical, teaching, and research skills; recurrent networking spaces; and reduced administrative or clinical expectations in order to facilitate scholarly productivity [30, 31]. They often include funds towards protected time and institutional seed money for pilot projects [31]. However, there is a limited number of programs tailored towards minoritized faculty and even less targeting LHS+ faculty.

In assessing the status of tailored programs for LHS+ faculty we recognize that many institutions have sponsored spaces and faculty communities for LHS+ faculty. However, a number of these spaces originate from grassroot efforts and the level of professional development opportunities vary greatly.

The professional development spaces developed for LHS+ faculty are few and far between. Colleges of Medicine in the U.S. are likely to have offices of diversity, many have active programs promoting compositional diversity and inclusive climates, and about half of them report hosting programs tailored to support historically underrepresented faculty (51.2% mentorship and 42.7% leadership development), few address specific populations such as LHS+ individuals [32], and the proportion of LHS+ faculty when reported tends to be modest.

The success of minoritized faculty development efforts when measured are highly variable and believed to be associated with the greater intensity (time and quality of commitment), broader scope (including mentoring, career development, social climate, pilot funding), and greater longevity (>5 years) of program activity [33]. Broad efforts to assess the impact of existing programs in LHS+ pre-faculty and faculty may help inform future LHS+ academic career development support design.

It is worth highlighting some of these programs. The Hispanic Center of Excellence at New Jersey Medical School provides a program dedicated to the advancement of Hispanic faculty

[34]. The Hispanic Center of Excellence Faculty Development Program at University of California, San Diego is designed to "improve recruitment, retention, and success of URM faculty in academic medicine at UC San Diego" [35]. At the national level, the Hispanic Association of Colleges and Universities offers a leadership development platform [36]. The American Association for Hispanics in Higher Education represents Hispanic academics, researchers, educators, and Hispanic students. Through their platform they offer several opportunities including a fellowship and leadership academy [37].

Institutions with external funding to support faculty development tend to be hosted at sites where the demographic representation of traditionally underrepresented individuals and impactful leaders from congruent backgrounds may coincide. The Health Resources and Services Administration (HRSA) Centers of Excellence are funded programs with comprehensive goals to advance the institution's ability to serve the needs of their diverse communities. Hispanic Centers of Excellence across the nation contribute locally to the recruitment, retention, and success of Hispanic Faculty members within specific colleges of medicine and at times collaborative consortiums [34]. The impact of these programs may be variable, and formal evaluation of broad impact is lacking.

Hispanic advancement organizations such as the National Hispanic Medical Association and the Hispanic Serving Health Professions Schools (HSHPS) have hosted professional development workshops and faculty development in support of Hispanic Medical (Health Professions) Faculty Development however they seem to be subjected to the time limitations associated with grant funding or short term collaborative opportunities. Similarly, AAMC Minority Faculty Leadership Development Seminar, and the AAMC Mid-Career Minority Faculty Leadership Development Program, although not specific for LHS+ faculty, they are designed to support individuals who aspire to leadership positions in academic medicine by helping individuals identify professional development goals and design a career path, learn the skills and tools to succeed, and expand their network of colleagues and role models. A number of scientific and professional societies, private research and benefit foundations also contribute to the piece meal opportunities described above. The National Institutes of Health have made important efforts to support the career development of individuals underrepresented in the biomedical sciences.

Funding support from mentored career awards (K-series), career development award (KL2) components of the Clinical and Translational Science Awards, multiple R25 funding mechanisms to support research career training and development. These are amazing opportunities for those who are competitively placed and seeking research careers. There is clearly a need for larger scale, durable, expert designed and longitudinally delivered faculty development program to support LHS+ faculty whose careers in academia may not follow the traditional independent investigator route, and who represent the overwhelming majority of LHS+ faculty serving in smaller, newer, educationally intensive institutions, or hospital based programs where opportunities for academic success are more limited.

Cultural values bring us together and there is great value in LHS+ tailored faculty development programs. In fact, LHS+ faculty conveyed these programs as important in several respects: tailored programs create spaces for networking, for relationship building, accountability and affirmation. Most importantly, these faculty development spaces reaffirm that microaggressions, discrimination and overt racism are not isolated events [12, 13]. Table 13.1 provides a sample of themes to be included in these training.

Table 13.1 LHS+ faculty development Topics [13]

Faculty development topics	
• Tenure and promotion criteria and strategies	• Leadership development
• Dealing with microaggressions	• Time management
• Bias in student evaluations	• Cultural taxation
• Importance of mentorship	• Dealing with hostile environments
• Impostor syndrome	• Cultural sensitivity/ inclusion
• Structural racism	• Difference between inclusion and diversity
• Cultural/intercultural competence	• Privilege
• Implicit bias	

Mentoring

Mentors are an essential component of the LHS+ and other minoritized in medicine faculty member's support-network impacting retention and advancement. Mentors may help demystify professional environments providing vital information and support to facilitate inclusion in important opportunities; they can help balance contributions to diversity efforts and ensure adequate compensation or acknowledgement; assist at dealing with internal conflict resulting from feeling responsible for serving their communities, and taking on too many service commitments; help understand the nuances of academic medicine culture and expectations; promote a sense of community decreasing feelings of isolation due to a lack of critical mass; and increase the sense of value minimizing stereotype threat, increasing resilience and improve coping with bias [38, 39].

Programs to enhance mentoring opportunities and skill development have been importantly promoted over the last decade. Of relevance, significant resources to develop and tailor specific trainings can be accessed from the University of Wisconsin-Madison Institute for Clinical and Translational Science. This team leads the coordination center for the National Research Mentoring Program (NRMN), an NIH consortium that strives to enhance diversity in the biomedical research workforce by serving mentors and mentees [40]. It is important to ensure that mentors and mentees receive training on various aspects of giving and receiving mentorship. Elements of training include the importance of developing a mentoring plan and contract, ideas for maintaining effective communication, aligning expectations, addressing equity and inclusion. A good mentee will have openness and desire to learn and benefit from the relationship, will take initiative, be prepared, responsible at completing tasks enthusiastically and in a timely fashion, and have a sense of ownership of the outcomes of the relationship dyad. A good mentor will be accessible, committed to the mentee and their relationship, eager to con-

tinually improve, embrace diversity, and have faith and respect for the mentee. A good mentoring contract includes descriptions of frequency and type of contact to be had, how the time will be utilized, what mechanisms for feedback and assessment of the dyad will be in place, among other commitments volunteered by the members. Although many of the above-mentioned approaches have been supported with data and observational reports, the effectiveness of NRMN and collaborative programs in the success of LHS+ faculty and trainees specifically has not been documented to this date.

Importance of Culturally Relevant Faculty Mentoring

As programs also focus on developing mentors, they need to also acknowledge that being mentored by someone from a similar LHS+ background might be at odds with what the representational numbers indicate. LHS+ faculty need more than career advice. Mentoring relationships must recognize the many assets that LHS+ faculty have to offer and their strong commitment to service. Mentors can practice cultural curiosity and familiarity in how they develop relationships. Mentors must socialize faculty into the academy, introduce them to the community, build mentoring networks of champions, sponsors, role models, advisors, institutional agents, etc. [41] This process should start as early along the LHS+ pre-faculty continuum as possible. LHS+ postgraduate trainees report less interest in academic medicine careers than their peers, report not having enough mentoring to pursue a career in academic medicine and are less likely to credit their mentors and role models with pursuit of academic medicine [17].

LHS+ students and faculty alike do not leave their cultural values "at the door" [42]. In order to persist, mentoring models should address collaborative relationships dealing with power, establishing connections among community and providing support to succeed [42].

Charting Your Course

Most academicians fill their days—often beyond work schedules—with urgent, dutiful, and exciting or rewarding experiences, many of which may have limited impact in the main academic outcomes of retention, promotion, and content related success. LHS+ faculty may benefit from carefully constructing an individual academic plan that is informed by the individual's values, and the articulation of their academic vision and mission. Once the values/vision/mission are clear, an intentional plan must be put in writing along with an timeline and metrics of success to include: Establishing career development goals; Identifying area of research/scholarship niche; Pursue/obtain grant funding; Improve skill set; Conduct ongoing studies/scholarly projects; Participate in education/teaching; Participate in outreach/service/professional network; and Life balance.

Informed by a clear understanding of the rules and practical options for promotion within assigned rank, faculty members must identify top priorities, set deadlines, and track metrics. Having a visible document with the timeline for one whole academic year allows us to plan the rhythm of national meetings, submission of abstracts, publication timelines, and facilitates the balance of teaching and service requirements which ideally should congruently flow. This is then converted to a monthly, weekly, and at times daily goals that inform our intentional investment of amount and quality of time, and effort. Adherence to such timeline allows us to separate the urgent from the important, the enjoyable from the relevant, and the distractors from the focused contributions that result in impactful coherent narratives of our value.

Strategies that allow us to maximize outcomes based on time is: organizing your office and outside life in addition to organizing your schedule, making lists, minimizing distractions, putting a time to each effort so keep meetings brief, having visible clocks and make others aware of the value of your and their time, learn to and practice delegating, support students and other team members to collaborate with you towards goal completion, align the various efforts so that it all counts towards your goals, manage email time, and be selective about what you agree to do [43]. As LHS+ faculty members master the skills listed above, they become a better equipped role model and can in turn work with trainees to guide them through similar process that matches their stage of pre-faculty development.

Career Advancement

Given the disparities in career retention and advancement in LHS+ faculty, faculty development efforts must be built upon a clear understanding of the value, process, and specific deliverables required for promotion in the individual faculty member's rank and track.

A very user friendly and valuable tool to use is "The Promotion Game" [44]. Early career faculty members often are ill informed about the tracks available at their institutions and unclear about the promotion timeline or targets associated with the track they agreed to be hired under or were assigned to without discussion. The implications of "playing the promotion game" before knowing the object of the game, the rules of engagement, and the cost of wining or loosing represents a major disadvantage, hence pre-faculty scholars would also benefit from having keen awareness of these rules. With a full appreciation of the criteria for promotion in their department, faculty must assess if the track is right for them, are the requirements consistent with how they spend their time, what activities and other requirements (scholarship, teaching, and service) fulfill those criteria.

With this knowledge aspiring and current faculty must revisit their personal/professional IAP goals paying attention to how achieving their individual goals moves them toward their target for initial appointment or promotion, and how their personal goals align with and support institutional and departmental roles, mission and goals. The ideal job lives at the intersection of the individual's values, preferences, passions, and ability to contribute.

Faculty progressing through the academic path should be encouraged to maintain a positive learning attitude, taking advantage of self- and external- assessments. Being an active seeker and participant during the Annual Reviews process with their Department Chairperson or Section Chief. In addition to obtaining feedback on accomplishments, as you talk through your plan for the year, use the opportunity to ask: Am I on track for promotion? Does my productivity and my workload assignment match my promotion targets? Are there areas in which I need to be more productive? What types of journals, conference presentations should I pursue? What service opportunities are most appropriate given my goals and interests? What else do I need to do? Similarly, pre-faculty scholars would benefit from assessing their progression and consider path adjustments to increase their competitiveness for faculty appointment and success.

Mid-Cycle Reviews are required for tenure track, but optional for other tracks. They tend to be a "Dress rehearsal" for promotion, it is an opportunity to update and assess if your CV is in the appropriate format, reflective of your efforts, and consistent with promotion requirements. This also allows you an opportunity to prepare and refine your candidate statement, including re-evaluating your workload assignments, and receive formal input from the departmental Promotion and Tenure committee about being on track for promotion, and suggestions to strengthen aspects that may require additional production or focus.

Academicians along the development continuum often wonder about how much to contribute to committee work. This is an important question since future and current LHS+ faculty members often are taxed with additional service demands. Although one must be vigilant not to be unduly burdened by committee work, this form of service can be an important avenue to learn about and be part of the institutional structure, expand networks, gain visibility and credibility, develop and practice governance skills, that open doors and leadership opportunities. In summary, some strategies to make this service stand out towards promotion and tenure involve the strategic and intentional participation in committees, outreach activities in our communities, and seeking to serve official positions within professional organizations.

It is important to note that in disrupting the current standards of promotion and tenure we should be engaging in conversations and action towards challenging colonial ideals in higher education. Higher education has evolved. Furthermore, in the context of academic medicine, our connection to education and health systems demands changes that push forward traditional areas: clinical, research and teaching and add service as an equal pillar. Hence, not small 's' for service, but large 'S'.

In relation to leadership, every aspiring and current faculty member should ask themselves "What leadership role(s) do I want to have in 5 years?" Whether content-based roles (research team leader), structured-based roles (section chief/department head), or group representative, you need to do a gut check to make sure you will be committed to the effort, and then accept or create leadership opportunities with incremental responsibility. Before you accept or develop an opportunity consider who do you want in your team/group, how can participation benefit them (not only the team), what will their questions/concerns be, what resources do we need, who can advise you? Individuals should continuously work on their accountability mechanisms, grow their leadership skills through training and the mentorship of successful leaders, and grow their credibility.

Credibility is supported by three components: trustworthiness (how likely you are to do what you say you will do), expertise (do you know what you need to know and do to accomplish the task), ethical integrity (do you behave in a manner consistent with your stated values, and with moral and ethical principles). Behaviors based in an asset-based model that builds credibility include: (1) do what you say you'll do, (2) honor appointments and be punctual, (3) prepare and be organized, (4) be present and pay attention during meetings, (5) model valuing yourself avoiding self-criticism, (6) being prudent with personal information, (7) be transparent and keep the team informed, (8) honor and acknowledge contributions of others, and (9) use graceful self-promotion [45, 46].

Successful Academic Writing

Academic writing is an often misunderstood and neglected skill that can certainly be developed. Given that writing is often seen as the thing we do when we find a big block of time, get inspired, face a deadline or other external pressure, or wait for everything else and everyone else to be done so we can "move to write", many academics engage in writing binges. Binge writing has disadvantages such longer periods without writing, more time required to warm up or catch up to previous progress, more fatigue and describe writing as grueling rather than enjoyable and have less creativity during their writing.

Empirical research supports the benefit of regular/scheduled writing in which near daily periods of less than 90 min are scheduled and honored as writing time [47].

Constancy with moderation matched with S.M.A.R.T. (small, measurable, achievable, relevant, time-based) writing goals leads to greater satisfaction, sense of accomplishment, greater productivity, and innovation. Additional strategies include dividing your efforts into generating versus editing minimizing perfectionism; writing something else of relevance even if altering the order or if it contributes to a different product; letting experience and past performances predict your realistic goals; defend your writing time within reason; measure your productivity for self-accountability, and assess your quality by inviting review and feedback from fair critics you trust [48].

The latter is particularly important for novice and non-native English speaker writers for whom being part of a peer writing group or formal skills development group can help develop confidence in writing conventions, linguistic knowledge, grammar, vocabulary, and thinking strategies that match academic expression.

Distinct Characteristics of Faculty Development in Puerto Rico

As previously noted throughout the book, Puerto Rico has 4 LCME accredited medical schools, San Juan Bautista School of Medicine, Universidad Central del Caribe School of Medicine, Ponce Health Sciences University School of Medicine, and the University or Puerto Rico School of Medicine. The experience of LHS+ faculty at the four medical schools in Puerto Rico is quite different than LHS+ faculty in the Mainland U.S. The majority of faculty at the four medical schools in PR are LHS+. Thus, socialization, mentoring, and support systems are developed and delivered by and between LHS+ faculty. The faculty development programs at each institution focus more on developing the teaching and research skills needed for retention, promotion, and tenure, and on specialty specific training. The four schools have different systems of assessing the needs of their faculty and, based on those needs and the current educational trends, they design their programs for each academic year. In addition, the fours schools have faculty with expertise, be it masters or Ph.D. degrees in education, educational technologists, and/or training in research and grant writing.

The Student as Teacher model has served a meaningful pathway for the development of skilled LHS+ faculty. Induction into the roles and responsibilities of a faculty member could begin as early as the first year of medical school. The Universidad Central del Caribe School of Medicine (UCCSoM) relies on a two-fold approach to enable the socialization of students into faculty roles. Early in the process faculty mentors identify students who demonstrate potential to become teachers. These students in turn are recommended to serve as classmate's tutors in addition to receive one-to-one advising on effective teaching methodologies. They are also invited to participate in faculty development activities aimed at helping them master best teaching practices. During the student's senior years, they participate in an elective course titled, "The Student as Teacher". This includes a one-to-one experience with a faculty member where the student is expected to demonstrate accomplishment of the course goals by designing educational objectives, a learning experience, and the corresponding assessment of the student learning.

Evaluations of these experiences suggest that effective mentoring plays a key role in supporting the development and strengthening diversity among medical educators. Opportunities to perform as effective teachers, in the safe environment of medical schools and under close guidance of a faculty mentor, reinforces self-reliance and confidence as medical students serve as residents and future faculty. Puerto Rico medical schools' model for medical student development presents a highly effective and meaningful pathway for the development of skilled LHS+ faculty.

In Closing

LHS+ pre-faculty- and faculty development efforts are important to ensure that LHS+ medical students receive optimal training delivered in part by culturally congruent individuals who are themselves successful in their academic careers and inspiring role models to medical students and members of the pre-health pathway, as we seek to address the health needs of LHS+ individualsş in this country. Although multiple examples exist of episodic and localized efforts to support LHS+ faculty development, little evidence exists for a one specific approach to enhance the skills, career success and impact of these faculty or pre-faculty. The opportunity exists to develop a carefully tailored longitudinal program of national scale to advance our ability to support LHS+ faculty through empirically validated interventions. Efforts beyond specific training programs are necessary to comprehensively address socialization and other topics identified as important for LHS+ faculty development [30] and individuals should feel encouraged to grow their developmental networks as they meet their identified needs. This includes finding a good team of mentors, sponsors and champions, as well as addressing cultural needs; develop a career development plan informed by personal values and mission; be

mindful and proactive at career and leadership advancement; be a successful writer of grants and scientific production; and keep committed to serving students and patients importantly supporting those of LHS+ origin.

References

1. Kaplan SE, Raj A, Carr PL, Terrin N, Breeze JL, Freund KM. Race/ethnicity and success in academic medicine: findings from a longitudinal multi-institutional study. Acad Med. 2018;93(4):616–22.
2. U.S. Census Bureau QuickFacts United States. https://www.census.gov/quickfacts/fact/table/US/PST045221. Accessed 10 Jan 2023.
3. AAMC 2022. Table 8. U.S. Medical School Faculty by Gender and Race/Ethnicity, 2021. https://www.aamc.org/media/9711/download. Accessed 10 Jan 2023.
4. AAMC 2022. Table 15: U.S. Medical School Faculty by Gender, Race/Ethnicity, Rank, and Tenure Status, 2021. Source: AAMC Faculty Roster, December 31, 2021 snapshot, as of December 31, 2021. https://www.aamc.org/media/9746/download. Accessed 10 Jan 2023.
5. AACOM. 2016-17 Osteopathic Medical College Faculty by Race/Ethnicity. https://www.aacom.org/docs/default-source/archive-data-and-trends/2016-17-osteopathic-medical-college-faculty-by-race--ethnicity.pdf?sfvrsn=1b12597_10. Accessed 10 Jan 2023.
6. Sánchez JP, Ellis D. Slide 13. Deans of U.S. Osteopathic or Allopathic Medical Schools of LHS+ Identity 2022. LMSA 50th Anniversary Reunion – Planning for the Next 50 Years Virtual Conference. December 3, 2022.
7. Ponjuan L. Recruiting and retaining Latino faculty members: the missing piece to Latino student success. National Education Association; 2011. https://vtechworks.lib.vt.edu/bitstream/handle/10919/84034/RecruitingLatinoFacultyMembers.pdf?sequence=1&isAllowed=y. Accessed 10 Jan 2023.
8. Guerrero JK. Latino Faculty at Research Institutions in the Southwestern United States. Education Resources Information Center, ED 420 261; 1998.
9. Contreras F, Gandara P. Latinas/os in the Ph.D. pipeline: A case of historical and contemporary exclusion. In: Castellanos J, Gloria AM, Kamimura M, editors. The Latina/o pathway to the PhD: Abriendo caminos. Stylus: Sterling, VA; 2006.
10. Rodríguez JE, Campbell KM, Pololi LH. Addressing disparities in academic medicine: what of the minority tax? BMC Med Educ. 2015;15:6.
11. Campbell KM, Rodriguez JE, Brownstein NC, Fisher ZE. Status of tenure among black and Latino faculty in

academic medicine. J Racial Ethn Health Disparities. 2017;4(2):134–9.

12. Sotto-Santiago S. What Gets Lost in the Numbers: A Case Study of the Experiences and Perspectives of Black and Latino Faculty in Academic Medicine (Doctoral Dissertation); 2017. Retrieved from: https://digitalcommons.du.edu/he_doctoral/1/. Accessed 10 Jan 2023.

13. Sotto-Santiago S, Vigil D. Racist nativism: an analysis of Latinx faculty credibility and accent modification program in academic medicine. Int J Qual Stud Educ. 2019, 2021; https://doi.org/10.1080/09518398.2021.1956617.

14. Verdugo RR. Racial stratification and the use of Hispanic faculty as role models. J High Educ. 2003;66(6):669–85.

15. AAMC. Table A-9: Matriculants to U.S. MD-Granting Medical Schools by Race, Selected Combinations of Race/Ethnicity and Gender, 2019–2020 through 2022–2023. https://www.aamc.org/media/6031/download?attachment. Accessed 10 Jan 2023.

16. AACOM. 2021-2022. Osteopathic Medical College Total Enrollment by Gender and Race/Ethnicity. https://www.aacom.org/docs/default-source/data-and-trends/2021-22_tenroll_gender_re_com.pdf?sfvrsn=9b020097_12. Accessed 10 Jan 2023.

17. Yehia BR, Cronholm PF, Wilson N, Palmer SC, Sisson SD, Guilliames CE, Poll-Hunter NI, Sánchez JP. Mentorship and pursuit of academic medicine careers: a mixed methods study of residents from diverse backgrounds. BMC Med Educ. 2014;14:26.

18. Villani J, Mortensen K. Decomposing the gap in satisfaction with provider communication between English- and Spanish-speaking Hispanic patients. J Immigrant Minor Health. 2014;16:195–203.

19. Tierney WG. Organizational socialization in higher education. The J High Educ. 1997;68(1):1–16. Retrieved from http://search.proquest.com/docview/205301259?accountid=7398

20. Figueroa JL, Rodriguez GM. Critical mentoring practices to support diverse students in higher education: Chicana/Latina faculty perspectives. New Dir High Educ. 2015;2015(171):23–32.

21. Núñez AM, Elizondo D. Institutional diversity among four-year Hispanic-serving institutions. In: Hispanic-serving institutions. London: Routledge; 2015. p. 65–81.

22. Turner CSV, González JC. Walking with company! /¡Caminando Acompañados!: Mentoring Latina/o students in higher education. In: Felder PF, St. John EP, editors. Supporting graduate students in the 21st century: implications for policy and practice, Readings on equal education, vol. 27. New York: AMS Press, Inc.; 2014. p. 177–95.

23. Espino MM. Exploring the role of community cultural wealth in graduate school access and persistence for Mexican American PhDs. Am J Educ. 2014;120(4):545–74.

24. Kegan R. In over our heads: the mental demands of modern life. Cambridge: Harvard University Press; 1994.

25. Sánchez JP, Peters L, Lee-Rey E, Strelnick H, Garrison G, Zhang K, Spencer D, Ortega G, Yehia B, Berlin A, Castillo-Page L. Racial and ethnic minority medical students' perceptions of academic medicine careers. Acad Med. 2013;88(9):1299–307.

26. Andriole DA, Yan Y, Jeffe DB. Mediators of racial/ethnic disparities in mentored k award receipt among U.S. medical school graduates. Acad Med. 2017;92(10):1440–8.

27. Flores G, Mendoza FS, DeBaun MR, Fuentes-Afflick E, Jones VF, Mendoza JA, Raphael JL, Wang CJ. Keys to academic success for under-represented minority young investigators: recommendations from the Research in Academic Pediatrics Initiative on Diversity (RAPID) National Advisory Committee. Int J Equity Health. 2019;18(1):93.

28. Hiemstra D, Van Yperen NW. The effects of strength-based versus deficit-based self-regulated learning strategies on students' effort intentions. Motiv Emot. 2015;39(5):656–68.

29. Gillespie KH, Robertson DL. A guide to faculty development. San Francisco, CA: Jossey-Bass; 2010.

30. Sotto-Santiago S, Saelua N, Tuitt F. All faculty matter: the continued search for culturally relevant practices in faculty development. J Faculty Dev. 2019;33(3):83–93.

31. Rodriguez JE, Campbell K, Fogarty JP, Williams RL. Underrepresented minority faculty in academic medicine: a systematic review of URM faculty development. Fam Med. 2014;46(2):100–4.

32. Page KR, Castillo-Page L, Wright SM. Faculty diversity programs in U.S. medical schools and characteristics associated with higher faculty diversity. Acad Med. 2011;86(10):1221–8.

33. Guevara JP, Adanga E, Avakame E, Carthon MB. Minority faculty development programs and underrepresented minority faculty representation at US medical schools. JAMA. 2013;310(21):2297–304.

34. Soto-Greene ML, Sanchez J, Churrango J, Salas-Lopez D. Latino faculty development in U.S. medical schools: a Hispanic center of excellence perspective. J Hisp High Educ. 2005;4(4):366–76.

35. UC San Diego, Health Sciences, Hispanic Center of Excellence. https://medschool.ucsd.edu/vchs/faculty-academics/faculty-affairs/development/hcoe/Pages/default.aspx. Accessed 10 Jan 2023.

36. Hispanic Association of Colleges and Universities. https://www.hacu.net/hacu/default.asp. Accessed 10 Jan 2023.

37. American Association of Hispanics in Higher Education Inc. https://www.aahhe.org/. Accessed 10 Jan 2023.

38. Beech BM, Calles-Escandon J, Bell RA. Mentoring programs for minoritized minority faculty in academic medical centers: a systematic review of the literature. Acad Med. 2013;88(4):541–9.

39. Pololi L, Cooper LA, Carr P. Race, disadvantage and faculty experiences in academic medicine. J General Intern Med. 2010;25(12):1363–9. https://doi.org/10.1007/s11606-010-1478-7.

40. Sorkness C, Pfund C, Ofili E, Okuyemi K, Vishwanatha J. A new approach to mentoring for research careers: training in the national research mentoring network. BMC Proc. 2017;11(Suppl. 12):14.

41. Sotto-Santiago S. A new framework for cross-culturally relevant mentoring in higher education. Paper presented at the Conference on Academic Research in Education, UNLV, Las Vegas, NV; 2018.

42. Torres V, Hernández E, Martínez S. Understanding the Latinx experience: Developmental and contextual influences. Sterling, VA: Stylus Publishing, LLC.; 2019.

43. Jackson VP. Time management: a realistic approach. J Am Coll Radiol. 2009;6(6):434–6.

44. Lane PH. The Promotion Game: Your Guide to Success in Academic Medicine; 2014. ISBN: 9781631922909.

45. Allgeier S. The personal credibility factor: how to get it, keep it, and get it back (If You've Lost It). Upper Saddle River, NJ: FT Press; 2009.

46. Huber K, Huber J, Zaidi Z. Graceful self-promotion: the impact of a short faculty development session. MedEdPublish. 2020;9(1):24. https://doi.org/10.15694/mep.2020.000024.1.

47. Boice R. Professors as writers: a self-help guide to productive writing. Stillwater, OK: New Forums; 1990. p. 80.

48. Gopalakrishnan K. The productive academic writer: an easy-to-read guide to low-stress prolific writing. Transdependenz LLC, USA; 2015

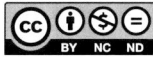

The Role of Offices of Diversity, Equity & Inclusion to the LHS+ Community

14

Francisco Lucio and David Acosta

Introduction

Academic health science centers (AHSCs) in the United States (U.S.) are positioned as leaders in health professions education, clinical care and biomedical health science research. AHSCs often comprise a medical school, other health professions programs (e.g. pharmacy, nursing, physician assistant, etc.), teaching hospital(s), and faculty heavily involved in biomedical, clinical, and medical education research [1]. Today, there are more than 150 allopathic medical schools and 36 osteopathic medical schools accredited in the U.S. as part of academic medicine [2, 3]. Many, but not all, of these institutions house an ODEI or equivalent (with alternative names including offices of diversity affairs, multicultural affairs, or minority affairs, among others). Historically, the Perelman School of Medicine at the University of Pennsylvania established the first office of minority affairs in 1968 to recruit and retain minority students [4]. The function of minority affairs offices began with—and, in large part, continues to be—the recruitment and retention of students underrepresented in medicine (UIM),

including LHS+ students. As described in earlier chapters, the representation of LHS+ medical students, about 11.3% in 2019, among all those enrolled in allopathic medical schools at the time of this chapter's writing [5], is sorely inadequate relative to the overall U.S. LHS+ population of ~18% [6]. Given this gap, many AHSCs in recent years have expanded the role of the ODEI beyond health professions trainee recruitment and retention to include more robust functions when working with the LHS+ community. These functions include, but are not limited to: sustaining comprehensive community engagement, assisting in cultural brokerage between the AHSC and the local LHS+ community, and creating strong partnerships in education and research with the LHS+ community.

Social Responsibility to Serve the LHS+ Community

AHSCs and ODEIs have a social responsibility to serve the LHS+ population that rises to the level of a social contract—that is, "social accountability [that] involves a commitment to respond as best as possible to the priority health needs of citizens and society." [7] This social responsibility should be reflected in the values and mission of each AHSC and ODEI and through the principles of health equity to address the unique language, cultures, socio-political history, and

F. Lucio (✉)
Obstetrics and Gynecology, University of Arizona College of Medicine-Phoenix, Phoenix, AZ, USA
e-mail: flucio@arizona.edu

D. Acosta
Association of American Medical Colleges, Washington, DC, USA

© The Author(s) 2024
J. P. Sánchez, D. Rodriguez (eds.), *Latino, Hispanic, or of Spanish Origin+ Identified Student Leaders in Medicine*, Sustainable Development Goals Series, https://doi.org/10.1007/978-3-031-35020-7_14

health disparities of the communities served by a given institution. To be clear, this expectation is not mutually exclusive to other marginalized populations, but merely the focus of this book.

LHS+ individuals are the largest racial-ethnic minority group in the U.S. and make up nearly half of all non-White people [6]. The distribution of LHS+ individuals is geographically widespread with particularly high densities in the West, Southwest, Northeast, and some parts of the South—most notably, Texas and Florida (see Fig. 14.1).

The projected increase of the LHS+ population in 2050 to nearly 100 million, representing 26% of the U.S. population (see Fig. 14.2), underscores the acute need for and special focus on AHSCs to ensure that the LHS+ population receives appropriate care and engagement. ODEIs at AHSCs are critical players in fulfilling this obligation, as they often serve as conduits between AHSCs and LHS+ communities, providing the latter with tailored services geared at improving health outcomes.

Since ODEIs reside within AHSCs, the core values of the institution should guide and shape the mission and vision for these offices. For example, at the University of Arizona College of Medicine—Phoenix, the college articulates "diversity" specifically as one of its core values [8]. This fundamental value is carried through to the mission of the ODEI:

> Through Inclusive Excellence, the University of Arizona College of Medicine—Phoenix is committed to and champions diversity and inclusion as core values central to its mission. Inclusive Excellence is the intentional driver of diversity and inclusion, which harnesses the differences, talents and unique qualities of all individuals at the College of Medicine—Phoenix. Inclusive Excellence engages the individual and system in practices that advance diversity in all that we do. Inclusive Excellence is inextricably linked to our pursuit of excellence in our research, clinical and educational missions to meet the needs of the students, faculty, residents, fellows, staff and the communities we serve.
>
> Moreover, through Inclusive Excellence and our tripartite missions, the College of Medicine—Phoenix is committed to mitigating health disparities, especially for marginalized groups and vulnerable populations, in order to improve community health outcomes, particularly in rural, inner-city and medically underserved areas [9].

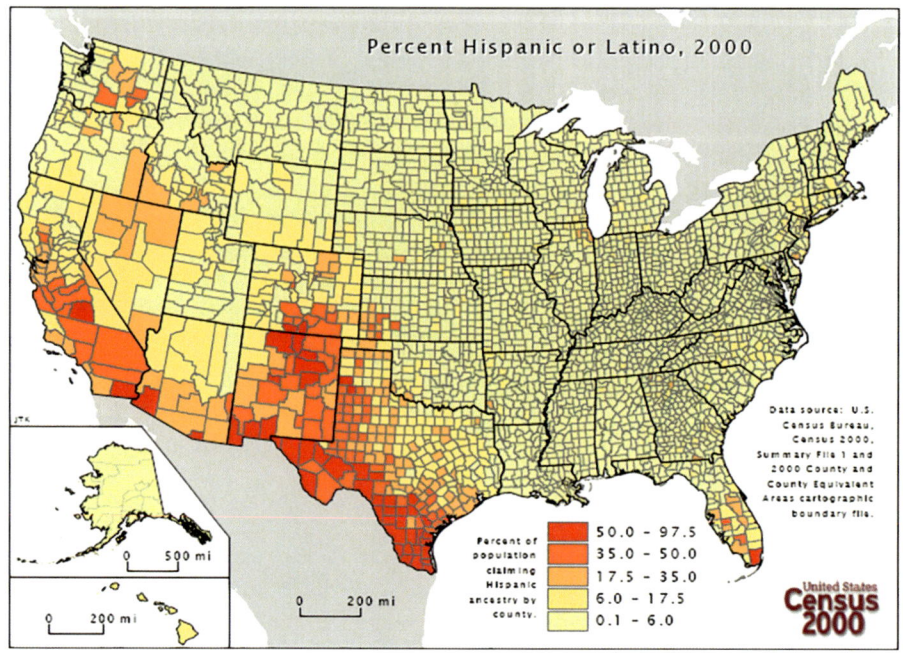

Fig. 14.1 Hispanic or Latino Population as a Percent of Total Population by County

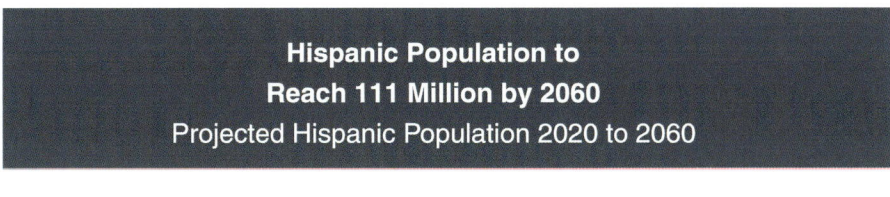

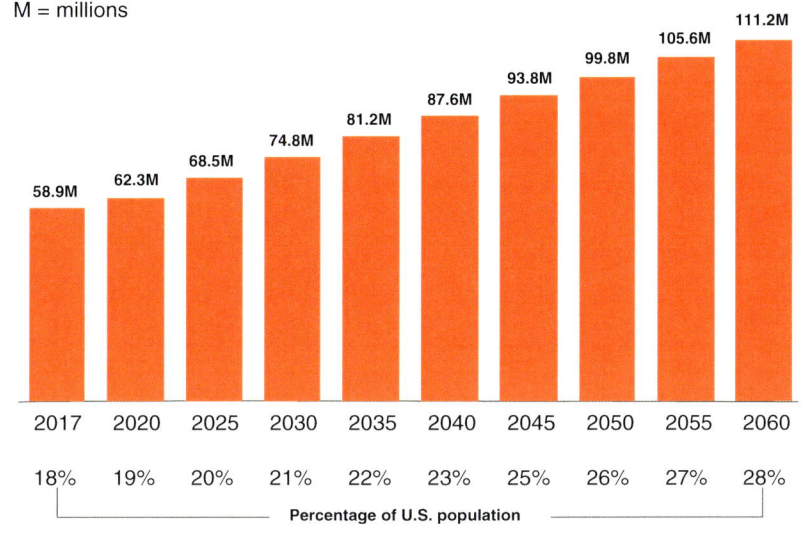

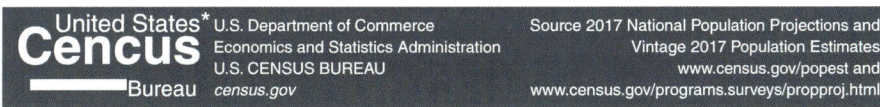

Fig. 14.2 Projected Hispanic Population 2020 to 2060

Some AHSCs may not explicitly state enumerated values but rely on guiding principles in their mission statements that connect to notions of excellence in the educational, clinical, research, and community engagement domains. The commitment to serving society and the community via some, or all, of the aforementioned domains creates an expressed social obligation for an AHSCs to care for the health and well-being of the population inclusive of the LHS+ community. Principles of health equity further focus this institutional responsibility to address the unique social determinants of health (SDOH) and associated health inequities faced by the LHS+ community to help the latter achieve its highest health potential.

Given the above, ODEIs have expanded their focus to help address the SDOH that lead to poorer health outcomes and contribute to health disparities for marginalized, disenfranchised and/or vulnerable communities. The LHS+ community—not being immune to the impacts of detrimental SDOH—unfortunately suffers from many health disparities. When compared to non-Hispanic Whites, for example, Hispanics are 23% more likely to be obese, die at a 50% higher rate from diabetes, and are 24% more likely to have uncontrolled high blood pressure [10]. Health disparities that particularly affect LHS+ patients can be attributed to a multitude of factors. As discussed in previous chapters, unique detriments to LHS+ health include insufficient attempts or resources to provide care in Spanish, a scarce LHS+ physician workforce, lack of health insurance coverage (especially for undocumented immigrants or mixed-status families), lack of culturally appropriate or sensitive care, and structural and societal inequities, among other factors [11]. While the faculty, staff, students, and other individuals affiliated with ODEIs strive to ameliorate the factors contributing to diminished health of medically underserved communities in their vicinity, ODEIs cannot tackle this challenge alone. Rather, to best serve a community in need, ODEIs must leverage other entities within and beyond their respective AHSCs—including members of the target community itself—to enact a multicomponent engagement strategy. This is discussed in greater detail below.

The Modern Role of Offices of Diversity, Equity and Inclusion

In the years preceding this chapter's writing, it has become increasingly common for ODEIs to serve many functions and roles both within and outside their respective institutions. ODEIs not only focus on the four standard mission areas of AHSCs—clinical care, medical education, research and community engagement—as pertaining to diversity, inclusion, and health equity efforts, but ODEIs also conduct work that overlaps with other domains of medical education and AHSC administration (see Fig. 14.3). To represent and amplify the voices of LHS+ students, residents, faculty, staff, patients, and communities, ODEIs must collaborate and synergize with other institutional offices. While the spe-

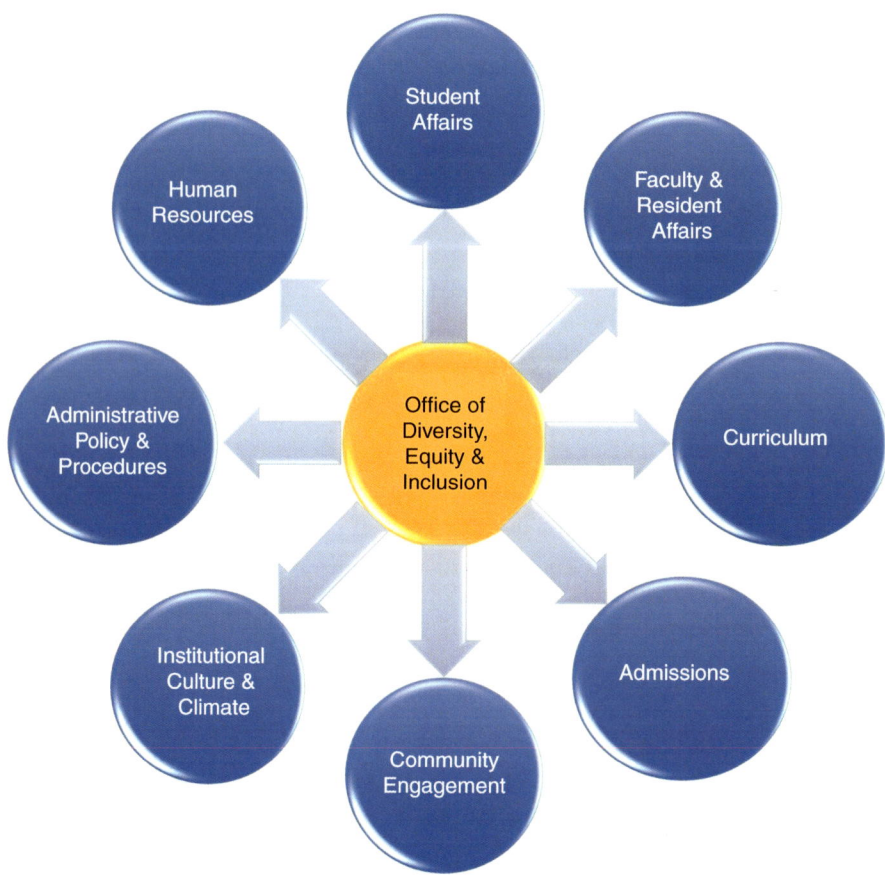

Fig. 14.3 Parts & Partners of Offices of Diversity, Equity and Inclusion

cific structure, charge, and duties of an ODEI may vary from one AHSC to another, the sections that follow will discuss general practices employed by and opportunities available to ODEI staff to promote the success of UIM groups.

Student Affairs

ODEI staff work closely and collaboratively with the staff of Student Affairs offices. While this work has been described earlier in this book, in general, ODEI officers and directors often serve as:

- Partners in addressing the needs of the LHS+ students, helping the latter navigate student life and personal concerns and issues, aspects of the institutional and local community, career choices in medicine, selection of elective rotations, and residency choice;
- Student advocates on committees for student evaluation and progress (CSEP) and commonly work with the student affairs dean on best strategies to support students;
  - ODEI officers often contribute their unique perspectives to the discussions about the student with other CSEP members when discussing external factors (cultural, traditions, beliefs) that have impacted the student's performance that are unfamiliar to most non-minority CSEP faculty.
- Writers of students' letters of recommendation for scholarship opportunities, grants, committee/student organization membership, and residency;
- Sponsors, advisors, and/or institutional representatives for UIM medical student organizations, including the Latino Medical Student Association (LMSA);
- Sponsors of student-run free clinics; and
- Liaisons between students, faculty, and communities external to the institution.
  - ODEIs often serve as the 'connectors' and trusted faculty and community liaisons to local racial-ethnic communities.

Faculty and Resident Affairs

ODEI staff work closely and collaboratively with the staff of Faculty Affairs offices, as well as staff affiliated with Graduate Medical Education (GME). While the work and impact of Faculty Affairs and GME offices have been discussed in previous chapters, ODEI officers/directors often serve as:

- Partners in addressing the needs of the LHS+ residents, fellows, and faculty members;
  - Such needs include, but are not limited to: helping these individuals navigate life in their current role(s), personal concerns or issues,, the healthcare system, their institution, their local community (especially the LHS+ community), career advice, and efforts to transform their activities into academic credit for appointment, promotion, and potential funding.
- Writers of letters of recommendation for grant opportunities, promotion, and internal and/or external leadership positions;
- Sponsors for advisory committees for UIM faculty and residents;
- Liaisons between faculty and to communities external to the institution;
  - ODEIs often serve as the 'connectors' and trusted faculty and community liaisons to local racial-ethnic communities.
- Connectors to mentorship opportunities and sponsorship opportunities;
- Connectors to precepting opportunities, such as student-run free clinics;
- Sources of funding for professional development opportunities, such as the AAMC Minority Faculty Leadership Seminar, and AAMC Women in Medicine Early and Mid-Career Leadership Seminars;
- Connectors to opportunities for teaching on the topics of health disparities, SDOH, and/or health equity;
- Members of and equity advisors for faculty search committees;
- Sponsors of second-look events for the recruitment of residents, especially those from UIM groups; and

- Content experts to assist Assistant, Associate, and Vice Deans of GME in meeting ACGME Core Requirements on diversity and inclusion, as well as ACGME's CLER Pathways to Excellence — specifically Pathways 5 and 6 regarding health disparities.

Curriculum

ODEIs can play important roles by engaging in, facilitating, and promoting education with the LHS+ community. Education can be in the form of informative presentations and topics specifically targeting the LHS+ community. Colloquially referred to as " mini-medical school," sessions that seek to raise awareness of type 2 diabetes, stress the importance of cancer screenings, and educate patients on heart disease—among other examples—have been offered in Spanish at meeting spaces frequented by the local LHS+ community. Moreover, ODEIs can play a role in assisting patient care facilities within the health system by (1) ensuring that patient education handouts and other materials are accessible in Spanish; (2) identifying Spanish-speaking experts at various levels and in various areas of medical practice at the institution; and (3) encouraging educational presentations and workshops to be given in Spanish. Not uncommonly, ODEIs deploy dedicated promotors—LHS+ community health workers—to develop and disseminate curricular content; this strategy may prove more effective in building trust and communicating with local LHS+ communities [12].

Ultimately, the success of educational initiatives and strategies developed by AHSCs for local LHS+ communities depends on collaboration with and guidance from trusted leaders within those communities [13]. Such leaders may be ministers or faith leaders, K-12 grade school teachers or administrators, civic leaders, or other prominent figures. For a given community, such individuals provide key insights into that community's historical and ongoing traumas or challenges; select examples include displacement of LHS+ community members through urban development projects, medical malfeasance or neglect of LHS+

community members, and troubled or harmful outreach efforts by an AHSC, among others. ODEIs are uniquely positioned within AHSCs to identify, connect with, and work alongside community leaders to understand any barriers to collaboration that may exist between the AHSC and the LHS+ community it serves. This work, often led by ODEI staff but requiring full commitment from the AHSC at large, is critical in cases where the AHSC seeks to establish a new relationship with its surrounding communities or rebuild previously existing but currently strained relationships.

Opportunities also exist for ODEIs to be involved in curriculum development. Examples of educational initiatives to which ODEIs contribute include, but are not limited to, the following:

- *Curricular pathways/tracks:* These programs usually involve structured course work that focus on LHS+ communities and their health, health inequities, health disparities, and SDOH. The purpose of these pathway/track programs is to better prepare medical students to provide comprehensive, culturally, and linguistically competent patient care and understand the importance of population health and population health management. Hispanic Centers of Excellence are a good resource, as well as the University of Washington's Latinx Health Pathway [14];
- *Courses on LHS+ health disparities:* These are common electives found in many medical schools that provide a substantial amount of health care to LHS+ communities. This is an opportunity to promote community-based participatory curriculum development that engages members of the LHS+ community to participate as partners in developing curricula that address LHS+ health and health disparities and serve as course instructors and panelists [15];
- *Student-run free clinics:* Some AHSCs leverage the expertise and community connections of ODEIs to establish and/or maintain clinics that provide free or heavily subsidized healthcare to indigent patients, often including undocumented immigrants or refugees of LHS+ descent; and

- *Medical Spanish courses:* Aimed at improving communication between healthcare providers and Spanish-speaking patients with non-English language preference, medical Spanish courses may achieve greater impact and longevity when implemented with input and assistance from ODEIs.

Admissions

ODEI staff work closely and collaboratively with the staff of undergraduate medical education admissions offices. In this capacity, ODEI officers/directors often serve as:

- Members (both voting and non-voting) of admissions committees;
- Application screeners and interviewers;
- Coordinators of outreach and recruitment efforts;
  - Commonly, ODEIs sponsor health career fairs that specifically target LHS+ and other UIM students in middle school, high school, and college.
- Designers, developers, and executioners of pipeline programming that specifically target LHS+ students in middle school, high school, and/or college interested in health careers;
- Coordinators of second look programs;
- Institutional ambassadors for the purpose of providing follow-up to prospective and admitted students; and
  - ODEI staff commonly reach out to LHS+ students on the admission's waitlist keeping the connection present and instilling patience and hope. That connection is sustained with both the students that have been accepted as well as those that have not been accepted.
- Presenters and contributors to onboarding at orientation.
  - ODEI are often asked to provide cultural competency training to all students, and frequently provide sessions for LHS+ students on how best to navigate the internal and external community.

Community Engagement

Community engagement describes the collaboration of institutions and their broader community for the mutual exchange of knowledge and resources rooted in partnership and reciprocity [16]. In their 2017 article, Ahmed et al. offer a paradigm for community engagement that has applicability for ODEIs. Their model separates community engagement into five distinct domains: (1) Community Outreach and Community Service; (2) Education; (3) Clinical Care; (4) Research; and (5) Policy and Advocacy. Each ODEI partakes in community engagement across these domains and others to varying degrees depending on its office structure, personnel capacity, financial resources, and expertise.

Community Outreach and Community Service

Community outreach and community service activities are often encouraged for medical students, faculty, residents and staff. The Liaison Committee on Medical Education (LCME), which sets accreditation standards for allopathic medical schools in the U.S. and Canada, requires "the faculty of a medical school [to] ensure that the medical education program provides sufficient opportunities for, encourages and supports medical student participation in service-learning and community service activities." [17] Community outreach refers to volunteer work that is related to an individual's professional appointment, such as serving on an organizational board. In contrast, community service refers to service that is unrelated to a professional appointment, such as volunteering to tutor students in an after-school program or helping to fundraise for a local charity. ODEIs are positioned to facilitate community service and outreach benefiting the LHS+ community through a number of avenues:

1. Keeping a running inventory of community service and community outreach opportunities that positively impact the LHS+ commu-

nity and making this available via newsletters, the college website, and social media outlets;

2. Connecting and recommending faculty, staff, and/or students to volunteer and leadership roles within organizations engaged in community outreach, acknowledging that some such organizations may make leadership opportunities available by invitation only; and

3. Bringing LHS+ community members into AHSCs as part of the mutual and bi-directional spirit of community engagement. In doing so, an ODEI can offer numerous benefits to LHS+ individuals, organizations, and communities at large by referring local candidates for employment at the AHSC, involving business executives in new and ongoing hospital advisory committees, and even enabling community members to contribute to the future physician workforce through a voting role on the medical school's admissions committee.

Assessments and Improvements of Institutional Culture and Climate

ODEIs are often engaged in assessments of the culture and climate of their respective institutions, or of departments and programs within the institution. Involvement of ODEIs in such efforts is critical for achieving a thorough evaluation of the learning or workforce environment and its inclusivity. As part of these efforts, ODEIs commonly collaborate with Human Resources departments to perform the assessment and monitor results and outcomes. Moreover, ODEIs use data derived from such assessments to drive institutional change to achieve inclusive environments. In partnering with their institutions' organizational development and human resource departments, ODEIs develop and/or deliver trainings and other educational programs designed to mitigate specific issues that threaten the learning and workplace environments. Examples of such programs include workshops on addressing microaggressions, implicit bias, mistreatment, abrasive behaviors (such bullying), sexual/gender harassment, and racial/ethnic discrimination.

Policy & Advocacy

Many AHSCs have offices of government affairs that directly engage with legislators and other policymakers and may discourage or prohibit other institutional offices from participating in certain policy and advocacy activities. However, ODEIs still have opportunities to influence institutional, local, and national policymaking. As discussed above, ODEIs play a vital role in ensuring that their respective institutions pursue policies and practices that advance racial/ethnic justice for all those served by the institution. In line with this charge, ODEI leadership may collaborate with the institution's office of governmental affairs and relations, as well as the institution's legal counsel and human resources department as needed, to participate in advocacy efforts geared at improving the health, wellbeing, and advancement of LHS+ communities. Such collaborations are evident in amicus briefs submitted to the U.S. Supreme Court regarding ongoing legal evaluations of race-conscious admissions in higher education. Moreover, through the relationships the office develops with its local LHS+ communities, an ODEI can provide critical information and understanding of pertinent issues that impact those communities. By engaging with internal entities and with external groups, such as the National Hispanic Medical Association, the Hispanic Chamber of Commerce, the Hispanic National Bar Association, local medical societies, and local Hispanic advocacy groups, ODEIs may provide additional expertise or perspectives that may enhance these groups' policy and advocacy agendas. Lastly, as a complementary strategy, ODEIs can contribute to advocacy efforts by financially supporting medical students to attend advocacy trainings, conferences, or similar initiatives, such as the LMSA National Policy Summit or other local advocacy activities.

Summary

Through community outreach and service, education, clinical care, research and policy and advocacy engagement activities, ODEIs can be seminal incubators of innovation, bridge-builders, and cultural brokers between academic medical institutions and the LHS+ community. These recommendations, however, should not be interpreted to mean that ODEIs are the sole unit of the AHSC responsible for advancing the health of the LHS+ community. On the contrary, the AAMC recommends the practice of diversity, inclusion excellence and equity mindedness, which requires all individuals and offices of the academic institution to advance these principles that lead to true institutional excellence [18].

Contributions of ODEIs to Other Mission-Related Domains of AHSCs

Clinical Care & Education

While direct clinical care will typically not be provided by the ODEI itself, there may be opportunities for the office to be involved with aspects of clinical care directed at the LHS+ community. The authors acknowledge that members of ODEI leadership, such as the director, Assistant Dean, Associate Dean, or equivalent, may be physicians or other healthcare professionals; these individuals' clinical appointment may require them to provide patient care on a part-time basis. However, as an office, ODEIs may be involved in the development and implementation of tailored communication strategies and cross-promotion of clinical information material to broaden the reach of AHSCs to the LHS+ community. Additionally, ODEIs may serve as activators to create and/or bolster medical Spanish offerings for trainees and faculty at AHSCs. For example, the University of Cincinnati College of Medicine created a Medical Spanish/Latino Health elective that is sponsored and operated by the College's ODEI. This longitudinal curriculum offers participants language instruction, simulated patient encounters, didactic sessions covering topics related to healthcare in LHS+ communities, and service-learning opportunities, culminating in course credit [19]. Based on a key 2015 survey enacted by scholars affiliated with LMSA, programs like the University of Cincinnati elective

remain rare. While 66% of surveyed medical schools actively provided some form of medical Spanish curriculum, most curricula were "not eligible for course credit" and were challenged by "lack of time in students' schedules… and a lack of financial resources." Thus, ODEIs have the opportunity to support and advocate for the incorporation of medical Spanish elements into medical school curricula in order for AHSCs to provide more culturally and linguistically appropriate clinical care [20].

Research

Although more and more medical research is focusing on the LHS+ community, there remains a dearth of research in many areas that address LHS+ health and health disparities. To address this gap, many ODEIs conduct their own research projects, collaborate on research projects, and/or consult with other departments and investigators to access diverse groups or to improve research projects targeting diverse groups. Moreover, the ODEI may leverage opportunities to expand ongoing research projects, improve research methodologies and data collection, and inspire new and more refined studies. For example, LHS+ individuals are often grouped together in research studies. LHS+ individuals constitute a heterogeneous group of a multitude of nationalities from various Latin American countries. Researchers may not always differentiate amongst these groups and, in doing so, may miss opportunities to distinguish important differences [21]. Moreover, there are many barriers related to participation of LHS+ individuals in research projects that may deter a focus on LHS+ communities. Some challenges include language barriers, patients' potential mistrust of healthcare institutions and providers (often related to the belief that experimentation occurs during health care visits), competing demands (such as conflicts with child care and work), stigma (as in cases of HIV positivity, mental health issues, etc.), and concerns related to immigration status (as undocumented individuals may fear deportation), among others [22]. Here lies an opportunity for ODEIs to help mitigate some of these issues, by serving as liaisons and partners on research projects to build trust, cultural awareness, unconscious bias training, cross-cultural communication skills, and cross-cultural confrontation/negotiation skills to better recruit and retain research participants. Moreover, utilizing and enabling others to engage in community-based participatory research can prove highly beneficial. Community-based participatory research elements involve:

- Fostering trusting relationships with community partners;
- Building on strengths and resources within the community;
- Promoting co-learning and capacity building among all partners;
- Utilizing equitable processes and procedures;
- Using cyclic and iterative processes to develop partnerships and build the research process;
- Disseminating results to all partners;
- Involving key stakeholders in all aspects of the research process from the outset; and
- Pursuing ongoing assessment and improvement of the partnership [23].

Engaging the LHS+ community through a community-based participatory framework will allow the AHSC to begin dialogue with and gain input from the LHS+ community about the specific health-related concerns the latter wants investigated. ODEIs can help orchestrate this valuable shift to improve research participation and research outcomes for the LHS+ community.

Collaboration with LMSA and other LHS+ Associations

ODEIs are a primary collaborator with LMSA at the institutional, regional, and national levels. Support of LMSA members and chapters may include recruiting prospective trainees at LMSA conferences, as well as funding students to attend such meetings for their professional development. At many U.S. AHSCs, ODEI leaders and staff members serve as formal advisors for LMSA chapters and/or work closely with LMSA chapters to support and advise students throughout medical training. There are several critical avenues for ODEI involvement in LMSA student chapters, including:

- Financial and logistical support for events, activities, and professional conference attendance;
- Advising on curricular and extra-curricular matters, including navigating the institutional culture;
- Advocacy on behalf of student interests to institutional leaders and the broader community;
- Psychosocial support or informal counseling to address the academic and non-academic challenges of medical school;
- Direct mentorship of students and/or creation/maintenance of a formal mentorship program;.
- Sponsorship of students to make opportunities accessible to students and allow them to further build their professional networks;
- Provision of nominations and letters of recommendation for scholarships and awards; and
- Service as a professional resource for students to use when lodging complaints related to mistreatment, discrimination, or bias.

Moreover, efforts by an ODEI to cultivate a network of external organizational partners serves the interests of the institution and its trainees. ODEIs may support local and national LHS+ professional associations, such as the National Hispanic Medical Association (NHMA), through opportunities for involvement in institutional initiatives, financial contributions, and in-kind support; doing so opens a mutual support system that grants access to potential mentors and advocates for medical trainees while encouraging the next generation of LHS+ physicians to become mentors and advocates for those behind them.

Planning Ahead for 2050

It is difficult to predict what healthcare and healthcare delivery will be like in 2050; however, we know that the needs of those receiving care will strongly influence the ways in which AHSCs and affiliated organizations will transform medical education, as well as the strategies such entities will employ to develop the healthcare workforce needed to address healthcare needs in a continually evolving society. Demographic projections from the U.S. Census Bureau, the Pew Research Center, and other groups clearly and consistently show that the U.S. LHS+ population will continue to grow. By 2050, LHS+ individuals may constitute 100 million individuals, comprising the majority racial/ethnic group in multiple U.S. states. How will the nation respond to the needs of this growing demographic? What will be the role of ODEI officers and directors? How will this role need to change?

Already, we are seeing forecasts of future healthcare trends that we must prepare for today. Artificial intelligence will be a mainstay, given the amount of 'big data' that we are accumulating with the rapid changes in medicine and science. Advanced technology will change the way that healthcare will be delivered. We have already seen the impact that telemedicine has had during the COVID-19 pandemic. Expertise in precision medicine continues to grow at a rapid pace and is predicted to change many of our diagnostic and treatment trends. The rising cost of healthcare will be unprecedented if we continue at the same pace that we are at today.

How will these trends impact LHS+ communities? How will these communities respond to such changes in healthcare? How can we be assured that artificial intelligence will assist in reducing or eliminating health disparities and inequities faced by the LHS+ population? Will every LHS+ patient have access to telemedicine? How will telemedicine guarantee culturally and linguistically competent care? In a world in which vulnerable populations and their suffering often remain invisible, and in which such communities harbor mistrust of the U.S. healthcare system, how will precision medicine be received by LHS+ communities? Will these communities have access to affordable and excellent precision medicine? Will the future bring universal health care coverage so that all LHS+ communities can achieve health equity?

There are no easy answers to any of these questions. But we, as ODEI officers, must begin to contemplate the future in order to better define our roles in the decades leading up to and beyond 2050. We cannot afford to wait to address the future. We need to begin thinking about what skillsets future ODEI directors and officers will need to better serve our faculty, staff, trainees, and stakeholders. At the same time, we need to be at the table with other medical educators and participate in the discussion of what additional skills our LHS+ medical students—and all medical students—will need to be successful as future physicians serving all demographics of our society. We need to be at the table with medical administrators and leaders and participate in the discussion of how healthcare and healthcare delivery must change to serve our new society's healthcare needs. Lastly, we need to engage the next generation of students and invite them to the table as well; as future medical professionals and academic faculty members, students have an extraordinary capacity to help institutional leaders keep the right focus looking forward and to drive us toward solutions. Although the means by which care is delivered to the LHS+ community will change, the paramount social obligation to provide the best care will remain steadfast for AHSCs and their ODEIs.

Personal Narratives:

- Francisco Lucio, JD | Associate Dean, Equity, Diversity and Inclusion
- The University of Arizona College of Medicine - Phoenix | LMSA FPAC Deputy Director

My mother immigrated to the United States from El Rodeo de San Antonio, a small rural town in Michoacan, Mexico. My father was born in Donna, Texas, but my paternal grandparents had roots in Matehuala, San Luis Potosi, Mexico. I was born and raised in Salinas, California, a migrant farm working community known as the "Lettuce Capital of the World." As social and structural factors would have it, both my parents were farm workers. My father did the dangerous work of spraying pesticides in the fields and my mother the back-breaking harvesting and packaging of lettuce. Growing up in a family and community of farm workers, I was privileged to have early exposure to the power of activism and workers organizing for fair wages and improved work-safety measures. Some of my earliest memories were attending United Farm Workers (UFW) rallies and seeing a sea of red from hundreds of farm workers demonstrating peacefully—but powerfully—for change. This grassroots and collective action left an indelible impression on me.

The pursuit for equity and justice led me to study political science at San Diego State University as a first-generation college student. While in San Diego, I had the opportunity to volunteer at a non-profit organization, Latino Health Matters, that engaged in improving the health of the Latino community as both local and transnational issues. Growing up with a father diagnosed with type 2 diabetes, along with other family members on dialysis due to complications from diabetes, I was keenly interested in health and how these outcomes were preventable. My studies, however, took me down a path to law school. After teaching middle school English as a Second Language for a year, I left the sunny coast of California and headed to New York City where I studied at St. John's University School of Law. Similar to the dearth of diversity in medical school, I was one of only two Mexican students in the school and without a faculty mentor from a similar background. Fortunately, there was the Latin American Law Students Association (LALSA) that was a supportive resource.

After graduating law school, I was drawn to use my legal training and background in education toward working with students. I cut my teeth in health care at the Manhattan Staten Island Area Health Education Center where I directed pipeline programs for underrepresented youth including many Latino students, advocated for health workforce policy reform to be more inclusive of underrepresented in medicine individuals, and gained a deeper understanding of health disparity issues afflicting the Latino and other communities. Eventually, I made my way to New York University School of Medicine (NYU SOM) where I was the

director in the office of diversity affairs. While at NYU SOM, I helped support students to attend and participate in LMSA activities and events.

In 2017, I became the inaugural Associate Dean of Diversity and Inclusion at the University of Arizona College of Medicine—Phoenix. In my years at the college, I helped create a culture of inclusive excellence and led important diversity initiatives for faculty, students, and staff that resulted in the Higher Education Excellence in Diversity (HEED) award in 2019. Many of these activities targeted the Latino community. I continued to support LMSA students through conference sponsorships, as well as scholarship and award nominations. In 2017, we hosted the LMSA Western Region Executive Board Leadership Retreat, where I gave a talk on integrating diversity and inclusion topics into the medical school curriculum. The following year, I had the privilege to begin serving on the LMSA National Faculty/Physician Advisory Board. And, in 2019, I was honored with the LMSA Regional Faculty Advisor Award. LMSA makes important impacts for Latino health issues that is in tune with my early-instilled drive to advance equity for marginalized and disenfranchised groups. I look forward to continued engagement and support of the organization.

David A. Acosta, MD | Chief Diversity and
   Inclusion Officer
Association of American Medical Colleges
   (AAMC) | LMSA Faculty Advisor, University
   of Washington School of Medicine LMSA
   Chapter (2010–2013) LMSA Faculty Advisor,
   University of California Davis School of
   Medicine LMSA Chapter (2013–2017)

Immediately following my family practice residency training, I was hired by Northeastern Rural Health Clinics, Inc. as one of the medical directors of a federally qualified health center (FQHC) system made up of three community health clinics (CHC) located in northeastern California (two of which were National Health Service Corp sites). The FQHC served a number of rural medically underserved communities that included a large migrant farmworker population and two American

Indian tribes (Northern Paiute and Maidu). My entry into academia was through the clinical educator pathway, where my colleagues and I served as clinical preceptors for the University of California Davis Department of Family and Community Medicine. Our CHC served as a clinical rotation site for family medicine for residents, medical/nursing/physician assistant students that had a major interest in serving rural underserved communities. After 8 years of service and teaching at the FQHC, I made the decision to follow my newly found passion as a medical educator and joined the faculty at the Tacoma Family Medicine (TFM) Residency Program, an affiliate of the University of Washington School of Medicine, Department of Family Medicine. At TFM, I was responsible for the development of curriculum in rural health, obstetrics, health care maintenance, procedural medicine, and health disparities. The residency was located in the heart of an underserved inner-city community that had a large population mix of African American/Black, Latinx, and Vietnamese patients. Our clinic functioned much like a CHC, so I felt right at home. There, I served as medical director of the residents/faculty clinic and was soon promoted to associate residency program director. After 2 years, I had the honor of developing the first rural medicine fellowship program in the U.S. for post-residency graduates that desired further training in rural family practice. This led to the development of a high-risk obstetrical clinic that served a large Hispanic population where the fellows worked. Speaking Spanish was a requirement for our fellows. I ultimately became residency director. After 13 years of service at TFM, I was recruited to the main campus at the University of Washington (UW) in Seattle to serve as the inaugural associate dean of multicultural affairs. It was there that I was first introduced to LMSA by our LHS+ medical students. The UW did not have a LMSA chapter when I arrived and, together with the medical students, we formed the inaugural chapter. I served as faculty advisor during my tenure at the UW and became the inaugural chief diversity officer. After 10 years of service, I was recruited to the University of California Davis School of Medicine, where I served as chief diversity officer and associate vice chancellor of equity, diversity and inclusion. I was honored to be asked to serve as the LMSA faculty advisor when I arrived and served in that capacity until I left for the AAMC. I had the pleasure and honor of attending many national and regional meetings and served as a keynote speaker and session lead. I continue to cherish the many LMSA mentees that I have mentored over the years and continue to mentor. LMSA provides me hope for the future as I witness the incredible leadership that will carry the torch forward with the sole purpose of being the voice for and providing the care for the communities we have all come from.

References

1. Anderson G, Steinberg E, Heyssel R. The pivotal role of the academic health center. Health Aff. 1994;13(3):146–58. https://doi.org/10.1377/hlthaff.13.3.146
2. AAMC Organization Directory Search Result; n.d.. Members.aamc.org. Retrieved 30 January 2023, from https://members.aamc.org/eweb/DynamicPage.aspx?site=AAMC&webcode=AAMCOrgSearchResult&orgtype=Medical
3. U.S. Colleges of Osteopathic Medicine – AACOM; n.d. https://www.aacom.org/become-a-doctor/u-s-colleges-of-osteopathic-medicine
4. University of Pennsylvania Medicine | Penn Medicine | Office of Diversity and Inclusion; n.d. Retrieved 22 March 2020 from https://www.med.upenn.edu/inclusion-and-diversity/medicaleducation.html
5. Association of American Medical Colleges. Total U.S. Medical School Enrollment by Race/Ethnicity (alone) and Sex, 2015-2016 through 2019–2020. AAMC.org. https://www.aamc.org/system/files/2019-11/2019_FACTS_Table_B-3.pdf.
6. QuickFacts: United States; 2018. Census Bureau QuickFacts; United States Census Bureau. https://www.census.gov/quickfacts/fact/table/US/RHI725218
7. Boelen C, Woollard B. Social accountability and accreditation: a new frontier for educational institutions. Med Educ. 2009;43(9):887–94. https://doi.org/10.1111/j.1365-2923.2009.03413.x.
8. Mission Statement | The University of Arizona College of Medicine – Phoenix, n.d. Retrieved 30 January 2023, from https://phoenixmed.arizona.edu/about/mission-statement
9. Office of Equity, Diversity and Inclusion | The University of Arizona College of Medicine – Phoenix; n.d. Retrieved 30 January 2023, from https://phoenixmed.arizona.edu/diversity

10. Centers for Disease Control and Prevention. Hispanic Health. Centers for Disease Control and Prevention; 2015. https://www.cdc.gov/vitalsigns/hispanic-health/index.html

11. Velasco-Mondragon E, Jimenez A, Palladino-Davis AG, Davis D, Escamilla-Cejudo JA. Hispanic health in the USA: a scoping review of the literature. Public Health Rev. 2017;37(1) https://doi.org/10.1186/s40985-016-0043-2.

12. McCloskey J. Promotores as partners in a community-based diabetes intervention program targeting Hispanics. Fam Community Health. 2009;32(1):48–57. https://doi.org/10.1097/01.fch.0000342816.87767.e6.

13. Huerta EE, Macario E. Communicating health risk to ethnic groups: reaching hispanics as a case study. JNCI Monographs. 1999;1999(25):23–6. https://doi.org/10.1093/oxfordjournals.jncimonographs.a024202.

14. Olson D. Latinx Health Pathway. Healthcare Equity; 2021, January 15. https://depts.washington.edu/hcequity/latinx-health-pathway/

15. Acosta D. Using a community-based participatory (CBP) approach to teaching medical students about minority health and health disparities: the CBP curriculum development tool. Hawai'i J Med Public Health. 2013;72(8 Suppl 3):11.

16. Ahmed SM, Young SN, DeFino MC, Franco Z, Nelson DA. Towards a practical model for community engagement: advancing the art and science in academic health centers. J Clin Transl Sci. 2017;1(5):310–5.

17. Liaison Committee on Medical Education. Functions and structure of a medical school: standards for accreditation of medical education programs leading to the MD degree. Association of American Medical Colleges; 2021.

18. Acosta DA. Achieving excellence through equity, diversity, and inclusion. Association of American Medical Colleges; 2020. https://www.aamc.org/news-insights/achieving-excellence-through-equity-diversity-and-inclusion

19. UC College of Medicine | Office of Diversity and Inclusion – MSLHE; n.d. Default. Retrieved 30 January 2023, from https://med.uc.edu/diversity/medicalspanishelective

20. Morales R, Rodriguez L, Singh A, Stratta E, Mendoza L, Valerio MA, Vela M. National survey of medical Spanish curriculum in US medical schools. J Gen Int Med. 2015;30(10):1434–9. https://doi.org/10.1007/s11606-015-3309-3.

21. Weinick RM, Jacobs EA, Stone LC, Ortega AN, Burstin H. Hispanic healthcare disparities: challenging the myth of a monolithic Hispanic population. Med Care. 2004;42(4):313–20. https://doi.org/10.1097/01.mlr.0000118705.27241.7c.

22. George S, Duran N, Norris K. A systematic review of barriers and facilitators to minority research participation among African Americans, Latinos, Asian Americans, and Pacific Islanders. Am J Public Health. 2014;104(2):e16–31.

23. Dulin MF, Tapp H, Smith HA, Urquieta de Hernandez B, Furuseth OJ. A community based participatory approach to improving health in a Hispanic population. Implement Sci. 2011;6(1):1–11.

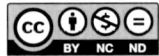

Looking Forward

Karina Diaz-Davis and Francisco Lucio

In this book, we describe the presence, activism and leadership of medical students, residents, fellows, physicians, faculty, and medical school staff in enhancing LHS+ diversity, equity, and inclusion in medicine, primarily through LMSA and antecedent organizations, over the past 50+ years. We highlight the changes that have occurred in medicine because we are here to advocate for the LHS+ community. With every year, we become more robust, and with every year we continue to see the ways in which the medical community still needs to change to provide better care and support for the LHS+ learners, faculty, and patients.

Although the future of the LHS+ medical pipeline is bright and built on a strong foundation of the past 50 years, there remain legal and political threats that could stymie progress. The authors in this book have covered in depth the underrepresentation amongst LHS+ physicians and trainees in the U.S. Ongoing developments in the legal and political landscape threaten to exacerbate an already dire situation.

K. Diaz-Davis (✉)
University of Colorado Pediatrics Residency,
Aurora, CO, USA
e-mail: karina.2.diaz@cuanschutz.edu

F. Lucio
Obstetrics and Gynecology, University of Arizona
College of Medicine-Phoenix, Phoenix, AZ, USA

Threats to LHS+ Advancement

Race-Conscious Admissions

At the time of this writing, the U.S. Supreme Court heard consolidated oral arguments for two cases: (1) Students for Fair Admissions, Inc. v. President and Fellows of Harvard College and (2) Students for Fair Admissions, Inc. v. University of North Carolina. Both cases are brought by petitioners who claim that the use of race in higher education admissions practices should be unconstitutional [1, 2]. Petitioners contend that the use of race as a factor in admissions practices is unfairly benefitting Black, Hispanic and Native American applicants to the detriment of White and Asian applicants. The petitioners are seeking to overturn Grutter v. Bollinger where the court upheld the use of race as a factor—amongst a multitude of factors—that institutions of higher education could use when making admissions decisions [3].

Overturning Grutter v. Bollinger and disallowing the use of race-conscious admissions practices would have a negative impact on the pipeline of LHS+ physicians already sorely needed in the U.S. We need only look at states where the use of race as a factor for admissions has been made illegal by state law to anticipate the calamitous results. In California for example, immediately after the 1996 passage of Proposition

© The Author(s) 2024
J. P. Sánchez, D. Rodriguez (eds.), *Latino, Hispanic, or of Spanish Origin+ Identified Student Leaders in Medicine*, Sustainable Development Goals Series, https://doi.org/10.1007/978-3-031-35020-7_15

209 that forbade the use of race in admissions decisions, there was a 32% decline in underrepresented in medicine (URM) students (inclusive of Main-Land Puerto Ricans and Mexican-American students) matriculating to California medical schools [4]. This decline is consistent when considering other states that have banned race-conscious admissions practices. A 2022 study examining eight states with bans on race-conscious admissions practices found an approximate 37% decline in URM (inclusive of LHS+) student enrollment [5]. Given that the LHS+ population is the largest minoritized group and one of the fastest growing populations in the U.S., a ban on the use of race-conscious admissions will only serve to further deepen the deficit of LHS+ physicians needed to proportionately reflect the U.S. population.

Whether the Court overturns or affirms the use of race-conscious admissions practices, it is imperative to advocate for the legality of race-conscious admissions practices as a tool to strive toward a racially/ethnically concordant physician workforce to care for the growing LHS+ population in the U.S. To this end, LMSA was a signatory to an amicus brief submitted by the Association of American Medical Colleges advocating for the preservation of precedent upheld in Grutter v. Bollinger for the continued use of race-conscious admissions practices [6]. Some key arguments advanced in the brief:

- Race-linked health inequities exist in the U.S. and require intervention
- Racially diverse medical teams improve health outcomes for minoritized patients
- Racially diverse physicians are more likely to work in medically underserved areas with minoritized patients
- Medical schools have a long history of highly individualized admissions practices
- Medical schools must consider applicants full background in order to achieve professional and educational aims

A clear need is tied to the diversity of the physician workforce and combating health inequities for minoritized populations including the LHS+ population. LMSA must remain steadfast and vigilant in helping to shape, block, and respond to legal threats that seek to erode and eliminate race-conscious admissions practices.

Deferred Action for Childhood Arrivals (DACA)

DACA was established by President Barack Obama in 2012 to allow individuals who were brought to the U.S. as children—and have known no other country as home—an opportunity to seek higher education or employment without fear of deportation [7]. DACA recipients are generally individuals who were not born in the U.S., but were brought to the U.S. as children, are enrolled or graduated from high school or obtained a general education degree or honorably discharged from the military, and have not been convicted of a felony or serious crime. [8] DACA represents a temporary solution in the absence of legislative action to reform current immigration law that carves out legal standing or a pathway to citizenship for DACA recipients or DACA-eligible recipients. DACA has had a politically charged and tumultuous history illustrated in the timeline below.

Year	Event
2001	DREAM Act (Development, Relief, and Education for Alien Minors Act) was introduced to Congress but fails to become law. DREAM Act would permit certain immigrant students who have grown up in the U.S. to apply for temporary legal status and to eventually obtain permanent legal status and become eligible for U.S. citizenship if they go to college or serve in the U.S. military; and the DREAM Act would eliminate a federal provision that penalizes states that provide in-state tuition without regard to immigration status [9]
2005–2010	Various DREAM Act and DREAM Act-like bills introduced to Congress but fail to become law [10–13]
2012	Given the inability to pass the DREAM Act in Congress, President Barack Obama issues a memorandum establishing DACA. A deferral of deportation for individuals and work authorization for those who meet criteria and submit an application for DACA [7]
2014	President Obama attempts to expand DACA for parents [14]
2014–2016	States sue and win an injunction to prevent the expansion of DACA to parents [15]
2017	President Trump rescinds DACA [16]
2018	Federal court issues injunction against President Trump's rescission of DACA [17]
2020	Department of Homeland Security v. Regents of the University of California holds that the manner in which DACA was rescinded was in violation of the Administrative Procedure Act (APA) and therefore unconstitutional, but the President has the authority to rescind DACA so long as it is done in line with the APA [18]
2022	President Biden's administration completes procedures to satisfy APA regarding DACA creation [19]
2022	Fifth U.S. Circuit Court Appeals court finds DACA creation unlawful and sends Texas v. United States case back to lower court for analysis given President Biden's administration's attempted satisfaction of APA regarding DACA creation [20]

Since the inception of DACA, more than 800,000 individuals have received DACA status of which 94% are LHS+ [21]. This large group of DACA recipients represents a contingent of individuals who may seek to enroll in medical school and practice medicine. To illustrate the point, of the estimated 188,000 DACA and DACA-eligible students in colleges and universities, 122,000 are LHS+ [21]. This pool must be tapped to cultivate and assist those interested in attending medical school. According to the American Association of Medical Colleges (AAMC), there are approximately 200 medical trainees and physicians that are DACA recipients [22].

Unfortunately, many medical schools do not currently accept DACA students [23]. Opportunities remain for LMSA to help advocate for the acceptance of DACA recipient applicants at all medical schools.

Until legislative action is taken to reform immigration law, DACA recipients remain suspended in uncertainty and vulnerable to legal challenges. LMSA should continue to advocate local respective medical schools, to state and federal legislators, and in collaboration with other professional organizations to support DACA recipient trainees, prospective trainees, and physicians.

LMSA Today

Truly, LMSA is always looking forward, because that is the only way we can continue to succeed in our mission. Every year, we continue some of our most successful programs and establish new ones to be the support, community, and validation that many of our members need. To tackle one of our top priorities, increasing the number of LHS+ physicians, we take a two-pronged approach: (1) increase recruitment of LHS+ medical students and (2) retention of LHS+ students through medical school.

Recruitment and Retention of LHS+ individuals:

1. Increase the number of LHS+ medical students
   (a) LMSA+: creation of a pre-medical branch of LMSA

(b) Mentorship program: organized pairing of pre-medical LHS+ students to current medical students

(c) National Conference: opportunities to present research, meet with mentors in person, and attend essential seminars for succeeding in medicine

(d) Monthly seminars through the application cycle: to guide and prepare students for medical school applications

2. LHS+ retention and success in medical school

(a) LMSA meetings: regional, quarterly, in-person sessions to meet with members and mentors across the country, establishing a sense of community

(b) Discounts/Partnerships with essential resources: including Canopy, Sketchy, and Magoosh for free MCAT prep and discounted study resources

(c) Mentorship program with Residents: direct pairing of senior medical students with current residents for guidance through and preparation for residency applications

(d) Leadership opportunities: with positions at the local, regional and national level

(e) Mentorship and training seminars through Residency applications

In addition to the focus we place directly on the LHS+ trainees across the country, we provide opportunities for the medical community as a whole to gain understanding of LHS+ struggles and, more importantly, provide tools and skills to aid in advocating and providing the support necessary to continue advancing the quality of medical education and health care.

Culturally competent care and improved quality of care to the LHS+ population:

- Medical Spanish courses with an integrated cultural understanding
- Policy and Advocacy Leadership Conference
- Research support
  - Partnership with IDSA
  - Annual Research symposium
  - Research-based scholarships

Finally, one of the ongoing projects is establishing national recognition of the LHS+ struggle in medicine by collaborating with numerous organizations such as AMA, ACGME, AOA, AACOM, AAMC, NHMA, BNGAP, and other organizations. For example, we have been working with the AAMC leadership for their support in publically acknowledging the LHS+ community as historically underrepresented and minoritized in medicine as they have with the Native American and African American populations of the United States. This identification will not only validate the healthcare insecurities and documented underrepresentation of LHS+ medical providers but will also bring awareness to the continued need for support from AAMC and other organizations heavily involved in the recruitment and training of future doctors.

The Next 50 Years

LMSA exists because our country needs it. The LHS+ population is growing and is nearly 19% of the total US population today. The number of doctors that identify as LHS+ does not reflect our country's population. The care that the Spanish-speaking population within the US receives still fails to meet the same standards as those whose primary language is English [24]. Given the health and healthcare disparities experienced by the LHS+ community, it is paramount that professional organizations such as the AMA, ACGME, AOA, AACOM, AAMC and other organizations center LHS+ needs in their advocacy, strategic planning, and other work toward health equity. Until then, it continues to be our responsibility to advocate for the changes necessary to train our doctors better, have a diverse team of doctors, and provide culturally competent care to our patients.

LMSA is poised to meet the needs of future student trainees. Our vast national network of chapter members and faculty-physician advisors covering every region of the country is a strength to build on. Given the growth and maturation of the LMSA, some areas of opportunity include:

- Establishment of paid professional staff members to help run the day-to-day operations of the organization
- Fortification and mentorship in grant writing and management for LMSA trainees
- Endowed scholarships for LMSA trainees
- Engagement in and publication of LMSA research and focused development of LHS+ researchers
- Creation of an LMSA Fellowship program to train future leaders
- Enhanced pathway program student national database and monitoring system
- Establishment of a support system for trainees and prospective trainees for success through the educational continuum (e.g. test prep, advising, coaching, shadowing and research opportunities, etc.)
- Growth and sustained chapter representation at every allopathic and osteopathic medical school in the country
- Expansion of resources and support to LHS+ international medical graduates
- Maintaining, expanding, and developing the network of LMSA alumni

Ultimately, the future leaders and members of LMSA will build on and continue to get better at leveraging new technologies, support programs and influencing policy for the betterment of the LHS+ community. Despite the challenges ahead, the 100th anniversary of LMSA promises to be bigger, more diverse and full of passionate individuals prepared to care for our growing LHS+ population.

References

1. Students for Fair Admissions, Inc. v. University of North Carolina at Chapel Hill, No. 21-707 (United States Supreme Court).
2. Students for Fair Admissions, Inc. v. President and Fellows of Harvard College, No. 20-1199 (United States Supreme Court).
3. Grutter v. Bollinger, 539 U.S. 306, 123 S. Ct. 2325 (2003).
4. Grumbach K, Mertz E, Coffman J. Underrepresented minorities and medical education in California. Center for California Health Workforce Studies: University of California, San Francisco; 1999. https://healthforce.ucsf.edu/sites/healthforce.ucsf.edu/files/publication-pdf/10.%201999-03_Underrepresented_Minorities_and_Medical_Education_in_California_Recent_Trends_in_Declining_Admissions.pdf.
5. Ly DP, Essien UR, Olenski AR, Jena AB. Affirmative action bans and enrollment of students from underrepresented racial and ethnic groups in U.S. public medical schools. Ann Intern Med. 2022;175(6):873–8. https://doi.org/10.7326/M21-4312.
6. Brief for Amici Curiae American Association of Medical Colleges et. al. in Support of Respondents, Students for Fair Admissions, Inc. v. President and Fellows of Harvard College, Students for Fair Admissions, Inc. v. University of North Carolina, et. al. No. 20-1199, No. 21-707. https://www.aamc.org/media/61976/download?attachment
7. Obama B. Remarks by the president on immigration [Transcript]. The White House Office of the Press Secretary; 2012, June 15. https://obamawhitehouse.archives.gov/the-press-office/2012/06/15/remarks-president-immigration
8. USCIS. DACA; 2022, Nov. 3. https://www.uscis.gov/DACA
9. Development, Relief, and Education for Alien Minors Act, S 1291, 107th Cong; 2001.
10. Development, Relief, and Education for Alien Minors Act, S 1545, 108th Cong; 2003.
11. Development, Relief, and Education for Alien Minors Act, S 2075, 109th Cong; 2005.
12. American Dream Act, H.R. 5131, 109th Cong. (2006).
13. Development, Relief, and Education for Alien Minors Act, S 3963, 111th Cong; 2010.
14. USCIS. 2014 Executive Actions on Immigration; 2014. https://www.uscis.gov/archive/2014-executive-actions-on-immigration
15. United States v. Texas, 136 S. Ct. 2271 (2016) (per curiam).
16. DHS. Memorandum for the Rescission of DACA. Department of Homeland Security; 2017, September 5. https://www.dhs.gov/news/2017/09/05/memorandum-rescission-daca#_ftnref5
17. Regents of the University of California, et. al., v. United States Department of Homeland Security, 908 F. 3d 476 (9th Cir. 2018).
18. Department of Homeland Security v. Regents of the University of California, 591 US__; 2020.
19. 87 FR 53152 https://www.federalregister.gov/documents/2022/08/30/2022-18401/deferred-action-for-childhood-arrivals
20. Texas v. United States, No. 21-40680. US Court of Appeals 5th Cir.; 2022.
21. Lucio F. COVID-19 and Latinx disparities: highlighting the need for medical schools to consider accept-

ing DACA recipients. Acad Med. 2022;97(6):812–7. https://doi.org/10.1097/ACM.0000000000004576.

22. AAMC. DACA students risk everything to become doctors; 2019. https://www.aamc.org/news-insights/daca-students-risk-everything-become-doctors

23. AAMC. Medical School Admissions Requirements Report for Applicants and Advisors. Deferred Action

for Childhood Arrivals; 2023. https://students-residents.aamc.org/media/7031/download

24. Cheng JH, Wang C, Jhaveri V, Morrow E, Li ST, Rosenthal JL. Health care provider practices and perceptions during family-centered rounds with limited English-proficient families. Acad Pediatr. 2021;21(7):1223–9. https://doi.org/10.1016/j.acap.2020.12.010. Epub 2021 Jan 9

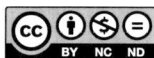

Index

© The Editor(s) (if applicable) and The Author(s) 2024
J. P. Sánchez, D. Rodriguez (eds.), *Latino, Hispanic, or of Spanish Origin+
Identified Student Leaders in Medicine*, Sustainable Development Goals
Series, https://doi.org/10.1007/978-3-031-35020-7